Clinical Scenarios in Thoracic Surgery

CLINICAL SCENARIOS IN SURGERY SERIES

Clinical Scenarios in Thoracic Surgery

Editor

Robert Kalimi, M.D.

Attending Surgeon
Minimally Invasive and Robotic Heart Surgery Center
Department of Cardiothoracic Surgery
North Shore University Hospital at Manhasset
Manhasset, New York

Associate Editor

L. Penfield Faber, M.D.

Professor
Department of Cardiovascular and Thoracic Surgery
Rush Medical College
Vice Chairman
Department of Cardiovascular and Thoracic Surgery
Rush-Presbyterian/St. Luke's Medical Center
Chicago, Illinois

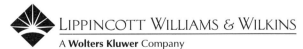
LIPPINCOTT WILLIAMS & WILKINS
A **Wolters Kluwer** Company
Philadelphia · Baltimore · New York · London
Buenos Aires · Hong Kong · Sydney · Tokyo

Acquisitions Editor: Brian Brown
Developmental Editor: Maureen Iannuzzi
Production Editor: Danielle Power
Manufacturing Manager: Colin Warnock
Cover Designer: Jeane E. Norton
Compositor: Lippincott Williams & Wilkins Desktop Division
Printer: Edwards Brothers

Library of Congress Cataloging-in-Publication Data
Clinical scenarios in thoracic surgery / editor, Robert Kalimi ; associate editor, L. Penfield Faber.
    p.;   cm. —(Clinical scenarios in surgery series)
  Includes bibliographical references and index.
  ISBN 0-7817-4797-X
  1. Chest—Surgery—Case studies.   I. Kalimi, Robert.   II. Faber, L. Penfield, 1930–
III. Series.
  [DNLM: 1. Thoracic Surgical Procedures—methods—Case Report.   2. Diagnostic Techniques, Surgical—Case Report.   3. Thoracic Diseases—diagnosis—Case Report.
WF 980 C641 2004]
RD536.C56 2004
617.5′4059—dc22

                                                                    2003066073

Care has been taken to confirm the accuracy of the information presented and to describe generally accepted practices. However, the authors, editors, and publisher are not responsible for errors or omissions or for any consequences from application of the information in this book and make no warranty, expressed or implied, with respect to the currency, completeness, or accuracy of the contents of the publication. Application of this information in a particular situation remains the professional responsibility of the practitioner.

The authors, editors, and publisher have exerted every effort to ensure that drug selection and dosage set forth in this text are in accordance with current recommendations and practice at the time of publication. However, in view of ongoing research, changes in government regulations, and the constant flow of information relating to drug therapy and drug reactions, the reader is urged to check the package insert for each drug for any change in indications and dosage and for added warnings and precautions. This is particularly important when the recommended agent is a new or infrequently employed drug.

Some drugs and medical devices presented in this publication have Food and Drug Administration (FDA) clearance for limited use in restricted research settings. It is the responsibility of the health care provider to ascertain the FDA status of each drug or device planned for use in their clinical practice.

10 9 8 7 6 5 4 3 2 1

To my lovely wife Lisa, who in our first year of marriage managed to make most of my dreams come true; and to my parents, Victoria and Mansour Kalimi, for giving me the opportunity to be a part of this wonderful profession.

R.K.

To Dr. Robert J. Jensik, a master surgeon, who taught us all the science and the art of thoracic surgery.

L.P.F.

contents

contributing authors

Emile Bacha, M.D.

Assistant Professor of Surgery and Pediatrics
Section of Cardiac and Thoracic Surgery
The University of Chicago
Director
Pediatric and Congenital Cardiac Surgery
Section of Cardiac and Thoracic Surgery
The University of Chicago Hospitals
Chicago, Illinois

L. Penfield Faber, M.D.

Professor
Department of Cardiovascular and Thoracic Surgery
Rush Medical College
Vice Chairman
Department of Cardiovascular and Thoracic Surgery
Rush-Presbyterian/St. Luke's Medical Center
Chicago, Illinois

Mark K. Ferguson, M.D.

Professor
Department of Surgery
The University of Chicago
Head
Thoracic Surgery Service
Department of Surgery
The University of Chicago Medical Center
Chicago, Illinois

Jonathan D. Hoffberger, D.O.

Attending Surgeon
Department of Cardiothoracic Surgery
Southeastern Michigan Cardiac Surgeons
Dearborn, Michigan

Lisa Khodadadian Kalimi, M.D., M.S.

Resident
Department of Nuclear Medicine
Albert Einstein College of Medicine/Montefiore
   Medical Center
Bronx, New York

Robert Kalimi, M.D.

Attending Surgeon
Minimally Invasive and Robotic Heart Surgery Center
Department of Cardiothoracic Surgery
North Shore University Hospital at Manhasset
Manhasset, New York

Fadi Munir Khoury, M.D.

Fellow
Department of Cardiovascular Surgery
Toronto General Hospital
University of Toronto
Toronto, Ontario, Canada

Jacques Kpodonu, M.D.

Fellow
Department of Cardiothoracic Surgery
University of Illinois Hospitals and Clinics at Chicago
Chicago, Illinois

Robert Gerard Kummerer, M.D.

Attending Surgeon
Department of Cardiothoracic Surgery
Condell Medical Center
Libertyville, Illinois

Rudy Lackner, M.D.

Associate Professor of Surgery
University of Nebraska
Omaha, Nebraska

Vassyl A. Lonchyna, M.D.

Chief
Division of Cardiothoracic and Vascular Surgery
Saint Mary of Nazareth Hospital Center
Chicago, Illinois

Mudiwa Munyikwa, M.D.

Attending Surgeon
Department of Thoracic Surgery
Beebe Medical Center
Lewes, Delaware

Jemi Olak, M.D.

Associate Professor of Clinical Surgery
Department of Surgery
University of Illinois at Chicago
Chicago, Illinois
Staff Surgeon
Department of Surgery
Lutheran General Hospital
Park Ridge, Illinois

Manisha A. Patel, M.D.

Attending Surgeon
Cardiac, Vascular, and Thoracic Surgeons, Inc.
Cincinnati, Ohio

Norman J. Snow, M.D.
Professor of Surgery
Division of Cardiothoracic Surgery
University of Illinois at Chicago
Chief
Section of Thoracic Surgery
Division of Cardiothoracic Surgery
University of Illinois Medical Center
Chicago, Illinois

Ozuru O. Ukoha, M.D.
Assistant Professor
Department of Cardiothoracic Surgery
Rush University
Senior Attending Physician
Division of Cardiothoracic Surgery
Cook County Hospital
Chicago, Illinois

The editors, Dr. Kalimi and Dr. Faber, have employed a unique approach to their presentation of the subject matter in their new text, *Clinical Scenarios in Thoracic Surgery*. The format of the text is that of a teaching conference based on the concept we all are familiar with—surgical grand rounds. These weekly conferences are both a highlight of the educational program as well as a bane to the uninformed or disinterested members of either the "house" or attending staffs. This text promotes the former (education) and diminishes the latter (the attendant chagrin of exposing one's ignorance of a given subject). In using this text, one can keep the latter to his or her self.

The text is set up quite simply. The subjects covered pertain to the pathologic involvement of the chest wall, diaphragm, pleura, tracheobronchial tree, congenital diseases and structural diseases of the lung, inflammatory disease of the lung, tumors and cysts of the mediastinum, malignant lung tumors, lesions of the esophagus, and the description of the pertinent surgical procedures for the management of the aforementioned disease processes. The text itself consists of the 58 scenarios, with each case presented initially as an unknown clinical problem. The history is presented and discussed as to what the possible diagnosis might be. To establish the diagnosis the appropriate diagnostic studies are presented (incidentally, the illustrations are excellent). Discussion of the entity and its ramifications follows, additional diagnostic procedures as indicated are outlined, and the therapeutic approach is selected. All these processes are described in appropriate detail. Additional cogent information is presented either relative to the disease entity or to the operative procedure, or both. Finally, the disposition of the case is given.

Overall, the amount of information presented, although in a concise manner, is more than satisfactory for the reader's understanding of the disease process and its present day treatment.

Lastly, the Index of Cases is presented. This contains the diagnostic topics discussed in the text. With this the reader, if so inclined, may explore a particular subject that is of immediate interest at a given time.

Thus, this volume may be used in one of two ways: as a testing tool to sharpen one's knowledge of an "unknown" clinical problem, or as an informational resource of an encapsulated but complete review of a given thoracic surgical subject. Surgeons in training or even throughout their careers will find this text a valuable addition to one's library.

Thomas W. Shields, M.D.
Professor Emeritus of Surgery
Northwestern University Medical School
Chicago, Illinois

preface

Clinical Scenarios in Thoracic Surgery is the first book of the Clinical Scenarios in Surgery series. The concept of editing a case-based textbook in which the information is presented in an interactive format greatly appealed to me. This unique format of clinical case presentation enables the reader to more effectively synthesize and integrate the information. In *Clinical Scenarios of Thoracic Surgery*, the reader is presented with a case-based review of general thoracic surgery patients. The authors were requested to create a clinical scenario based on radiographic images and to then provide the reader a differential diagnosis, treatment plan, and discussion of the disease process. Cases were chosen to provide a global overview of the subject, such as the chest wall, diaphragm, pleura, trachea and bronchus, congenital diseases of the lung, structural diseases of the lung, inflammatory diseases of the lung and mediastinum, lung disease, and esophageal disease. Clinical scenarios involving new technology such as laser and stent treatment of tracheal obstruction and video-assisted thoracoscopic surgery (VATS) are also included.

For many years attending and resident surgeons of the Thoracic Surgical Department at the Rush University Medical Center have met each Saturday morning to discuss interesting cases. Other surgeons and physicians from the Chicago area were invited to participate and present cases from their respective institutions. Traditionally, radiographic images were presented to a thoracic resident and heated, but quite informative discussions soon emerged. The success of the Saturday morning conference was due to the fact that the cases were interesting, the radiographic images were classic for the disease pathology, and the audience who participated were knowledgeable and experienced in the field of thoracic surgery.

This book was put together with the intention of providing the reader with a stimulating and interactive case-based discussion of the disease processes. The reader can review case scenarios without prior knowledge of the disease pathology and then follow the radiographic interpretation, diagnostic tests, operative approach, and postoperative management. In turn, one can refer to the table of contents or the index of cases and review a particular case for a disease process that may be of interest.

I had the pleasure of editing this book with my mentor and colleague, Dr. L. Penfield Faber. During his career in thoracic surgery at the Rush University Medical Center, Dr. Faber has assisted in the training of approximately 80 thoracic surgeons who are now practicing in the United States and abroad. His suggestions and comments in editing this manuscript were invaluable, and I am indebted to him for his contribution.

I would like to thank the authors, many of whom have had the opportunity to participate in the Saturday morning conferences, for providing numerous radiographic images, meticulously researching the information, and promptly submitting the scenarios for editorial revisions. I would also like to thank my colleague, Dr. Robert Bojar, also a graduate of the Rush University Medical Center's Thoracic Surgical Residency Training Program, for providing me with the necessary guidance and for encouraging me in this endeavor.

Finally, I would like to thank Lisa McAllister, Acquisitions Editor at Lippincott Williams & Wilkins, for her diligence and effort in getting this book to publication and Dr. Thomas Shields for providing useful suggestions and for writing the foreword for this book.

Robert Kalimi, M.D.

Presentation

A 27-year-old student is admitted to the hospital complaining of dyspnea and cough occurring over the past 6 weeks. The patient has no significant medical problems and does not smoke. He has no family history of malignancy. He has not traveled outside the United States in 20 years. On physical examination, vital signs are stable, heart sounds are normal, and there are decreased breath sounds over the right chest.

■ Chest X-rays

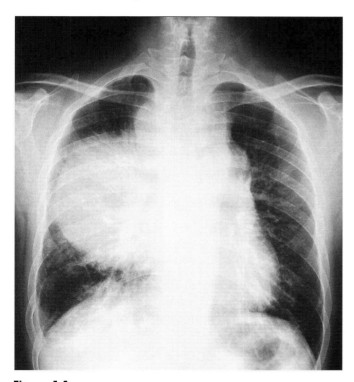

Figure 1-1

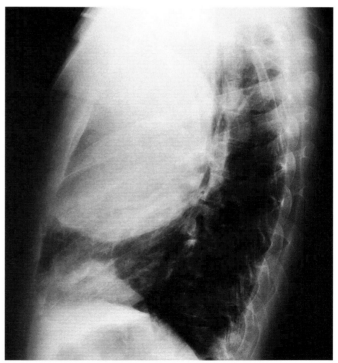

Figure 1-2

Chest X-ray Report

The chest x-rays demonstrate a large anterior mass located in the mediastinum and the right chest. The heart is not enlarged. There are no pleural effusions. There are no masses in the left lung field. ▪

Discussion

The differential diagnosis of anterior mediastinal masses includes thymoma, lymphoma, thyroid goiter, and germ cell tumor. In a patient who presents with an anterior mediastinal mass, a complete history and physical examination is important. A history of ptosis, dysarthria, and muscle weakness, particularly if the weakness increases with increased activity, suggests the diagnosis of mediastinal thymoma associated with myasthenia gravis. Patients with enlarged axillary, supraclavicular, and cervical lymph nodes may have lymphoma. About 60% of patients with mediastinal germ cell tumors are asymptomatic, and 40% have dyspnea and chest pain.

In a young man with a mediastinal tumor, a computed tomography (CT) scan of the chest, as well as tumor markers, should be obtained. Tumor markers include α-fetoprotein, β-human chorionic gonadotropin, and lactate dehydrogenase.

▪ CT Scans

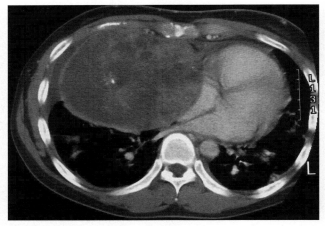 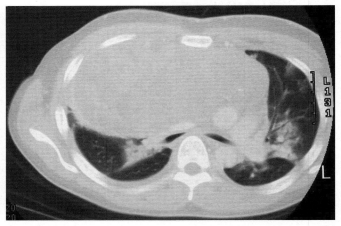

Figure 1-3   **Figure 1-4**

CT Scan Report

The chest CT demonstrates a heterogeneous 18-cm × 8-cm × 9.8-cm mass with calcifications and multiple areas of necrosis and hemorrhage. The mass extends into the neck and right pleural space. There is compression of the trachea and both main-stem bronchi. ▪

Case Continued

Tumor markers are submitted, and the α-fetoprotein is 437 ng/mL; the β-human chorionic gonadotropin level is slightly elevated.

Discussion

Elevated α-fetoprotein and β-human chorionic gonadotropin levels in a young man are highly suggestive of the diagnosis of germ cell tumor. About 10% of germ cell tumors are extragonadal; they can be benign (such as teratomas or epidermoid cysts) or malignant. The mediastinum is the most common extragonadal site of germ cell tumors. Malignant germ cell tumors are further categorized into seminomas and nonseminomatous germ cell tumors. Malignant germ cell tumor is a possible diagnosis when either the α-fetoprotein or β-human chorionic gonadotropin tumor marker is elevated. In most pure mediastinal seminomas, α-fetoprotein and β-human chorionic gonadotropin levels are normal. Serum α-fetoprotein is never elevated, and β-human chorionic gonadotropin is mildly elevated in about 10% of patients with mediastinal seminomas. Germ cell tumors are believed to arise from totipotential cells in the thymus. In the past, some believed that these tumors represented metastases from occult gonadal tumors. However, pathologic examination of scrotal contents of patients with mediastinal tumors has not substantiated this theory. Thus, in patients with mediastinal germ cell tumor and a normal testicular examination, ultrasonography of the testis is not necessary. Because the treatments of benign and malignant germ cell tumors differ, tissue diagnosis is necessary for determining therapeutic plans. Tumor marker (e.g., α-fetoprotein or β-human chorionic gonadotropin) levels higher than 500 ng/mL are diagnostic of nonseminomatous germ cell tumors, and the chemotherapy regimen should commence without awaiting histologic diagnosis.

In patients with elevated tumor markers, histologic and cytologic methods have been used to determine the histologic subtype. CT-guided core needle biopsies may provide adequate sampling. If core needle biopsy does not yield a diagnosis, open biopsy by anterior mediastinotomy (Chamberlain's procedure) is performed to provide sufficient tissue for diagnosis.

Case Continued

The patient undergoes Chamberlain's procedure through an incision over the second costal cartilage, and histologic evaluation reveals endodermal sinus (yolk sac) tumor.

Discussion

Only about 10% of germ cell tumors are extragonadal, and the mediastinum is the most common extragonadal site. Other extragonadal sites include the retroperitoneum and pineal gland. Germ cell tumors account for about 10% of mediastinal tumors. About 10% of mediastinal germ cell tumors are benign (teratomas); the rest are malignant tumors, which are categorized into seminomatous and nonseminomatous tumors and which respectively account for 30% and 70% of the malignant mediastinal germ cell tumors. The histologic subtypes of nonseminomatous germ cell tumors include (a) teratocarcinoma, (b) endodermal sinus (yolk sac) tumor, (c) choriocarcinoma, and (d) embryonal carcinoma. The incidence of malignant germ cell tumors of the mediastinum appears to be increased in patients with Klinefelter's syndrome (hypogonadism, XXY, azoospermia). These patients develop germ cell tumors about 10 years earlier than patients without Klinefelter's syndrome. Malignant germ cell tumors of the mediastinum are unusual in women.

The clinical presentation is dependent on the histology. Benign tumors (teratomas) are usually incidental radiologic findings. Malignant tumors usually cause symptoms, often owing to compression or invasion of mediastinal structures such as the airway, the esophagus, or the superior vena cava. Compared with seminomatous tumors, nonseminomatous tumors have a propensity to grow rapidly; thus, prompt diagnosis and initiation of therapy are important. Up to 85% of patients may present with metastatic disease to the lung, pleura, retroperitoneal lymph nodes, liver, bone, brain, and kidneys. Hematologic malignancy may also be associated with nonseminomatous mediastinal germ cell tumor and is usually diagnosed within 1 year of the diagnosis of nonseminomatous germ cell tumor. Treatment of nonseminomatous germ cell tumors includes cisplatin-based chemotherapy regimen.

Case Continued

Abdominal and brain CT scans demonstrate no evidence of metastatic disease. The patient undergoes four cycles of cisplatin, etoposide, vinblastine, and bleomycin in various combinations.

Although the patient's serum α-fetoprotein markers decrease to normal levels, the tumor does not shrink and continues to cause progressive dyspnea and chest pain. The patient undergoes surgical resection through a median sternotomy. Surgical dissection permits total removal of the mass with its capsule intact. Care is taken to avoid injury to the recurrent laryngeal nerves and the phrenic nerves. Because the mass is adherent to the right upper lobe, a small rim of lung is stapled and resected with the mass. Pathologic examination reveals mature teratoma with no evidence of malignancy.

▌ Intraoperative Photograph

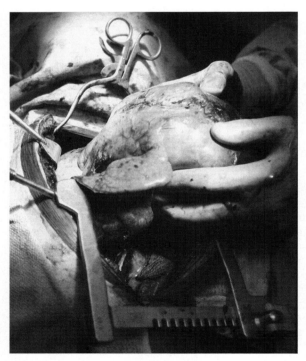

Figure 1-5 See Color Plate 1 following page 114.

Discussion

In contrast to pure mediastinal seminomas that are sensitive to radiation and cis-platin-based chemotherapy, nonseminomatous mediastinal tumors are treated by a variety of cisplatin-based chemotherapy regimens without radiation. After a 3-month cycle of chemotherapy, the patient is restaged by CT scan of the chest and abdomen and by reevaluation of serum markers. If tumor markers normalize and there is no radiographic evidence of tumor, no further intervention is necessary, and the patient is evaluated monthly with physical examination and a chest x-ray for the first 2 years. If tumor markers remain elevated after a chemotherapy regimen, higher-dose chemotherapy or other chemotherapy regimens are used. If tumor markers normalize but the tumor is present radiographically (as in the scenario described), surgical resection should be performed if tumor fails to regress on serial CT scans. Usually, the residual tumors are benign teratomas and necrotic tumors. Benign teratomas after successful chemotherapy treatment should be resected because of the possibility of increased size of the teratoma, with subsequent compressive effects. Furthermore, teratomas may undergo malignant degeneration. Finally, if the resected specimen includes viable germ cell tumor, additional cycles of chemotherapy should be administered.

case 2

Presentation

An 85-year-old woman with a 50-pack-per-year history of smoking has been treated with antibiotics for the past 2 weeks for symptoms of bronchitis. After a 2-week course of antibiotics, the patient's cough persists, and a chest x-ray is obtained. The chest x-ray demonstrates a nodule in the right lung, and computed tomography (CT) scans are obtained for further evaluation.

CT Scans

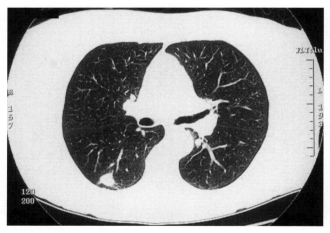

Figure 2-1

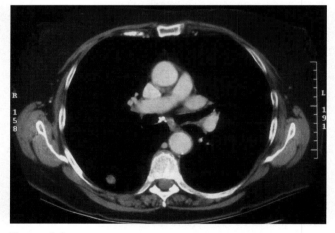

Figure 2-2

CT Scan Report

The CT scans demonstrate a 2-cm solitary nodule in the superior segment of the right lower lobe. The mass is spiculated and extends to the pleura. There is no mediastinal adenopathy. Mild emphysematous changes are present. There are no pleural effusions. ▉

Case Continued

The patient undergoes a bronchoscopy, and brushing of the superior segment is negative for malignancy. Pulmonary function tests (PFTs) show a forced expiratory volume in 1 second (FEV_1) of 73% of predicted and a diffusing capacity of lung for carbon monoxide (D_{LCO}) of 60% of predicted. This is followed by video-assisted thoracoscopic biopsy and frozen section. Frozen section demonstrates squamous cell carcinoma, and the patient undergoes thoracotomy, right lower lobectomy, and mediastinal lymph node dissection.

At surgery, the cancer is defined as T2 N0 M0, stage IB. No radiation or chemotherapy is administered.

The patient stops smoking and returns to the clinic for surveillance chest x-ray and physical examination. Three years after surgery, the physical examination is normal, but the chest x-ray reveals an abnormality that prompts further CT scans.

CT Scans

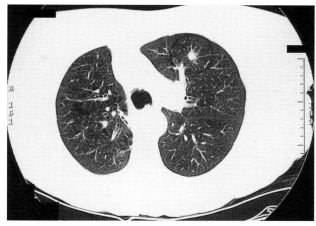

Figure 2-3

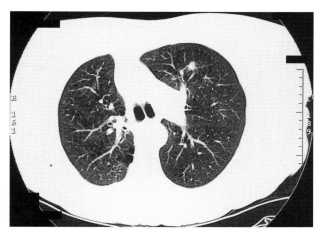

Figure 2-4

CT Scan Report

The CT scans demonstrate a nodule 8 mm in diameter in the lingular portion of the left upper lobe. There is volume loss in the right hemithorax owing to previous right lower lobectomy. There is mild centrilobular emphysema throughout. There is no mediastinal adenopathy or pleural effusions.

Differential Diagnosis

A new lung mass presenting several months after resection of a primary cancer can be a metachronous, metastatic, recurrent, or benign lesion. A second primary tumor occurs in 6% to 8% of patients treated successfully for lung cancer.

Metachronous lesions are defined as new and separate lesions and can be of different or similar histology. Metachronous lesions may be of the same histology if there is a disease-free interval of 2 years, if the lesion originates from carcinoma *in situ*, or if the lesion originates in a separate lobe, with no involvement in common lymphatics and no extrapulmonary metastases.

Surgery for synchronous or metachronous lesions is practically limited to two lesions. If three or more sites are involved—especially if the patient reports a significant weight loss and general debility—metastatic disease is highly likely, and surgery is not indicated. Recurrent disease usually occurs in the region of the original tumor. A second primary should be treated as a new lesion. When the tumor is defined as stage I or II, consideration for appropriate anatomic resection should be made if the patient has sufficient pulmonary reserve and adequate cardiac function to tolerate the procedure. Lung-sparing procedures are particularly appropriate in this situation.

Recommendation

This patient has been disease-free for 3 years. A new lesion in the contralateral lung is suggestive of a second or metachronous lung cancer. Positron-emission tomography (PET) scanning can determine evidence of metastatic disease in regional lymph nodes and other parts of the body. A CT scan of the brain is obtained only if symptoms warrant it. Physiologic performance status is evaluated by PFTs, split-function ventilation-perfusion ratio (V/Q) scan, and cardiac evaluation. Bronchoscopy is performed to assess the previous surgical site and to exclude endobronchial pathology.

PET Scan

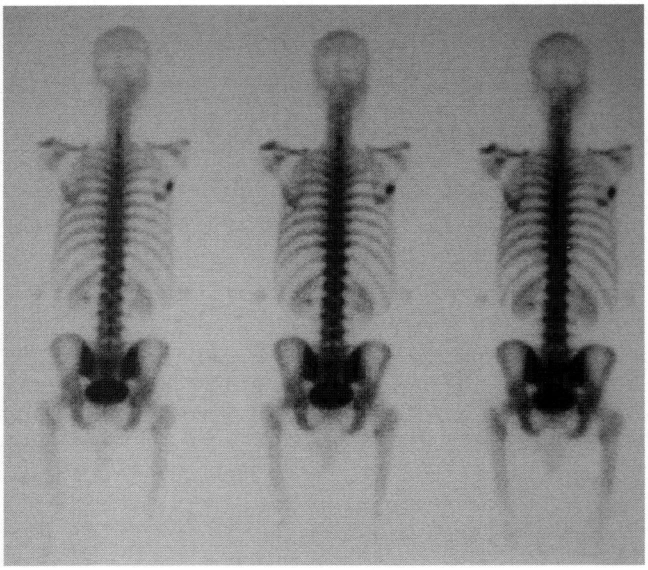

Figure 2-5

PET Scan Report

The PET scan demonstrates uptake in a mass in the left lung field, SUV 3.2. No other metabolically active sites were demonstrated. ▮

Case Continued

The patient lives by herself and is entirely self-sufficient. She walks to the grocery store daily and walks up a flight of stairs to her apartment. She has a good appetite, and her weight has been stable for years. The PET scan demonstrates uptake only on the left lung lesion. Laboratory data are normal. PFTs show an FEV_1 of 1.35 L. The V/Q split function is 35% on the right and 65% on the left. Bronchoscopy is negative. Dobutamine stress test shows nonreversible ischemic changes of the inferior wall.

Recommendation

The patient has been tumor-free for 3 years and physiologically is a good surgical candidate. Because she is an octogenarian, and for the purpose of preserving pulmonary parenchyma, a limited resection is appropriate. A wedge resection is adequate for a benign lesion or a metastatic implant. An anatomic segmentectomy would be a more appropriate resection for a malignant lesion. The long-term survival rates of segmentectomy and lobectomy for cancer are equivalent. However, there is a higher local recurrence rate with segmentectomy.

▮ Surgical Approach

A left lateral thoracotomy is performed. The latissimus dorsi muscle is spared. With the left lung collapsed, the nodule is palpated in the lingular segment of the left upper lobe. A needle biopsy is performed, and the pathology of adenocarcinoma is established on frozen section.

The oblique fissure is developed, and a GIA stapler is used to dissect the fissure fully. The distal pulmonary artery is dissected within the fissure, and the branches of the inferior and superior lingular arteries are isolated. Level 11 and 12 lymph nodes are removed, and frozen-section analysis is obtained to exclude nodal involvement before proceeding with a segmentectomy. Pulmonary artery branches are then ligated and divided. The bronchus to the lingular segment is identified, divided, and closed using interrupted polyglyconate sutures. Venous drainage of the lingular segment is dissected free, ligated, and transected. The intersegmental plane is clearly identified, and the stapling device is used to transect the lung parenchyma. After the segmentectomy is completed, removal of mediastinal lymph nodes is performed. ▮

Discussion

Segmentectomy is a procedure used traditionally for resection of tuberculous and bronchiectatic segments. It is also an acceptable procedure for lung cancer, especially in patients with diminished pulmonary reserve and in those with a second primary tumor. In patients of advanced age or compromised cardiac function, segmentectomy is an appropriate procedure that provides a curative resection with minimal loss of pulmonary parenchyma. This procedure is performed through a muscle-sparing or limited thoracotomy.

The major complications of segmentectomy are prolonged air leak and bronchopulmonary fistula. The use of a tissue sealant can minimize air leak from the area of dissection. Locoregional recurrence may be as high as 15% after segmentectomy for primary lung cancer.

Presentation

A 64-year-old man presents with a 4-month history of solid food dysphagia associated with a 12-pound weight loss. He also complains of excessive belching and regurgitation within 1 hour of meals. He reports a 40-pack-per-year smoking history and no history of alcohol abuse. He presents with a chest x-ray that was obtained by his primary medical physician.

▨ Chest X-ray

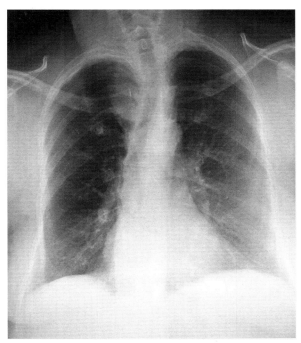

Figure 3-1

Chest X-ray Report

There are no lung masses or pleural effusions. The trachea is shifted to the right. The heart size is normal. ▨

Discussion

The differential diagnosis for dysphagia includes obstructive etiologies as well as etiologies from neuromuscular disorders. Obstructive etiologies include causes such as cancer of the esophagus, Schatzki's ring, peptic strictures, and webs. Neuromuscular etiologies include achalasia, diffuse esophageal spasm, and the nutcracker esophagus. Other rare etiologies of dysphagia include those associated with extrinsic compression of the esophagus, such as with aberrant vasculature, lymphadenopathy, and mediastinal masses.

The history and physical examination are important in evaluating patients for dysphagia. Many of the signs and symptoms that can be elicited from the patient by careful and detailed history and physical examination will aid in determining the most likely diagnosis. An upper gastrointestinal (GI) study provides an excellent diagnostic evaluation for patients who present with dysphagia and symptoms of esophageal obstruction. This study also provides some information on esophageal motility. A double-contrast study better demonstrates esophageal mucosa. Other studies, such as endoscopy, manometry, and 24-hour pH monitoring, may be needed after upper GI studies demonstrate an esophageal pathology.

Upper GI Studies

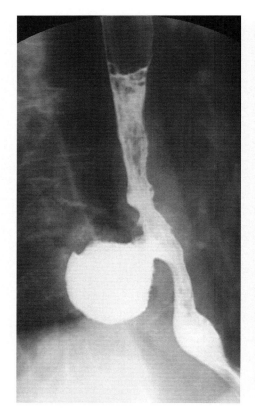

Figure 3-2

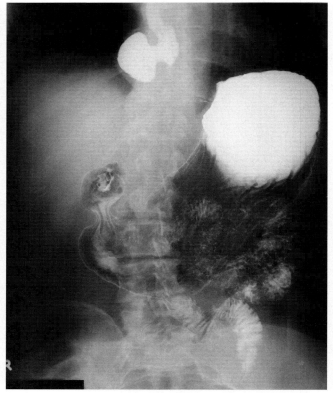

Figure 3-3

Upper GI Study Report

There is a 5-cm × 5-cm epiphrenic diverticulum with a 2-cm orifice. Fluoroscopy reveals tertiary contractions within the esophagus. Gastroesophageal reflux, to the level of the thoracic inlet, is also demonstrated. ▪

Recommendation

An upper endoscopy should be performed to assess for ulceration and inflammation within the diverticulum and for reflux esophagitis or hiatal hernia. Although malignancy within an epiphrenic diverticulum is rare, endoscopic evaluation can assess for malignancy as well.

Case Continued

Upper endoscopic examination confirms the presence of a wide-mouthed diverticulum proximal to the gastroesophageal junction (GEJ). The esophageal mucosa is normal in appearance. There is a small hiatal hernia, and the stomach and duodenum appear normal.

Recommendation

An esophageal manometry is necessary to assess for motility disorder and to plan for operative intervention. Manometric information is important in deciding on the length of myotomy to be performed during surgical intervention.

Esophageal Manometry Results

A water-perfusion manometry catheter is placed under direct vision to avoid coiling of the catheter in the diverticulum. Fluoroscopy is used to confirm the position of the catheter within the stomach. The stomach, lower esophageal sphincter (LES), esophagus, and upper esophageal sphincter (UES) are examined using the slow pull-through technique. The LES is characterized as follows:

LES length: 3.7 cm
LES intraabdominal length: 2.0 cm
LES resting pressure: 48.4 mm Hg

The LES response to wet swallows is variable—some complete relaxations, some 50% to 75% relaxations. The resting LES pressure is above the upper limit of normal (14.3 to 34.5 mm Hg).

The distal one third of the esophagus demonstrates high-amplitude (up to 320 mm Hg) peristaltic waves highly suggestive of the nutcracker esophagus. The proximal two thirds of the esophagus show normal peristaltic activity. UES resting pressure is 38.4 mm Hg (normal range, 70 to 94 mm Hg) with normal relaxation with wet swallows.

Case Continued

Based on the above results, it is recommended that the patient undergo a left thoracotomy, diverticulectomy, extended myotomy, and partial fundoplication (Belsey Mark IV).

■ Surgical Approach

Intraoperatively, a thoracic epidural catheter is placed for postoperative pain control. The patient is intubated with a left-sided double-lumen endotracheal tube. An 18-French nasogastric (NG) tube is placed into the stomach, and the patient is positioned in the right lateral decubitus position. A left posterolateral thoracotomy is performed, and the chest cavity is entered through the seventh intercostal space. The inferior pulmonary ligament is divided to the level of the inferior pulmonary vein, and the esophagus is encircled with a Penrose drain at that level. The esophagus distal to the Penrose drain is mobilized using sharp and blunt dissection, taking care to avoid injury to the vagus nerves. The diverticulum is dissected from the surrounding tissues. A 50-French bougie is then guided down the esophagus, and the diverticulum is resected over the bougie using a TA-60 stapler with 3.5-mm stapler leg length. The staple line is oversewn with an interrupted 4-0 polydioxanone suture (PDS). An extended esophageal myotomy is then performed 180 degrees away from the staple line. The myotomy extends from the level of the inferior pulmonary vein to a point 1.5 cm onto the stomach. Crural approximation sutures of number 1 Ethibond are then placed but not tied. A Belsey Mark IV fundoplication is then performed. The first layer of horizontal mattress sutures of 2-0 silk is placed on the stomach 2 cm distal to the GEJ and 2 cm proximal to the GEJ after first resecting the fat pad at the GEJ. The second row of horizontal mattress sutures of 2-0 silk includes bites on the diaphragm, then on the stomach 2 cm distal to the first suture line, then on the esophagus 2 cm above the first suture line, and finally back on the diaphragm. This maneuver creates a 4-cm segment of intraabdominal esophagus. The operative field is checked for mucosal leaks by submerging the myotomized esophagus in water and insufflating air through the NG tube. Air is aspirated from the stomach, and the NG tube is fixed to the nostril. A chest tube is placed, and the thoracotomy incision is closed in standard fashion. ■

▦ Operative Diagram

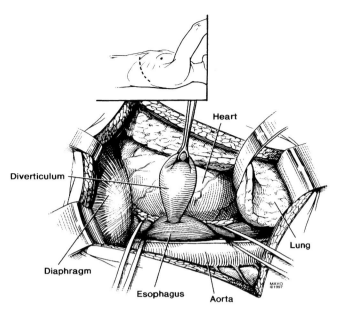

Figure 3-4 Surgical management of epiphrenic diverticulum. (Reprinted from Deschamps C, Trastek VF. Esophageal diverticula. In: Shields TW, LoCicero J, Ponn RB, eds. *General thoracic surgery*, 5th ed. Philadelphia: Lippincott Williams & Wilkins, 2000:1846.)

Discussion

Epiphrenic diverticula are located within 10 cm of the GEJ. They represent about 20% of all esophageal diverticula and are more common in men than in women (male-to-female ratio of 2:1). Most patients (42%) with epiphrenic diverticulum are asymptomatic; thus, the exact prevalence of these pulsion diverticula is unknown. Between 58% and 90% of patients have other associated functional abnormalities of the esophagus. These include diffuse esophageal spasm, achalasia, vigorous achalasia, and hypertensive lower esophageal sphincter.

A contrast esophagram is used to identify the location, number, and size of the diverticula as well as the presence of an associated hiatal hernia. Endoscopy should be obtained to evaluate for esophagitis and cancer. Esophageal scintigraphy is performed when assessment of the emptying capacity of the esophagus is required. Manometric assessment of the esophagus is necessary to determine the nature and extent of a coexisting motor disorder. Surgical management is planned based on the results of these investigations.

Surgical management is recommended for all symptomatic diverticula, for diverticula that are increasing in size, and for diverticula that are associated with an esophageal motor disorder. Most surgeons advocate performing an esophagomyotomy with resection or suspension of the diverticulum. When the myotomy extends onto the stomach, a partial fundoplication should be performed to avoid postoperative reflux.

case 4

Presentation

A 46-year-old man with no significant past medical history presents to your office complaining of a nonproductive cough accompanied by dull pain in the right chest for the past 2 weeks. The patient is a sheep farmer on a trip from New Zealand who is visiting friends in your area.

On examination, he is noted to be febrile (temperature of 100.8°F), and the lungs are clear to auscultation.

Chest X-rays

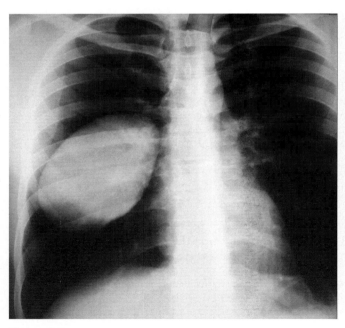

Figure 4-1

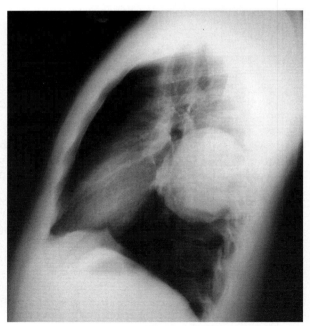

Figure 4-2

Chest X-ray Report

There is a smooth, dense, spherical opacity in the right lower lobe and no effusions. The heart is of normal size.

Differential Diagnosis

The differential diagnosis for chest masses of this type includes malignancy and infectious etiologies. In a patient from an endemic area, dry cough, fever, and pain with a smooth, round lesion are associated with echinococcosis. Endemic areas other then New Zealand include South Africa, Australia, South America, and Mediterranean countries.

Several radiographic signs that can further suggest the diagnosis include the following:

Escudero-Nenerow sign: a spherical to oval shape change observed with deep inspiration

Notch sign: an indentation in the bronchus from a centrally located cyst

Moon, crescent, or pulmonary meniscus sign: a crescent-shaped shadow from air between layers of the cyst indicating impending rupture

Double-domed arch sign: a result of air entering the cyst after rupture

Water lily sign: a result of an air and fluid layer produced by the floating membrane of the cyst

If the echinococcal cyst ruptures, a loculated hydropneumothorax may be present.

Discussion

Hydatid disease, caused by the *Echinococcus granulosus* tapeworm, is often found in cattle- and sheep-raising regions of the world. It should therefore be considered in a patient presenting with a well-defined round pulmonary density who has spent time in an endemic area. The organism is usually found in dogs, coyotes, and wolves that ingest echinococcal cysts from the intestines of their prey. The ova from the cysts are released in the feces, thereby contaminating water and vegetation.

In humans, once ingested, the parasite typically penetrates the small bowel mucosa, entering the portal system. However, entry by way of intestinal lymphatics or direct inhalation has also been suggested. The most common site of lodgment is the liver. The lung may be involved in 10% to 30% of cases and is usually accompanied by synchronous hepatic lesions. As the cysts rupture, ova enter the venous circulation and can result in secondary cyst formation.

Pulmonary echinococcosis usually affects the lower lobes and is more common on the right side. Cysts are multiple in 30% of cases and bilateral in 20% of cases and may develop more quickly and extensively in children.

Two types of cysts exist: unilocular and alveolar. The unilocular type is found in the lung. These cysts are thick walled and are filled with clear hydatid fluid. The wall has three layers: a germinal layer and laminated membrane from the parasite, surrounded by a pericystic zone or adventitia from the host. The inner germinal layer is a thin, transparent layer lined with capsules containing larvae, which can form daughter cysts suspended in the fluid. The laminated membrane is 1 to 3 mm in thickness and forms the plane for surgical dissection. The outer pericystic layer is formed by local reaction against the parasite, with infiltration by leukocytes and fibroblasts. Hepatic cysts usually calcify, although this is rarely seen in pulmonary cysts.

Intact or simple cysts are usually asymptomatic. Cysts enlarge up to 5 cm per year, until either size produces compressive symptoms or rupture occurs. Typical symptoms include dull, aching pain or pressure sensation in the chest; nonproductive cough; and occasionally blood-tinged sputum. Patients also note a chronic cough and repeated fevers. Rupture may be spontaneous or may occur during coughing or sneezing and may be contained by the pericystic layer. If the cyst ruptures into the bronchus, the patient will suddenly produce a large amount of salty sputum containing mucus, hydatid fluid, and fragments of the laminated membrane that look like grape skins and can result in airway obstruction. Cyst rupture into the pleural space is heralded by pleuritic chest pain and dyspnea and usually results in formation of dense adhesions, which complicate subsequent surgical intervention. Rupture, whether spontaneous or iatrogenic, may be accompanied by an anaphylactic reaction, rash, fever, pulmonary congestion, and bronchospasm.

Recommendation

Laboratory tests: white blood cell count with differential, indirect hemagglutination test, and computed tomography (CT) scan of the chest.

Case Continued

A presumptive diagnosis can be made based on the history of exposure to an endemic area with the classic chest x-ray findings noted above. Additional diagnostic tests should include a CT scan of the chest and abdomen to define the extent of involvement. Magnetic resonance imaging (MRI) can be used to delineate cyst membrane layers and communications between the cyst and bronchial tree as well as to assess ring enhancement, which may indicate a local host inflammatory reaction.

Laboratory studies usually reveal a normal white blood cell count with eosinophilia in 20% to 30% of cases. Several serologic tests have been used in the past, including Casoni's test, Weinberg's complement fixation test, indirect hemagglutination test, latex and bentonite flocculation tests, and immunodiffusion and immunofluorescence tests. The hemagglutination test has emerged as the clinical test of choice, with a sensitivity of 66% to 100% and a specificity of 98% to 99%.

Needle biopsy or aspiration should be avoided because of danger of spillage with accompanying anaphylaxis and subsequent difficulty during operative excision of the cyst.

This patient had a normal white blood cell count with marked eosinophilia, a positive hemagglutination test, and the following CT scans.

■ CT Scans

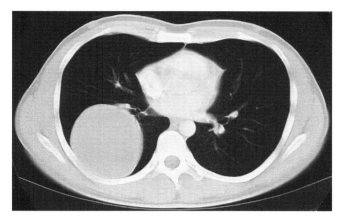

Figure 4-3

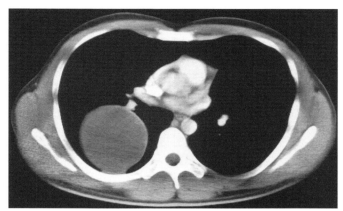

Figure 4-4

CT Scan Report

There is a 6-cm × 8-cm homogeneous mass in the right lower lobe, no pleural effusions, and no other nodules in the lung field. ■

Diagnosis

Intact echinococcal cyst in the right lower lobe.

Discussion

Benzimidazole compounds, of which albendazole is the least toxic, have a 36% to 94% partial to complete response rate. Young patients and those with thin cysts tend to do better. Because side effects are considerable, failure and recurrence rates are high, and course of treatment is lengthy (months to years), this is typically indicated for inoperable cysts (widely disseminated, difficult locations, contraindication for surgery).

Historically, these cysts were approached through the chest wall in one or two stages. However, problems with secondary cysts developing in the wound and chronic bronchocutaneous fistulae were encountered. This led to the recommendation for complete excision or enucleation of the cyst, preserving surrounding lung tissue if possible; in many cases, capitonnage of the cavity and closure of an opened bronchus is also performed. Lobectomy is indicated for greater than 50% lobar involvement, severe pulmonary suppuration, multiple cysts, or sequelae of the disease such as pulmonary fibrosis, bronchiectasis, and hemorrhage.

■ Surgical Approach

Preoperatively, postural drainage and antibiotics (albendazole, 400 mg given twice daily) should be employed to minimize the suppurative process. If the disease is bilateral, excision should be done in two stages, 2 to 4 weeks apart, and the side with larger, intact, or multiple cysts should be excised first to prevent rupture.

Intraoperatively, airway compromise may occur by cyst matter or anaphylaxis. Cyst rupture occurs during induction or resection. A posterolateral thoracotomy is performed, and the surgical field is packed with gauze soaked in hypertonic saline, which will be scolecoidal in the event of rupture. A cruciate incision is made in the outer portion of the cyst, and blunt dissection is used to separate the laminated membrane from the pericystic layer, taking care not to rupture the cyst. Airway pressures are minimized during the dissection and raised at the end to deliver the cyst into a basin filled with normal saline. Any patent bronchial openings in the residual cavity should then be closed.

Other surgical options include (a) needle aspiration or injection of scolecoidal agents before cyst excision, and (b) pericystectomy, excising pulmonary tissue around the cyst.

Case Continued

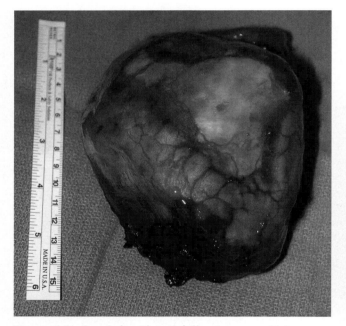

Figure 4-5 See Color Plate 2 following page 114.

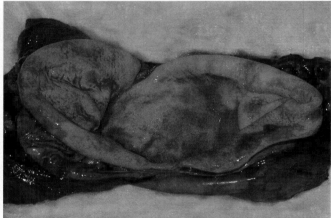

Figure 4-6 See Color Plate 3 following page 114.

The right lower lobe is removed in total with the cyst. The cyst is then opened (the inner surface of the cyst is depicted in the second photograph).

Discussion

In a case in which the surgeon ruptures the cyst during the dissection from the lung, most of the hydatid fluid should be absorbed by the hypertonic saline soaked gauze, destroying the scolices. Some fluid may come into contact with the patient, and it is necessary to suction as much fluid as possible to minimize exposure. If the rupture is intrabronchial, a bronchoscopy may be required to clear the airway. The patient should be monitored carefully for signs of anaphylaxis.

Case Continued

The remainder of the cyst is excised, the rest of the operative course is uneventful, and the patient makes a full recovery.

All patients should be maintained on oral albendazole for several weeks after surgery.

case 5

Presentation

A 42-year-old man presents to the emergency department complaining of sudden onset of right-sided chest pain accompanied by shortness of breath and cough. His symptoms started 3 days ago and have gradually worsened. The patient denies any history of trauma before the onset of symptoms. The physical examination is significant for mild distress, tachypnea, and absent breath sounds over the right chest with normal breath sounds over the left chest. The patient denies any similar history. His past medical history is negative. The patient says he presented to the emergency department because his symptoms have not improved.

▓ Chest X-rays

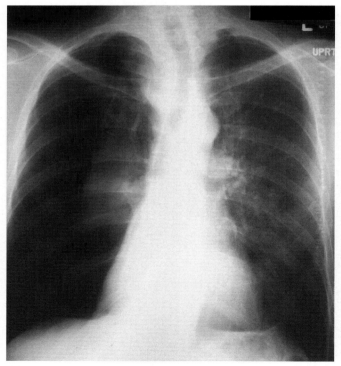

Figure 5-1

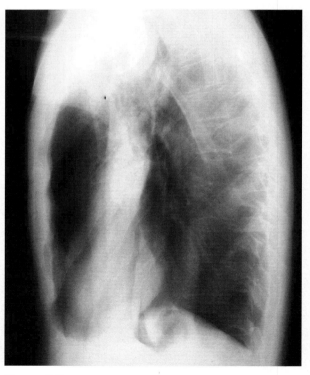

Figure 5-2

Chest X-ray Report

The posteroanterior and lateral chest x-rays reveal a right pneumothorax with complete collapse of the right lung. There is no evidence of mediastinal shift. The trachea is midline in position, with a depression of the right main-stem bronchus. The left lung is well inflated without any pathology. The heart size is normal.

Discussion

A spontaneous pneumothorax is one that occurs without any antecedent traumatic or iatrogenic cause. Spontaneous pneumothoraces can be categorized into primary or secondary types. A primary spontaneous pneumothorax occurs without any clinically apparent underlying lung disease known to promote a pneumothorax. The most common cause of primary spontaneous pneumothorax is an apical subpleural bleb. The typical patient is young, tall, and thin, and in late adolescence or early adulthood. The male-to-female ratio is 6:1. Clinical presentation may vary from asymptomatic (other than the initial chest pain episode) to tension pneumothorax with hemodynamic compromise or collapse. A secondary spontaneous pneumothorax occurs in lungs with underlying pathology that predisposes to a pneumothorax, such as cystic fibrosis, Marfan's syndrome, metastatic osteosarcoma, *Pneumocystis carinii*, and asthma. Bullae are larger than blebs, usually larger than 1 cm. Rarely, a spontaneous pneumothorax may present with hemothorax due to disruption of vascular adhesions. The most common presentation, however, is without progression to tension pneumothorax. Symptoms also depend on the underlying baseline condition of the lungs, or of the remaining inflated lung. The plain chest x-ray is the standard diagnostic modality, preferably in the upright posteroanterior projection.

Recommendation

Right tube thoracostomy.

Treatment Approach

The treatment options for a pneumothorax include observation in selected cases, percutaneous catheter drainage, tube thoracostomy, tube thoracostomy with instillation of a pleural irritant, video-assisted thoracic surgery (VATS), and thoracotomy. The choice of treatment largely depends on the clinical scenario. A clinically stable patient with a small pneumothorax may be observed in the emergency room for 3 to 6 hours and discharged home if a repeat chest x-ray demonstrates no progression of the pneumothorax. A follow-up chest x-ray should be obtained during the next 24 to 48 hours. A clinically stable patient with a large pneumothorax should be hospitalized and undergo a procedure to reexpand the lung. A chest tube is inserted and connected to water-seal drainage.

Case Continued

A right tube thoracostomy is placed with prompt evacuation of air from the right chest and resolution of the patient's distress, shortness of breath, and tachypnea. The chest tube is placed on 20-cm H_2O negative suction. An hour later, you are called to the bedside. The patient has recurrence of distress and shortness of breath. Physical examination reveals tachypnea with labored respirations, tachycardia, subcutaneous emphysema, and crackles over the right lung with normal breath sounds over the left lung. The patient is placed on oxygen first by nasal cannula with progression to 100% oxygen by mask. The patient's condition continues to deteriorate and progresses to severe distress, labored breathing, mild hypotension, and persistent desaturation.

Recommendation

Immediate orotracheal intubation and mechanical ventilation.

Case Continued

A supine chest x-ray is performed.

▫ **Chest X-ray**

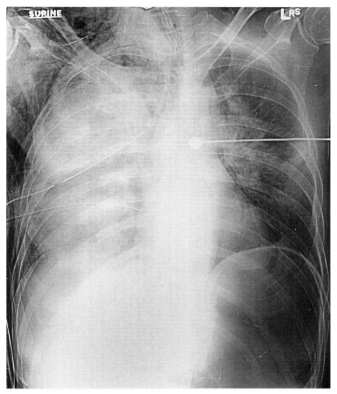

Figure 5-3

Chest X-ray Report

Right-sided chest tubes are present. The right lung is expanded; however, there is a unilateral right pulmonary edema with sparing of the left lung. There is also subcutaneous emphysema, mostly on the patient's right side. An endotracheal tube is identified above the level of the carina. There is significant gastric distention. ▫

Discussion

Reexpansion pulmonary edema (REPE) is a rare condition. It is most often reported after reexpansion of the lung following a sudden decompression of pneumothorax of several days' duration. This complication can also occur with reexpansion of the lung following drainage of large pleural effusions. The mechanism of REPE is poorly understood. The clinical presentation ranges from minimal appearance of unilateral pulmonary infiltrates to severe respiratory compromise accompanied by cardiovascular manifestations. Treatment is mainly supportive to the patient's clinical condition. REPE is more likely to occur when the lung has been collapsed for an extended period of time. Radiographic evidence or clinical manifestations of REPE occur within minutes to hours after lung reexpansion. With decompression of a pneumothorax, it is recommended to avoid immediate intrathoracic suction. In patients with a large pleural effusion, a gradual drainage of the effusion over time and avoidance of immediate total evacuation has been recommended.

Early surgical treatment is recommended in patients with a persistent air leak or prior pneumonectomy and in high-risk patients, such as divers and airplane pilots. In low-risk patients, an intervention to prevent recurrence of primary spontaneous pneumothoraces should be performed after a second pneumothorax. This recommendation stems from the fact that the chance of recurrent pneumothorax after the first incident is about 20%, whereas the chance of a third pneumothorax after a second pneumothorax is about 50% in low-risk patients.

VATS is an alternative to thoracotomy. Some authors have reported a higher recurrence rate with VATS than with a limited thoracotomy. The goal of surgery is excision of the bleb or bulla with the establishment of pleural adhesions by pleural abrasion (with a sponge) or by apical pleurectomy. The instillation of sclerosing agents, such as talc and doxycycline, through a chest tube can be acceptable in patients for whom surgery poses a high risk and for those who refuse surgery. Success rates with chemical pleurodesis are reported to be 78% to 91%, in contrast to 95% to 100% with surgical intervention.

Case Continued

This patient has significant clinical deterioration requiring intubation and mechanical ventilation. With positive-pressure ventilation, the patient develops significant subcutaneous emphysema, most likely from a persistent air leak from the right lung.

The patient is managed in the intensive care unit. The REPE slowly resolves, and the patient is extubated and transferred to the floor on the fifth hospital day. The right chest tube remains in place, and the air leak resolves after 3 days. The chest x-ray demonstrates a completely expanded right lung.

Presentation

A 14-year-old boy presents to the emergency department complaining of a cough and dyspnea for the past 2 weeks. The patient does not report elevated temperature, chills, or sweats. An evaluation performed in the emergency department includes a chest x-ray, which is interpreted as showing right lung pneumonia. Oral antibiotics are administered, and the patient is discharged home. Over the next few weeks, the patient's symptoms fail to improve, and a repeat chest x-ray is performed. Physical examination is significant for diminished breath sounds and wheezing at the right lung base.

Chest X-rays

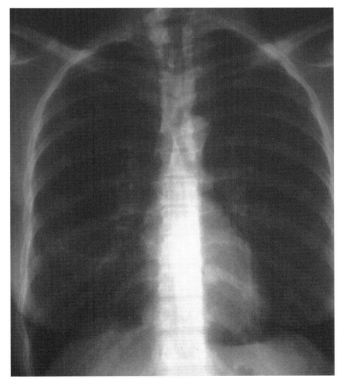

Figure 6-1

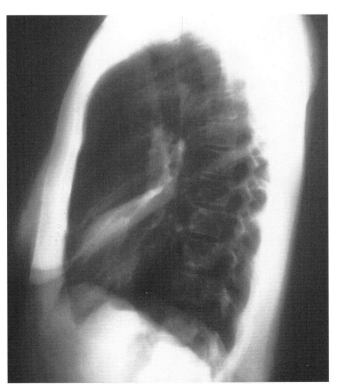

Figure 6-2

Chest X-ray Report

This study demonstrates a right middle lobe atelectasis. The heart size is normal. There are no effusions.

Case Continued

Based on the chest x-rays, a different course of antibiotics is instituted with some mild improvement. A Mantoux purified protein derivative (PPD) skin test is obtained but is nonreactive. The radiographic abnormality does not resolve after the second course of antibiotics, and chest computed tomography (CT) scans are obtained to delineate the findings on chest x-rays.

CT Scans

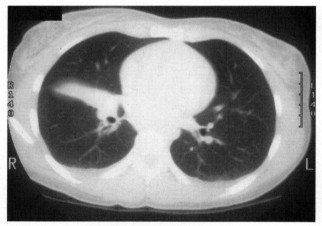

Figure 6-3

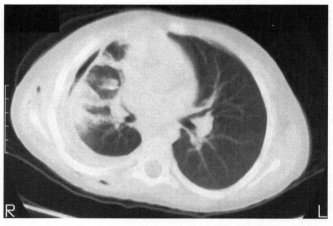

Figure 6-4

CT Scan Report

The scan demonstrates a right hilar density measuring 3 cm with no evidence of calcification. No other enlarged hilar or mediastinal nodes are identified. The lung windows show segmental atelectasis of the right middle lobe. On additional images, right hilar adenopathy with segmental atelectasis of the right middle lobe is noted. These findings are consistent with right middle lobe syndrome.

Discussion

Right middle lobe syndrome is a bronchial compressive disease assumed caused by extrinsic compression of the airway by peribronchial adenopathy. Symptoms typically include productive cough, hemoptysis, recurrent fever, and chest pain. Chest x-ray studies demonstrate a collapsed middle lobe, with or without associated adenopathy. Because other causes of bronchial obstruction exist, a definitive diagnosis needs to be established.

Recommendation

Flexible bronchoscopy.

▪ Flexible Bronchoscopy Photograph

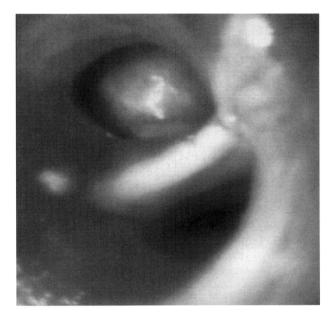

Figure 6-5

Bronchoscopy Findings

At bronchoscopy, a smooth, red-tan tumor is identified obstructing the right middle lobe bronchus. A biopsy is performed. ▪

▪ Histologic Photograph

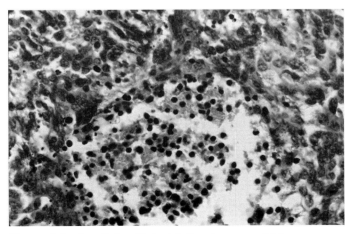

Figure 6-6 See Color Plate 4 following page 114.

Histologic Report

Hematoxylin and eosin preparation demonstrate pleomorphic cells with cytologic atypia and mitotic activity greater than 2 to 10 mitoses per 10 high-power fields (HPFs), consistent with atypical carcinoid tumor. ▪

Discussion

Carcinoid tumors make up less than 1% of all tumors of bronchial origin. Initially believed to be benign, they are now known to exist in a spectrum of neuroendocrine tumors. The malignant potential varies with the degree of differentiation and stage at diagnosis. Although most carcinoid tumors are asymptomatic, presentation of carcinoid tumors depends on their location, with the peripheral tumors being less likely to cause symptoms and with the more centrally located tumors causing symptoms associated with partial or complete bronchial obstruction. Symptoms include cough, wheezing, stridor, hemoptysis, and infection. Carcinoid syndrome is rare, occurring in patients with large tumors or with hepatic metastases. Right-sided cardiac valvular abnormalities are associated with carcinoid hepatic metastases, whereas left-sided cardiac abnormalities are associated with large carcinoid tumors of the lung. As a neuroendocrine tumor, carcinoid can be associated with Cushing's syndrome and the multiple endocrine adenomatosis syndrome. Hormones that can be increased include adrenocorticotropic hormone (ACTH), inappropriate antidiuretic hormone (IADH), and melanophore-stimulating hormone (MSH). Patients with the carcinoid syndrome may have elevated levels of serotonin and 5-hydroxyindoleacetic acid in the blood and urine. This syndrome is rarely seen in patients with tracheobronchial carcinoid.

Bronchoscopy identifies the tumor in 75% of patients. Frozen section should not be obtained because the tumor has similarities to small cell carcinomas. Surgical resection remains the treatment of choice for patients diagnosed with carcinoid tumors in the absence of distant metastatic disease. Surgical resection should be guided by the principle of lung conservation whenever oncologically feasible.

Endobronchial therapy with neodymium:yttrium-aluminum-garnet (Nd:YAG) laser has been suggested as an alternative form of therapy; however, because the tumors are often locally invasive, the risk for recurrence is higher, and this form of therapy should be reserved for nonoperative candidates. Chemotherapy, etoposide (VP-16), and cisplatin are administered to patients with metastatic carcinoid, with less than 50% of patients demonstrating a major response to the chemotherapeutic regimen. The prognosis for typical carcinoid is excellent, with greater than 90% 5-year survival rates with or without lymph node involvement. In comparison, atypical carcinoids have a 60% 5-year disease-free survival rate.

Recommendation

Thoracotomy and lung resection.

Case Continued

At thoracotomy, the middle lobe is consolidated, with some adhesions to the pericardium and diaphragm. The tumor itself is about 3 cm in diameter. Adjacent to the bronchus is a small but abnormal-appearing lymph node. This lymph node undergoes biopsy for frozen-section analysis, which shows carcinoid tumor. Because of the size and location of the tumor and a positive hilar lymph node, bilobectomy and mediastinal lymph node dissection are performed. There is minimal intraoperative blood loss, and the patient is extubated in the operating room.

The patient is transferred to the pediatric intensive care unit for postoperative monitoring. Overnight, the patient's vital signs are stable, but during the first post-operative day, he begins to complain of respiratory distress with decreasing oxygen saturation. Diuretics and aerosolized bronchodilators are administered. The chest x-ray shows increasing interstitial edema. Despite these maneuvers, the oxygen saturations continue to decline, and the patient is reintubated. Over the next few hours, despite an increased fraction of inspired oxygen (FIO_2) and a positive end-expiratory pressure (PEEP) of 20, the patient requires 100% FIO_2. Broad-spectrum antibiotics and steroids are administered. With the oxygenation remaining marginal (82%), the use of extracorporeal membrane oxygenation (ECMO) is considered. The patient is switched to an oscillating ventilator, which improves oxygen saturation by recruiting atelectatic lung. Using this modality, lung barotrauma is reduced by means of very low tidal volumes. Gradually, the oxygen saturation improves, and within several days, the patient is switched back to a conventional ventilator for the remainder of his weaning. All cultures drawn during this time show no growth.

Chest X-rays

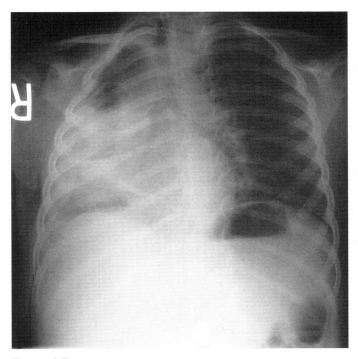

Figure 6-7

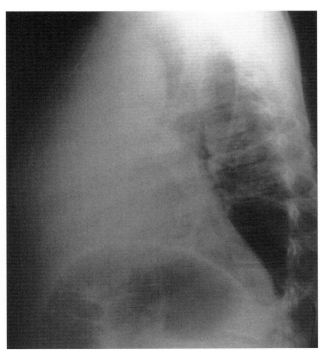

Figure 6-8

Chest X-ray Report

Partial consolidation of the right upper lobe is present. There are no effusions. The heart is shifted slightly to the right.

Discussion

Respiratory complications are a significant cause of morbidity and mortality following thoracic surgical procedures, in some series representing more than 50% of the complications identified. It has been estimated that 40% to 70% of the postoperative deaths are due to pulmonary complications. Risk factors for the development of respiratory complications include smoking, cardiovascular disease, obesity, older age, and preoperative performance status.

After respiratory distress has developed, multiple therapeutic options exist for management. Treatment goals include limiting F_{IO2} and avoiding hyperinflation and alveolar derecruitment. Therapeutic strategies include the use of PEEP, inverse ratio ventilation, high-frequency and jet ventilation, and in some cases extracorporeal support. These major strategies are in addition to appropriate fluid, pharmacologic, and nutritional management.

Pathology Report

The final pathologic study revealed an atypical carcinoid tumor based on the presence of coarse chromatin, hyperchromatism, and small nucleoli. There were also 3 to 4 mitoses per 10 HPFs. Tumor extended into the peribronchial lymph nodes. ▨

Discussion

Atypical carcinoids constitute about 10% of the carcinoids reported in most series. Because of the greater frequency of lymph node involvement and distal metastases, disease-free survival and overall survival rates are decreased in comparison to those of patients with typical carcinoids. Octreotide therapy has been used with some success in patients with distant metastatic disease.

▨ Histology of Typical Carcinoid

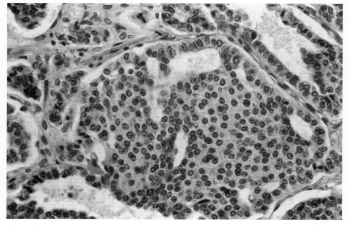

Figure 6-9   See Color Plate 5 following page 114.

Hematoxylin and eosin preparation demonstrating nests of polygonal cells arranged in a rosette-like fashion with less than 2 mitoses per 10 HPFs, consistent with typical carcinoid tumor.

Presentation

A 60-year-old woman presents to her family doctor complaining of a persistent cough for the past 3 weeks. After a short course of antibiotics, the following chest x-rays are obtained.

Chest X-rays

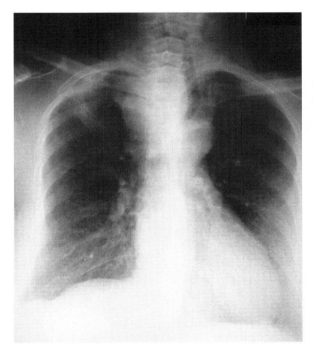 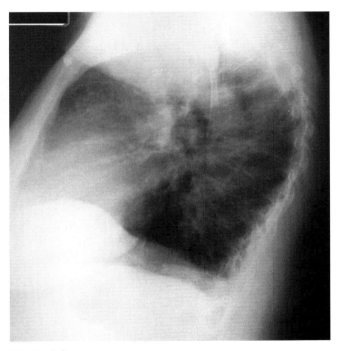

Figure 7-1   **Figure 7-2**

Chest X-ray Report

A mass is present in the anterosuperior mediastinum displacing the trachea to the left. The anterior mediastinum is enlarged. The cardiac silhouette is normal. The lung fields are clear, and there are no pleural effusions.

Case Continued

The patient's family doctor orders a computed tomography (CT) scan of the chest and refers her to a thoracic surgeon. Upon questioning, she admits to having some difficulty swallowing solid food. The patient denies stridor, wheezing, hoarseness, weakness, and flushing. On examination, she has no respiratory distress. There is an enlarged right lobe of the thyroid gland, without any cervical adenopathy. The rest of the examination is unremarkable.

Discussion

This patient has a mass in the anterosuperior mediastinum. The mediastinum is composed of three regions: the anterosuperior, middle, and posterior compartments. Common tumors arising in the anterosuperior mediastinum include thymoma, lymphoma, germ cell tumor, and substernal thyroid.

The clinical presentation of a patient with a mediastinal tumor varies. About 50% of patients with mediastinal tumors are asymptomatic. Others may experience symptoms related to mass effect, tumor invasion, or hormonal production. Hoarseness and Horner's syndrome are usually associated with malignancy. Superior vena cava syndrome and airway compression may be caused by large tumors.

▨ CT Scans

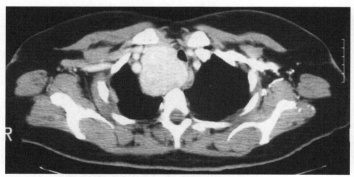
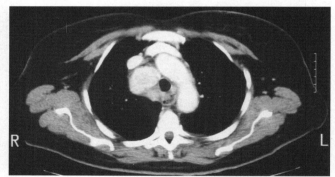

Figure 7-3   **Figure 7-4**

CT Scan Report

There is a large mass to the right of the trachea, extending from the sternoclavicular joint to the vertebral body. This mass extends posteriorly and inferiorly along the trachea to the aortic arch. The mass is displacing the trachea anteriorly and to the left. ▨

Discussion

The most common mediastinal mass arising from the cervical region is the substernal extension of a thyroid goiter. Most of these tumors are nonfunctioning and benign. Most extend into the anterosuperior compartment, but they may extend behind the trachea as well. Usually, the tumor can be palpated in the neck, and tracheal deviation may be present. Some, however, may be isolated completely within the thorax. The arterial circulation most often arises from the inferior thyroid artery in the neck. In advanced stages, these tumors may cause symptoms of compression (such as airway compression, hoarseness, or superior vena cava syndrome). In contrast, malignancy may demonstrate invasion rather than compression of surrounding structures. Substernal thyroid goiters are usually nontoxic, multinodular goiters. Many have areas of calcification on chest x-ray or CT scan. Needle biopsy is generally not necessary before removal. These tumors should be removed, even if asymptomatic, because of potential for airway compromise.

Chest x-rays and CT scan are usually diagnostic, and additional evaluation is rarely necessary. Contrast used during CT scan provides iodine load and may produce thyrotoxicity. Nuclear scanning cannot be performed after contrast CT scan for several weeks. However, negative thyroid imaging, before iodinated contrast load, does not exclude the diagnosis of intrathoracic thyroid goiter. Magnetic resonance imaging (MRI) offers enhanced resolution and may be valuable if vascular or tracheal invasion is suspected. Diagnostic bronchoscopy is not necessary in this situation and, in fact, may precipitate airway compromise. An esophagram may show extrinsic compression but is not necessary. Mediastinoscopy is also not necessary to establish the diagnosis.

Recommendation

Mediastinal tumors, with the exception of lymphomas and germ cell tumors, are generally treated surgically. Because of cervical involvement of the thyroid gland, the most likely etiology of the substernal mass is direct extension of this tumor. Preoperative thyroid function tests should be obtained.

In this situation, careful preoperative evaluation of the airway is essential. An experienced anesthesiologist must be prepared for an awake, fiberoptic intubation. A wire-reinforced endotracheal tube can be beneficial in maintaining tracheal stability. Rigid bronchoscopic instrumentation should be available. Arterial blood pressure measurements and large-bore peripheral intravenous lines are necessary.

The patient is positioned supine with shoulder padding to extend the neck. Many thyroid tumors with substernal extension can be safely removed from the standard cervical approach. If there is a large substernal component and concern that the tumor's blood supply arises from an intrathoracic source, or if the tumor appears to be invading surrounding structures, partial or complete sternotomy should also be performed. A combined right thoracotomy and cervical approach can also be considered. Ectopic intrathoracic goiters (no cervical component) and substernal goiters in patients who have previously undergone cervical thyroidectomy receive blood supply from intrathoracic sources. These patients should be approached by sternotomy or thoracotomy.

Postoperatively, the patient should be monitored for airway compromise from swelling, recurrent laryngeal nerve injury, and hematoma. More remotely, signs of hypothyroidism and hypoparathyroidism should be monitored.

Case Continued

The patient is taken to the operating room where a collar incision is performed. The strap muscles are retracted laterally, the thyroid is identified, and the middle thyroid vein is ligated. After identification of the parathyroid and recurrent laryngeal nerve, an attempt is made to deliver the substernal portion of the thyroid through the neck incision; however, this is unsuccessful. A median sternotomy is performed, and the thyroid is carefully dissected and removed. At the conclusion of the procedure, the patient is extubated and transferred to the recovery room, where calcium levels are monitored. On postoperative examination, the patient is noted to be hoarse but is able to breathe without difficulty.

Discussion

Recurrent laryngeal nerve injury is a complication of thyroid surgery and may result in hoarseness and aspiration. Less commonly, bilateral recurrent nerve injury may cause airway compromise and an aspiration risk. Otolaryngology consultation should be obtained in patients with suspected vocal cord paralysis. Several management options are available to medialize the paralyzed cord. Such treatments are performed under local anesthesia and involve injection of Gelfoam, which will medialize the cord for 4 to 12 weeks, or Teflon, which provides long-term medialization but can be associated with granuloma formation. Other agents that may be injected include fat, silicone, and bovine collagen. Laryngeal framework surgery may be necessary in some patients who do not have an appropriate result with vocal cord injection; in some centers, this surgery has become the primary method for treating vocal cord paralysis.

Case Continued

Laryngoscopy is performed, which demonstrates paralysis of the right vocal cord. Vocal cord injection with Gelfoam is performed with excellent results. The remainder of the patient's postoperative course is unremarkable.

Presentation

A 74-year-old woman is referred to you by her primary medical doctor. She had been living independently up until recently but now requires supervision for progressive somnolence and intermittent confusion. Past medical history is significant for hypertension. She quit smoking 10 years ago after a 50-pack-per-year smoking history. On physical examination, there are no neck masses, the lungs are clear, the heart is regular, and there are no focal neurologic deficits.

Chest X-rays

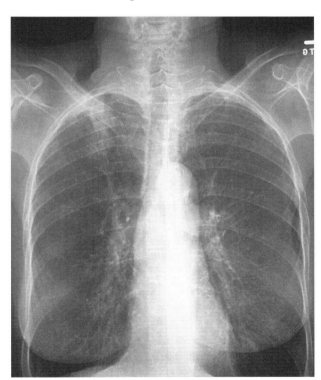

Figure 8-1

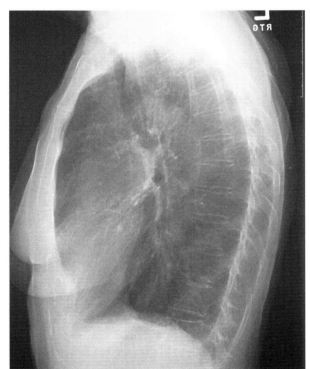

Figure 8-2

Chest X-ray Report

There is an irregular density in the right upper lobe. There are no other lung masses. The heart size is normal, and there are no pleural effusions. ▪

Differential Diagnosis

The presenting symptoms of change in mental status could be due to a variety of etiologies, including primary brain lesions, metabolic disturbances, medications, hypoxia, and infection. In this patient with neurologic symptoms and a lung nodule, brain metastases or hypercalcemia as part of a paraneoplastic syndrome should be considered.

Computed tomography (CT) scans of the chest should be obtained to delineate the chest mass. In addition, serum chemistries and a CT scan of the head are required.

Serum Chemistry Results

Serum calcium is elevated at 11.5. CT scan of the head shows no mass lesions.

▪ CT Scans

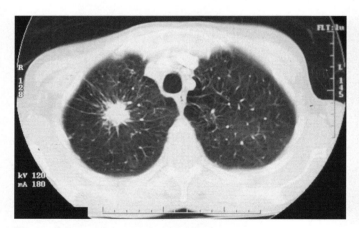

Figure 8-3

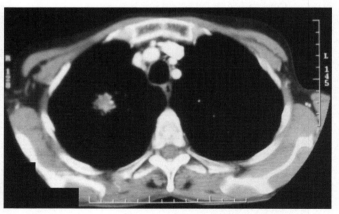

Figure 8-4

CT Scan Report

CT scans of the chest demonstrate a 3-cm spiculated mass in the right upper lobe. There are no enlarged mediastinal lymph nodes or pleural effusions.

Discussion

Lung cancer is the leading cause of cancer death in the United States. Although the incidence of lung cancer in men has stabilized, the rates continue to escalate in women, with overall 5-year survival rates of only 10% to 15%.

Tobacco use has been identified as a major risk factor for development of lung cancer by activating oncogenes. Other risk factors include female gender, a diet low in β-carotene, bullous disease, airway obstruction, previous lung cancer, and environmental factors such as secondhand smoke and occupational carcinogens.

In large studies, screening chest x-rays did not improve survival and are not recommended in asymptomatic patients. Presenting symptoms of patients with lung cancer are variable depending on location of the primary lesion and presence of metastatic disease. Most patients are asymptomatic in the early stages. Generally, the disease is advanced if significant symptoms are present. The initial symptoms are usually cough, hemoptysis, wheezing, stridor, dyspnea, or recurrent infections. Extrapulmonary signs and symptoms such as hoarseness, chest pain, dysphagia, pleural effusion, Horner's syndrome, Pancoast's syndrome, and superior vena cava syndrome are present in more advanced disease.

Paraneoplastic syndromes can be the first sign of disease. Hypercalcemia, the syndrome of inappropriate antidiuretic hormone (SIADH), and Cushing's syndrome are the most common. In addition, gynecomastia, galactorrhea, excess growth hormone, increased calcitonin, increased thyroid-stimulating hormone, and hyperglycemia or hypoglycemia can be a manifestation of lung cancer. Squamous cell lung cancer can be associated with hypercalcemia either from bone metastases or parathyroid hormone (PTH)-related protein secretion, although Cushing's syndrome, SIADH, and gynecomastia can also be associated with squamous cell lung cancer.

Recommendation

Radiographic evaluation of this patient indicates a possible neoplasm of the right upper lobe; clinical staging is indicated. After history and physical examination are performed, bronchoscopy and transthoracic needle biopsy are recommended.

Discussion

Clinical staging includes histologic confirmation of cancer, assessment of hilar and mediastinal lymph node involvement, and evaluation of metastatic disease. The plain chest x-ray and CT scan of the chest are the best tools for evaluating tumor size and location. Lung cancer occurs more frequently on the right side and in the upper lobes more often than in the lower lobes; 50% to 60% of lung cancer nodules are peripheral lesions. Because lesions that have been stable in size and shape over time are unlikely to be malignant, previous radiographic studies are important for comparison. Squamous cell cancer is found centrally in 65% of patients and may be associated with obstructive pneumonitis and consolidation.

Staging by radiographic techniques is most accurate for tumor size (T). CT scan can separate T1 (less than 3 cm) from T2 (greater than 3 cm) lesions; however, visceral pleural involvement (T2) can be difficult to evaluate. CT scans do not readily assess chest wall invasion (T3 lesions). Definite rib destruction or chest wall mass greatly increases accuracy of CT scan staging.

Mediastinal lymph node involvement greater than 10 mm in greatest diameter, on CT scan, may indicate metastatic spread to the lymph node. Mediastinoscopy in such instances is indicated for staging.

Other modalities can be employed to evaluate the extent of mediastinal involvement. Positron-emission tomography (PET) can identify areas of high metabolism throughout the body with 94% sensitivity and 82% specificity for malignancy. The false-positive results are usually due to infectious or inflammatory disease, and false-negative results are found in tumors with low metabolic activity such as carcinoid or bronchoalveolar cancer. PET scans are less accurate for lesions smaller than 1 cm.

Transthoracic CT-guided fine-needle biopsy has become the procedure of choice for peripheral lesions and can be 80% to 95% accurate. Needle biopsies are well suited to situations in which a mass extends to the chest wall or in which mediastinal disease is present. This diagnostic modality is indicated when the patient has a high operative risk and the lesion is considered benign by radiographic evaluation. If the patient is not an operative candidate, histologic confirmation of cancer is required to proceed with chemotherapy, radiation, or both.

The presence of enlarged lymph nodes or distant metastases can be suggested by the previously mentioned imaging modalities. Mediastinoscopy is the most accurate method for lymph node staging, with a false-negative rate of 10% and no false-positive findings. However, the use of routine mediastinoscopy in patients with lung cancer remains controversial. Most surgeons use mediastinoscopy selectively in patients with enlarged lymph nodes (larger than 10 mm), T3 tumors, and central cancers. Anterior mediastinotomy has been used when the subaortic and lateral aortic area nodes are enlarged in a patient with lung cancer.

When bronchoscopy and needle biopsy are not diagnostic, video-assisted thoracic surgery (VATS) can be used to excise peripheral nodules. In addition, VATS sampling of lymphadenopathy can also be performed. If the lung mass is not accessible by VATS, thoracotomy and wedge excision should be performed.

Recommendation

A CT-guided biopsy is performed. The needle biopsy and postprocedure x-ray are shown.

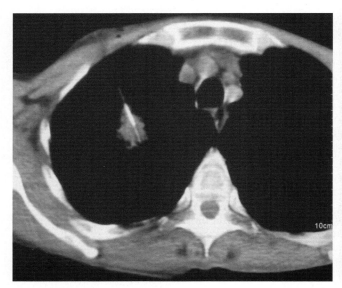

Figure 8-5

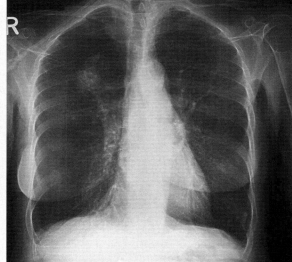

Figure 8-6

The postprocedure x-ray shows a right pneumothorax. Pneumothorax as a complication of transthoracic CT-guided needle biopsy is present in 20% to 25% of the patients who undergo the procedure. About half of the patients who have a pneumothorax require catheter drainage.

A pigtail catheter is placed in the right chest, and the lung reexpands, as shown in the chest x-ray that follows. The histologic diagnosis of the tissue sample demonstrates squamous cell cancer.

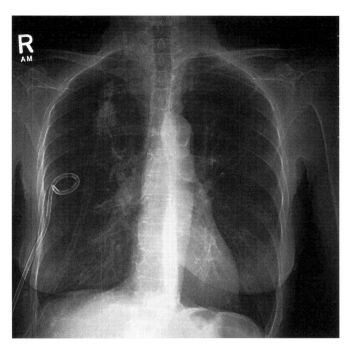

Figure 8-7

Discussion

Lung cancers are separated into two main groups: the small cell type and the non–small cell type, the small cell type belonging to the neuroendocrine set of tumors. The classification for lung cancer, therefore, includes the following:

1. Squamous cell
2. Adenocarcinoma
   a. Bronchoalveolar (highly differentiated form)
3. Large cell
4. Adenosquamous
5. Small cell
   a. Pure small cell
   b. Small cell–large cell
   c. Combined small cell

Squamous cell cancer represents 20% to 35% of all lung cancers. Two thirds of such masses are found centrally and are characterized by slow growth and late metastasis. Central necrosis and cavitation are seen in 10% to 20% of cases. The tumors extend endobronchially, producing obstructive pneumonitis and consolidation, as well as peribronchially, resulting in constrictive symptoms.

When metastatic disease is present, it generally occurs in adjacent pulmonary or thoracic tissue. Lymphatic spread is initially to lobar or hilar nodes, followed by the ipsilateral mediastinal nodes. In this case scenario, the tumor should drain to levels 4, 3, and 2 on the right, and contralateral involvement would be quite unusual. Distant metastases are usually found in the brain, liver, lungs, skeletal system, adrenals, kidneys, or pancreas and are due to hematogenous spread. At the time of presentation, 15.5% of these patients are asymptomatic.

Case Continued

The patient recovers from the needle biopsy and pigtail placement. Based on the radiographic findings, this case represents a stage I squamous cell lung cancer, and surgery would be recommended.

Discussion

The treatment of lung cancer can involve surgery, chemotherapy, and radiation. However, less than 15% of patients diagnosed with non–small cell lung cancer are candidates for resection. Stage I node-negative cancers are divided into two groups based on size: T1 N0 and T2 N0. In this case, the tumor is T1 N0, which is associated with excellent 5-year survival rates of 60% to 80% for all types. Squamous cell cancer patients have the best outcomes, with 90% free of recurrence 5 years after surgery. Adjuvant therapies have not been shown to offer any advantage to surgical resection.

Case Continued

After pulmonary function tests are obtained, the patient undergoes a right upper lobectomy and mediastinal lymphadenectomy through a lateral thoracotomy through the fourth intercostal space.

Discussion

Placement of an epidural catheter is recommended for postoperative pain control. Intraoperative bronchoscopy should be performed, if it was not performed previously. The patient is then intubated with a double-lumen endotracheal tube and placed in the lateral decubitus position. A lateral thoracotomy is made in the fourth intercostal space, using a muscle-sparing thoracotomy.

Upon entering the chest, ventilation of the ipsilateral lung is stopped, and the location of the mass is examined. Central tumors have a homogeneous whitish cut surface and are usually irregular firm masses that may occlude the bronchial lumen. Peripheral tumors may have puckering of the overlying visceral pleura and may show central necrosis on cut section. Intraoperative staging should be performed by assessing the tumor for extension into adjacent structures. In addition, absence of pleural studding, satellite nodules, and obvious mediastinal lymph node metastases should be confirmed. Some surgeons advocate intraoperative VATS to evaluate patients for pleural studding before performing a lateral thoracotomy.

The goal is complete resection by lobectomy. Sleeve lobectomy or pneumonectomy can be employed as needed to achieve complete resection. Segmentectomy would be indicated for patients with poor pulmonary reserve and compromised cardiac status. If the tumor is adherent to the chest wall, an attempt at extrapleural dissection should be made. If the tumor extends to the chest wall, *en bloc* lobe and rib resection should be performed.

The need for mediastinal lymph node sampling or complete lymphadenectomy is controversial. The advantage is histologic verification of staging without significantly increasing operative morbidity or mortality and perhaps removing microscopic disease. Disadvantages include technical difficulties involved in complete dissection with associated surgical risks and the fact that survival may not be increased because the disease is possibly systemic. Mediastinal lymphadenectomy should include levels 2, 4, 7, 8, and 9, including lymph nodes at levels 5 and 6 for left-sided cancers.

Case Continued

The patient has an uneventful postoperative course. Final pathology confirms a T1 N0 (stage I) squamous cell cancer.

Discussion

Because this patient has fully resected node-negative disease, there is no benefit of adjuvant therapies. However, given the risk for recurrence, there is a need for lifelong surveillance. Most failures occur within the first 3 years and usually occur as distant metastases affecting the brain, bone, liver, or contralateral lung. Follow-up should include a chest x-ray, which is performed every 3 to 4 months for the first year, every 6 months through the third year, and annually thereafter.

case 9

Presentation

A 65-year-old man with no significant past medical history presents to your office with symptoms of dysphagia and regurgitation. He reports difficulty initiating swallowing both solids and liquids. He also experiences occasional spontaneous regurgitation of undigested food into the back of his throat. There is no history of cough or pneumonia. His wife reports that in recent months she noticed that her husband has bad breath. He has had no weight loss, and his physical examination is normal.

Differential Diagnosis

The differential diagnosis for dysphagia includes malignant obstruction, benign stricture, leiomyoma, extrinsic compression, motility disorder, diverticulum, disorders of the nervous system producing discoordinated swallowing, and congenital abnormalities of the esophagus such as duplication cyst. The history in this patient of difficulty initiating swallowing suggests a disorder of the cervical esophagus or a nervous system disease.

Recommendation

Options for initial investigation include endoscopy or a contrast x-ray of the esophagus and stomach. In this case, because the most likely diagnoses include a motility disorder, a contrast esophagram is the best initial test. If the patient has an unexpected diverticulum, there is an increased risk for perforation during an initial endoscopic examination.

Esophagogram

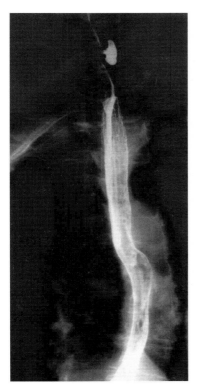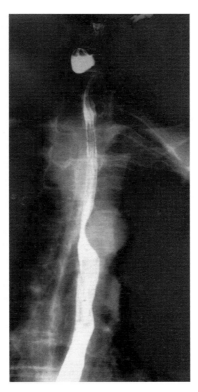

Figure 9-1

Esophagogram Report

The barium swallow demonstrates a mild nonspecific motility disorder of the esophageal body, a small hiatal hernia, and a pharyngoesophageal diverticulum.

Discussion

A pharyngoesophageal, or Zenker's, diverticulum usually occurs in patients older than 50 years of age, and results from discoordination between the inferior pharyngeal constrictors and the cricopharyngeus muscle. In some patients, the only manifestation of this discoordination is the presence of a poorly relaxing cricopharyngeus muscle (cricopharyngeal bar) that impinges on the hypopharyngeal lumen. Long-standing excess pressure ultimately causes the development of a diverticulum in the region between the two muscles that has a paucity of overlying muscle, known as Killian's triangle. These diverticula can become quite large, extending into the mediastinum.

Patients with pharyngoesophageal diverticula are at risk for regurgitation and aspiration, particularly if the diverticulum is large. In patients with symptoms, correction of the abnormality is recommended. Endoscopy and manometry are not necessary components of the preoperative evaluation because they rarely have an impact on the management of this diagnosis.

The main therapeutic objective is the interruption of discoordinated activity between the inferior pharyngeal constrictor muscle and the cricopharyngeus muscle. This is accomplished by division of the cricopharyngeus muscle (myotomy). Management of the diverticulum may include excision or plication to the prevertebral fascia in an inverted orientation. For diverticula that are moderate in size (2 to 4 cm in length), endoscopic management may be considered. A linear cutting stapler is placed transorally, with the staple cartridge in the esophagus and the anvil in the diverticulum. Firing the stapler divides the cricopharyngeus and creates a common cavity between the esophagus and the diverticulum. This procedure is not recommended for very small or very large diverticula.

Recommendation

Cricopharyngeal myotomy and diverticulopexy.

Case Continued

You perform a left neck incision and a cricopharyngeal myotomy that extend several centimeters down the esophagus. During efforts to dissect the investing fascia off of the diverticulum, a small defect is created in the diverticulum.

Discussion

Endoscopic stapling of the diverticulum is not considered in this patient because the diverticulum is too small to permit the stapler to accommodate the entire cricopharyngeus muscle. An open myotomy is therefore performed. The primary advantage of performing a diverticulopexy is that no suture or staple line is created, eliminating the possibility of leakage. This permits the patient to be fed liquids on the same day as the operation and allows discharge the morning after the operation.

In this patient, the location of the defect in the diverticulum does not permit stapling across the neck of the diverticulum. Rather than creating a long suture line, you elect to repair the defect with a few interrupted sutures and to proceed with diverticulopexy.

Case Continued

The patient's initial postoperative course is unremarkable. He complains of right pleuritic chest pain 8 hours after surgery and has a low-grade temperature during the night after his operation. The next morning, his examination reveals decreased breath sounds at the right base and a small amount of cloudy drainage from the lower part of the neck incision.

Diagnosis and Recommendation

The findings suggest the possibility of a leak from the hypopharynx or esophagus. A chest x-ray is ordered, and antibiotics are administered.

Chest X-ray

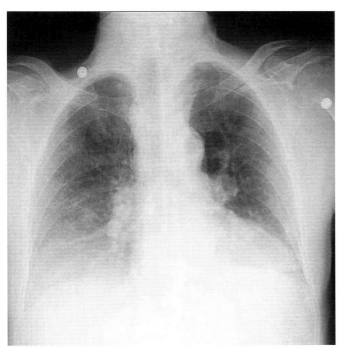

Figure 9-2

Chest X-ray Report

The chest x-ray shows right pleural effusion and a small amount of subcutaneous emphysema in the left neck.

Recommendation

The history and the physical and radiographic findings are suggestive of a leak. Broad-spectrum antibiotics should be administered. A right thoracostomy tube is placed that yields serous fluid. The patient should be returned to the operating room for neck exploration.

Discussion

Morbidity associated with surgery for Zenker's diverticulum includes vocal cord paralysis, wound infection, suture line leak, and recurrence of the diverticulum. A suspected leak from the hypopharynx or esophagus requires urgent diagnosis and management. In this patient, endoscopy and contrast esophagram are not necessary because there is already a region of high suspicion for leak based on the findings during the initial operation. The pleural fluid represents a sympathetic effusion based on chemistries. Thoracostomy tube insertion is sufficient management as long as the effusion is adequately drained. At the time of neck exploration through the original incision, a small amount of cloudy fluid is evident, but the tissues are otherwise healthy, and there is no obvious defect in the mucosa.

An appropriate amount of concern is necessary in managing suspected leaks. In this patient, even though no obvious leak is identified, reinforcement of the region of suspected leakage with healthy tissue and proper drainage is appropriate.

Recommendation

Sternocleidomastoid muscle flap to cover the region of leakage and flat suction tube to drain the neck and upper mediastinum.

▦ Chest X-ray

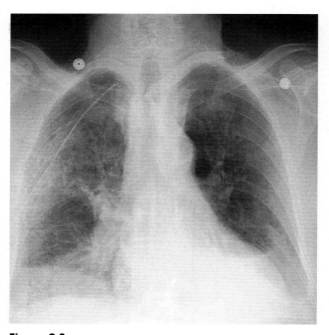

Figure 9-3

Chest X-ray Report

The patient has a new right thoracostomy tube with reduction in the size of the right pleural effusion. A drain is present in the left neck extending into the upper mediastinum. ▦

Case Continued

The patient is not allowed oral intake for several days, during which time he has no fever or leukocytosis. His neck drain and thoracostomy tube yield very little fluid. He is started on a clear liquid diet on the fifth postoperative day, and there is no increase in drainage from either of the tubes. The thoracostomy tube is discontinued the following day, and the neck drain is incrementally withdrawn over 3 days, permitting discharge on the eighth postoperative day on a full liquid diet. A follow-up chest x-ray is obtained at the time of his outpatient clinic visit 1 week later.

Chest X-ray

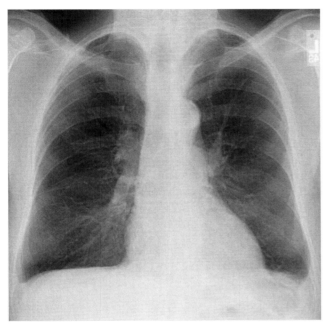

Figure 9-4

Chest X-ray Report

Normal chest x-ray.

case 10

Presentation

A 56-year-old truck driver has been incapacitated for several years because of chronic obstructive pulmonary disease (COPD). The patient reports having shortness of breath while walking from the bedroom to the bathroom. Recently, he was prescribed oxygen at 3 L/min to use continuously.

Past medical history includes hypertension and moderate peripheral vascular disease. The patient has a 40-pack-per-year history of smoking. On physical examination, the vital signs are stable; oxygen saturation is 91% on 3-L nasal cannula. There are decreased breath sounds and fine crackles bilaterally. Diagnostic tests include a chest x-ray, which demonstrates hyperinflated lungs compatible with COPD. There are no infiltrates or masses. The heart size is normal, and there are no pleural effusions. Pulmonary function tests reveal a forced expiratory volume in 1 second (FEV_1) of 0.67 L and a forced vital capacity (FVC) of 1.86 L.

Discussion

Medical therapy for end-stage COPD consists of bronchodilators, expectorants, pulmonary care, steroids, and prevention and treatment of pulmonary infection. Lung transplantation should be considered in patients for whom lifestyle is severely restricted and life expectancy is diminished.

Lung transplantation is a treatment option for many end-stage pulmonary diseases. It is specifically performed in patients who have a life expectancy of less than 1 to 2 years and are severely debilitated. Single-lung transplantation is performed in patients with obstructive or interstitial lung disease, whereas bilateral sequential lung transplantation is performed in patients with infectious pulmonary processes, such as cystic fibrosis and bronchiectasis, and for young patients with emphysema. Combined heart-lung transplantation is reserved for end-stage lung and heart disease.

Candidates for lung transplantation are patients with diminished exercise capacity, poor pulmonary function, and in most cases, oxygen dependency. Contraindications for lung transplantation include acute infection; malignancy; irreversible dysfunction of renal, hepatic, cardiac, or nervous system; and psychiatric conditions such as addiction or noncompliance. Relative contraindications to lung transplantation include ventilator dependency, prior thoracic surgery, and advanced age. In a candidate for single-lung transplantation, the side chosen to transplant is the one that has the worst function as measured by ventilation-perfusion mismatch.

Case Continued

Assessment of the patient by the lung transplantation team includes an echocardiogram, cardiac catheterization, ventilation-perfusion scan, pulmonary function tests, bronchoscopy, and surveillance for infection. The patient is referred to a pulmonary rehabilitation program to maximize his physical condition, and he is provided with information about transplantation procedure, immunosuppression, and risks. The following computed tomography (CT) scans are obtained in the preoperative evaluation.

CT Scans

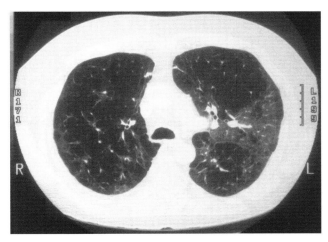 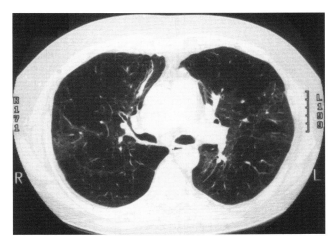

Figure 10-1   **Figure 10-2**

CT Scan Report

The CT scans demonstrate numerous confluent bullae with little normal lung parenchyma. There are no lung masses or enlarged mediastinal or hilar lymph nodes.

Case Continued

After 4 months, the transplantation coordinator receives a call that a lung is available for this patient. Most organ donors are victims of trauma or cerebral catastrophe. Before an organ can be accepted for harvesting, brain death must be established. An acceptable donor should be younger than 55 years of age and must have ABO compatibility with the recipient. Donor operation coordinates multiple teams for multiple organ harvesting. To be an acceptable organ, the lung should not have incurred direct trauma, contusion, or hemorrhage. On 100%

fraction of inspired oxygen (FiO_2) and positive end-expiratory pressure (PEEP) of 5 cm, the partial pressure of arterial oxygen (PaO_2) should be at least 300 mm Hg. The chest x-ray of the donor must be clear of masses and infiltrates, serology of the donor [human immunodeficiency virus (HIV), hepatitis C, and cytomegalovirus (CMV)] is checked, and any history of previous lung disease is ascertained. The size match should be within 15% to 20% of the calculated total lung capacity (TLC) of the patient. Measurements of the circumference as well as vertical and horizontal lengths are also used in the assessment of the fit for the recipient. Finally, bronchoscopy at the time of harvesting is essential to exclude purulent bronchial secretions and aspiration, either of which contraindicates use of the lung as an acceptable donor organ.

Surgical Technique: Donor

After bronchoscopy of the donor, the chest is opened through a median sternotomy, and the lung is inspected for adhesions, contusions, and hemorrhage. The lung is mobilized; the trachea is dissected, and a tape is placed around it. The superior vena cava (SVC) is mobilized, and a tape is placed around it. After the abdominal organ team completes their dissection, 30,000 units of heparin are administered intravenously to the patient. In addition, 500 µg of prostaglandin E_1 (PGE_1) are injected directly into the pulmonary artery. PGE_1 causes systemic hypotension, at which time the aorta is cross-clamped and cardioplegia is administered for cardiac preservation. Cold pulmoplegia (3 L of Euro-Collins solution) is delivered into the pulmonary artery. The effluent is vented through the left atrial appendage and the inferior vena cava at the level of the diaphragm. Ice and cold saline are placed in the chest cavity to provide topical cooling. Simultaneously, the SVC is ligated (to prevent warm blood from entering the right heart), and the innominate artery and vein are stapled to facilitate exposure of the trachea. Ventilation is maintained with 100% oxygen, keeping the lungs gently inflated. After the heart and lungs are preserved, the endotracheal tube is pulled back, ventilation is maintained to keep the lungs at least two thirds inflated, and the trachea is stapled and transected. The heart is excised, taking care to leave a sufficient left atrial cuff with sufficient length on the pulmonary veins. The pericardium is cut from the diaphragm, behind the hilum, and continuing beneath the trachea. Dividing the posterior wall of the remaining left atrial cuff separates the pulmonary veins, and the pulmonary artery is bisected at the bifurcation. The left main bronchus is doubly stapled and transected, keeping both donor lungs inflated. The donor lung is placed in a sterile bag, ice and cold saline are placed into the bag, and the bag is tied securely. After double bagging, the lung is placed in a cooler filled with ice and taken expeditiously by the harvesting team to the recipient hospital. Ischemia time begins with the cross-clamping of the aorta and infusion of pulmoplegia.

Surgical Technique: Recipient

As soon as a donor lung is available, the patient is admitted to the hospital and assessed for surgery. Intraoperatively, the patient is positioned in a modified decubitus position, with rotation of the ipsilateral hip to enable access to the femoral area for possible use of cardiopulmonary bypass (CPB). A transesophageal echocardiogram probe is used in all lung transplantations to assess ventricular function, evaluate adequacy of de-airing, and verify integrity of the vascular anastomosis after transplantation.

A standard pneumonectomy is performed when the donor lung arrives in the operating room. Generous cuffs of the pulmonary artery and the pulmonary veins are left with the staple line. The left main-stem bronchus is transected two cartilaginous rings proximal to the origin of the upper lobe bronchus without dissecting the peribronchial tissue, which includes the blood supply of the bronchus. The cartilaginous ring is cut, the membranous portion of the bronchus is cut with some redundancy, and the bronchial stump is cleared of secretions. The pericardium around the veins is incised widely and the pulmonary veins mobilized. The pulmonary artery is prepared intrapericardially.

Surgical Technique: The Transplantation

The superior and inferior pulmonary veins of the donor lung are connected to provide one orifice for the anastomosis. The pulmonary artery is inspected for emboli, and the bronchus is trimmed flush at the second cartilaginous ring proximal to the takeoff of the upper lobe bronchus. Secretions are cultured, and the bronchial tree is suctioned. The bronchial anastomosis is performed first using a running 4-0 polyglyconate suture on the membranous portion, everting the edges. Simple interrupted sutures are used to complete the anastomosis of the cartilaginous wall. In cases in which there is a size discrepancy, a telescoping anastomosis is performed. The peribronchial tissues are wrapped around the suture line for reinforcement.

The pulmonary venous anastomosis is performed next. A vascular clamp is placed on the left atrium, encompassing both the superior and inferior veins. The bridge between them is cut to form a single orifice for anastomosis. Cardiopulmonary bypass may have to be instituted if hemodynamic instability occurs when the clamp is placed on the left atrium.

The left atrial cuff of the donor is aligned with the orifice of the recipient left atrial pulmonary venous orifice, and a direct anastomosis with a 4-0 polypropylene suture is performed in a continuous manner, everting the edges.

Next, the vascular clamp is placed on the pulmonary artery, and the end is spatulated. The clamp is opened momentarily to flush debris from the pulmonary artery. A 5-0 polypropylene suture is used for the end-to-end anastomosis. One gram of methylprednisolone is administered intravenously before allowing perfusion of the lung with warm blood. The pulmonary artery clamp is removed momentarily to perfuse the lung and to de-air the vessels through both untied anastomotic suture lines. The clamp is replaced, and the sutures are tied. The left atrial clamp is removed first, followed by the arterial clamp. The integrity of both anastomoses is checked, and the lung is ventilated. The bronchial stump is checked for air leaks by increasing the airway pressures. The pericardium of the donor lung is trimmed and wrapped around the bronchial suture line for additional protection.

The ischemia time for this organ is less than 6 hours. Optimal ischemia time for lung transplantation is 6 to 8 hours. The patient is reintubated with a single-lumen endotracheal tube at the end of the procedure, and bronchoscopy is performed to check the integrity of the bronchial anastomosis and to clear away blood and secretions.

Postoperative Care

After surgery, excessive fluid administration is minimized. Pulmonary care in lung transplant recipients is essential, and early extubation is preferred. If the patient requires ventilation, pressures are kept low to minimize barotrauma (tidal volume less than 10 mL/kg; PEEP less than 5 cm H_2O). Chest tubes are removed when the air leak seals, and the drainage is minimal.

Immediate Postoperative Chest X-ray

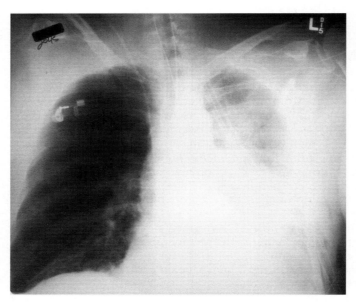

Figure 10-3

Case Continued

The postoperative chest x-ray demonstrates an infiltrate compatible with reimplantation response of the newly transplanted lung. The chest x-ray is consistent with noncardiogenic pulmonary edema that may occur within the first few days after transplantation and may last for several days. Ventilatory support is required for 3 days, during which time fluid intake is restricted, and diuresis is pharmacologically achieved.

▓ Chest X-ray: Fifth Postoperative Day

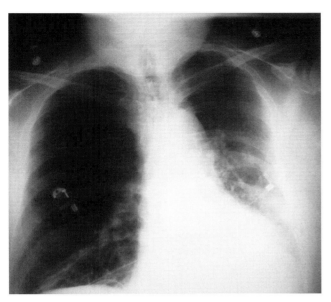

Figure 10-4

Chest X-ray Report

The chest x-ray demonstrates absence of an endotracheal tube that was present on previous x-rays. In addition, there is a resolution of reimplantation response with only minimal patchy infiltrate remaining in the left mid-lung and basilar regions. A small apical pneumothorax is present, the native right lung is hyperinflated, and the mediastinum is shifted to the left. ▓

Recommendation

Triple-drug therapy immunosuppression (steroids, azathioprine, and cyclosporine) is initiated preoperatively. Prophylactic antibiotic, antifungal, and antiviral medications are administered. These include cephalosporin, itroconazole, trimethoprim-sulfamethoxazole (Bactrim; for *Pneumocystis* species prophylaxis), and ganciclovir.

The patient's immediate postoperative spirometric study showed an FEV_1 of 1.67 L and a FVC of 2.55 L. The patient is discharged home on the tenth postoperative day. He is followed frequently in the lung transplantation clinic with physical examinations, chest x-rays, spirometry, laboratory work, and surveillance bronchoscopy.

Case Continued

Five months after transplantation, the patient complains of tiredness, low-grade fever, and decreasing exercise capacity. Serial pulmonary function tests in the clinic show a progressive decline of the FEV_1 to 800 mL. The following chest x-ray is obtained.

Chest X-ray

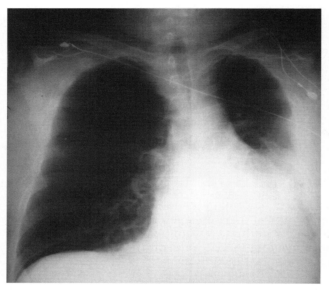

Figure 10-5

Chest X-ray Report

The chest x-ray demonstrates that the left lung is expanded and there is an infiltrate in the left lower lobe. The left main-stem bronchus is narrowed proximally.

Discussion

The most common complications following lung transplantation are infections and rejection. Symptoms are similar in both cases. Objective data are collected to establish a diagnosis, and empiric therapy often has to be initiated. If infection is suspected, antiinfective drug therapy is started after cultures are obtained. If rejection is suspected, the patient receives steroids for 3 days (1 g of methylprednisolone given as an initial bolus). Steroids are continued until the patient improves or another diagnosis is made and specific treatment is given.

Airway complications, such as stenosis, dehiscence, and malacia, occur in up to 15% of lung transplant recipients. The most frequent cause of ischemia of the bronchus following harvesting is disruption of the blood supply. Early after transplantation, the transplanted bronchus has to rely on retrograde perfusion from the lung until revascularization occurs over the course of weeks. Symptoms of shortness of breath and decreasing exercise tolerance, along with radiographic, spirometric, and bronchoscopic evidence, should raise suspicion of this complication.

Case Continued

The patient undergoes rigid bronchoscopy with a 10.5-mm scope. Copious secretions are aspirated. The anastomosis of the left main-stem bronchus is severely narrowed with granulation tissue.

A flexible bronchoscope is introduced through the rigid scope and used to maneuver a guidewire past the obstruction. A 12-mm balloon is placed across the stricture and inflated to 10 atm for 30 seconds. This is repeated, and a 12-mm × 40-mm Wall stent is placed across the anastomosis and deployed. The stent is situated between the origin of the main-stem bronchus and just before the bifurcation of the lobar bronchi. The postoperative FEV_1 is 1.67 L.

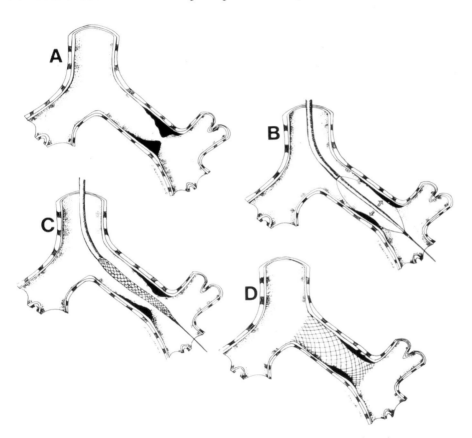

Figure 10-6 From Lonchyna VA, Arcidi JM Jr, Garrity ER Jr, et al. Refractory post-transplant airway strictures: successful managements with wire stents. *Eur J Cardiothorac Surg* 1999;15(6):842–849. Copyright 1999, Elsevier Science. Reprinted with permission.

Case Continued

A follow-up chest x-ray and CT scan show the bronchus to be widely patent and the lung well aerated.

Chest X-ray and CT Scan

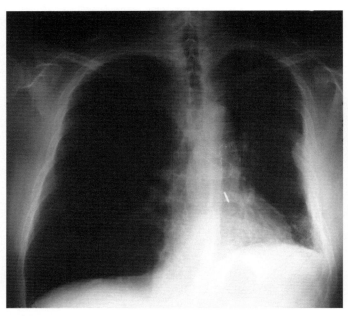

Figure 10-7

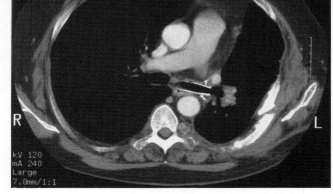

Figure 10-8

Presentation

A 62-year-old man is admitted to the medical service with complaints of dry cough, chest discomfort, and dyspnea for the past 3 months. The chest discomfort is mildly painful, is localized to the left side of the chest, does not radiate, and involves the left shoulder. The patient reports a fever (oral temperature of 101.5°F) but no night sweats or chills. On physical examination, vital signs are stable, and oxygen saturation is 93%. Examination of the chest reveals dullness and diminished breath sounds on the left side. The patient denies weight loss. Social history reveals a nonsmoking patient who for 24 years worked in dismantling old buildings and construction. You are being consulted after the following chest x-rays and computed tomography (CT) scans are obtained.

■ Chest X-rays

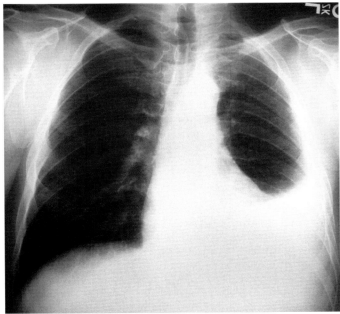

Figure 11-1

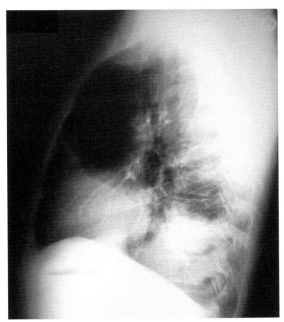

Figure 11-2

Chest X-ray Report

The chest x-ray demonstrates a left pleural effusion. There are no lung nodules in both lung fields. The heart is not enlarged. ■

■ CT Scans

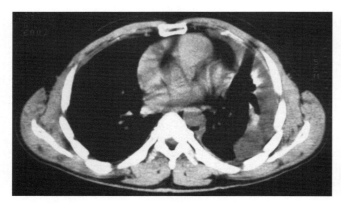

Figure 11-3

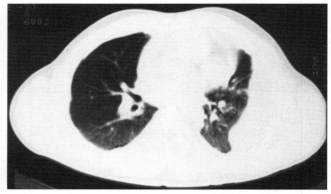

Figure 11-4

CT Scan Report

The CT scans demonstrate a loculated effusion encasing the left lung, with a significant volume loss. There is no evidence of lung nodules.

Case Continued

A diagnostic thoracentesis is performed. The fluid is amber and exudative. The glucose level is 60 mg/dL, and the pH is 7.15. Cytologic examination demonstrates mesothelial cells, lymphocytes, and polymorphonuclear leukocytes. Some cells appear suspicious for malignancy. The patient's symptoms of dyspnea improve minimally.

Discussion

Given the patient's occupational history and the possibility of exposure to asbestos, mesothelioma should be strongly considered. Adenocarcinoma of the lung with involvement of the pleura is also in the differential diagnosis. Infectious causes are less likely given the clinical presentation of this patient. Thoracentesis demonstrates positive cytology in 30% to 50% of patients with mesothelioma. In comparison, needle pleural biopsy is positive in only 30% of the patients. It is often not feasible to confirm malignancy on cytologic specimens in this setting. Furthermore, distinguishing between mesothelioma and adenocarcinoma is difficult by light microscopy alone. Early mesotheliomas may not be easily distinguished from benign mesothelial hyperplasia or severe fibrosis because of the cell types found in such tumors. Because the treatment is dependent on a definite diagnosis, a more substantial quantity of a specimen should be obtained to perform immunohistochemical assays and electron microscopy. Furthermore, diffuse malignant mesothelioma can be histologically confused with metastatic adenocarcinoma or sarcoma. Several histologic stains that enable differentiation of mesothelioma from other diagnoses are available to the pathologist. Adenocarcinomas usually stain with mucicarmine, whereas mesotheliomas do not. Mesotheliomas stain for certain cytokeratins, which may differentiate them from sarcomas, whereas they do not stain for carcinoembryonic antigen (CEA), which is usually seen with adenocarcinoma. Electron microscopy displays the numerous long sinuous microvilli of mesothelioma or the short straight microvilli of an adenocarcinoma as well as the presence of intracellular desmosomes, junctional complexes, and characteristic microvilli. Proper preparation of the specimen is essential when mesothelioma is suspected. Part of the specimen is fixed in neutral buffered formalin, and the rest is fixed with glutaraldehyde preparation for electron microscopy examination.

To confirm the diagnosis, either thoracoscopy with histologic biopsy or open pleural biopsy should be performed. If the pleural space is obliterated by a tumor, thoracoscopy will be difficult to perform. The incisions must be carefully planned so that they can be included in either a surgical incision or the radiation field because mesothelioma has a predilection for seeding the biopsy tract, needle tracts, or chest tube sites. Thoracoscope with adequate pleural tissue usually provides the correct histologic diagnosis.

Case Continued

A pleural biopsy confirms the diagnosis of mesothelioma of epithelial variety.

Discussion

Mesothelioma is classified into localized and diffuse. Histologically diffuse malignant mesothelioma may be of epithelial type, sarcomatous type, or mixed. The epithelial type is most common. Prognosis and management of patients with mesothelioma depends on the stage of the tumor. The staging process has undergone many changes and is currently still under discussion. More recently, positron-emission tomography (PET) is being investigated as an adjunct to chest computed tomography (CT) in evaluating tumor extension. Recognition of diaphragmatic penetration, mediastinal invasion, and mediastinal lymphadenopathy is necessary in assessing candidacy for surgical treatment and for preoperative planning.

The original staging system is the one proposed by Butchart:

Stage I: tumor confined within capsule of parietal pleura—ipsilateral pleura, lung, and diaphragm
Stage II: involving chest wall or mediastinal structures; intrathoracic lymph node involvement
Stage III: penetrating diaphragm involving peritoneum, contralateral pleura; extrathoracic lymph node involvement
Stage IV: distant metastases

A TNM classification has been proposed as well because recent studies have shown that involvement of mediastinal lymph nodes by mesothelioma has prognostic implications.

Treatment is dependent on the extent of the disease, the predominant cell type of the tumor, and careful assessment of the patient's ability to undergo an operative resection of the tumor. Palliative care with control of the malignant pleural effusion in elderly patients and in those who cannot withstand an operative procedure can be of benefit. Thoracoscopic drainage of the pleural effusion followed by talc insufflation can usually control the pleural effusion. Newer chemotherapeutic agents have recently shown benefit and can also be considered. Palliation can achieve a median survival time of about 18 months. Trimodality therapy consisting of extrapleural pneumonectomy followed by chemotherapy and radiation has recently been shown to increase survival. Median survival can approximate 24 months, with 2- and 5-year survival rate of 45% and 22%, respectively. Patients with epithelial histology and negative mediastinal nodes have the best prognosis. Full-thickness diaphragmatic invasion, sarcomatous and mixed histology, and positive lymph nodes are associated with a worse prognosis. Pleurectomy and decortication may be a treatment option in patients with early-stage disease who are unable to tolerate a pneumonectomy. Postoperative radiation and chemotherapy are administered after this procedure. Although complete resection enhances survival, there have been no large-scale studies comparing treatment options in a randomized fashion.

Recommendation

CT of the chest demonstrates no mediastinal adenopathy or invasion through the diaphragm. Pulmonary and cardiac function should be assessed, and a left extrapleural pneumonectomy is planned.

Case Continued

A left posterolateral thoracotomy is performed; the sixth rib is resected along with the left lung, parietal pleura, pericardium, and diaphragm *en bloc*. A mediastinal lymph node dissection is also performed. The diaphragm is repaired with a Gore-Tex patch (W. L. Gore & Associates, Flagstaff, AZ).

Twelve hours after surgery, the patient is hypotensive with a systolic blood pressure of 82 mm Hg and a heart rate of 124 beats/min sinus tachycardia.

Recommendation

Fluid bolus, auscultation of the chest. Immediate chest x-ray and complete blood count to evaluate for bleeding, mediastinal shift, right-sided pneumothorax, and cardiac herniation.

Case Continued

On the chest x-ray, the heart is elevated and positioned posteriorly. These findings suggest herniation through the pericardial defect. The patient is emergently returned to the operating room, where the thoracotomy is reentered and the pericardial defect enlarged to reduce the heart. The defect is repaired with a Gore-Tex patch. After surgery, the patient recovers uneventfully and is discharged on the sixth postoperative day.

Discussion

Failure to repair a pericardial defect may result in cardiac herniation more commonly on the right side where the heart can rotate on its axis and occlude caval inflow, which may result in acute decrease in cardiac output and cardiac arrest. Although rare, left-sided herniation results in hemodynamic compromise by strangulating the left ventricle and compromising blood flow to the myocardium. Right pericardial defects are always repaired with a patch, whereas left-sided defects are not, especially in cases in which the pericardium is opened to the level of the diaphragm and in which the risk for herniation cannot occur because of the large amount of pericardium resected. Most cardiac herniations occur in the first 24 hours after surgery and are associated with the patient's change in position. Cardiac herniation has a high mortality rate, and prompt diagnosis and emergent thoracotomy with reduction of the herniated heart are necessary.

case 12

Presentation

A 48-year-old male presents with a 6-month history of progressive dysphagia. He first noted difficulty swallowing solids and liquids on occasion but now has difficulty with every meal. He has nocturnal regurgitation of undigested food. There is no history of heartburn. He has experienced a 10-pound weight loss in the past 2 months. He is a nonsmoker and nondrinker. On physical exam, the patient is afebrile, the lungs are clear to auscultation, and there are no heart murmurs. The abdomen is soft, nontender, and nondistended. Pulses are equal bilaterally. Several weeks before presenting to you, he was seen in the emergency department where the following chest x-ray was taken.

▓ Chest X-ray

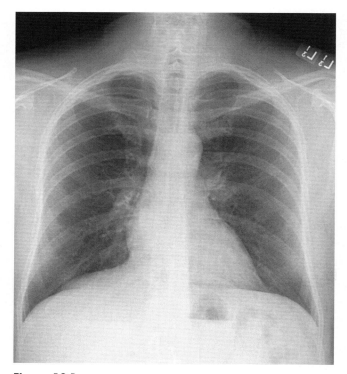

Figure 12-1

The lung fields are clear. The heart is of normal size. There are no pleural effusions.

Differential Diagnosis

Signs and symptoms of dysphagia and weight loss raise concerns regarding esophageal cancer. The nature of this patient's dysphagia, which involves solids and liquids equally, is more suggestive of a benign process. A peptic stricture might be considered, but the lack of a history compatible with gastroesophageal reflux disease makes this diagnosis unlikely. Endoscopy is necessary to evaluate for malignancy as a cause for the dysphagia the patient is experiencing. If no mass is seen, and if the lower esophageal sphincter is easily traversed with the endoscope, pseudoachalasia can be ruled out as well. The clinical signs and symptoms are then most consistent with a motility disorder.

When motility disorder is suspected, a contrast esophagram is usually helpful in confirming the diagnosis. Manometry is always necessary to diagnose diffuse esophageal spasm and high-amplitude peristaltic contractions of the esophagus (nutcracker esophagus). Manometry is sometimes necessary to diagnose achalasia conclusively when the clinical presentation is questionable. In patients with a typical clinical picture, a normal endoscopic examination, and a typical barium swallow, the clinical diagnosis of achalasia usually is certain, and recommendations regarding therapy can be made without the need for manometry.

Recommendation

Esophagogastroduodenoscopy (EGD) and a contrast esophagram.

EGD Report

Mild distal esophagitis with a moderate amount of retained food in the distal esophagus. Absence of motility in the distal esophagus. Tight mucosal rosette at the lower esophageal sphincter, which permits easy passage of the endoscope. Normal stomach, pylorus, and first portion of the duodenum.

◼ Barium Swallow

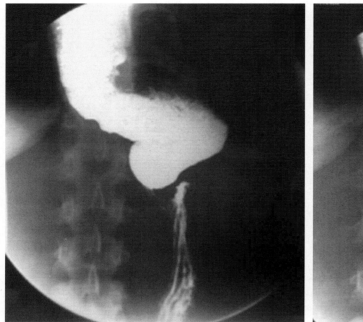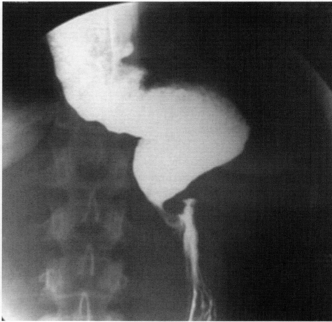

Figure 12-2

Barium Swallow Report

Mild esophageal dilation. Absence of peristaltic activity in the lower esophagus. Air–fluid level in the mid-esophagus due to retained fluid and food. "Bird's beak" abnormality at the level of the esophagogastric junction with incomplete opening of the lower esophageal sphincter (LES). ◼

Diagnosis

Achalasia.

Discussion

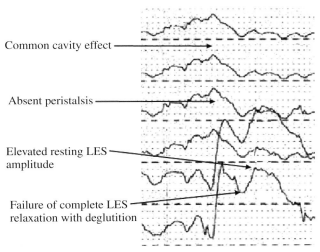

Common cavity effect

Absent peristalsis

Elevated resting LES amplitude

Failure of complete LES relaxation with deglutition

Figure 12-3 Manometric findings in a patient with achalasia.

Patients with symptoms of achalasia, such as severe dysphagia, regurgitation, reflux, and chest pain, usually require therapy on an elective basis. A traditional management option includes pneumatic dilation, which has a success rate of 75% over a period of several years and a perforation risk of 3% to 5%. A newer endoscopic technique is botulinum toxin injection, but the symptomatic recurrence rate after this therapy is more than 50% within 6 months of treatment, and 80% of patients have recurrent symptoms at the end of 2 years.

Minimally invasive esophageal myotomy achieves a 95% rate of symptom resolution in patients with achalasia and is considered an excellent form of therapy in otherwise healthy patients. The antireflux mechanism of the esophagogastric junction is often destroyed by the myotomy, leading to the recommendation by most surgeons that, in addition to the myotomy, a partial fundoplication is also performed to help prevent postoperative acid reflux symptoms.

Recommendation

Laparoscopic myotomy and partial anterior fundoplication.

Case Continued

You perform a laparoscopic myotomy, and intraoperatively the results of the myotomy are evaluated endoscopically. During air insufflation, bubbles are seen emerging from a small tear in the distal esophageal mucosa.

Discussion

During the myotomy, a perforation in the esophageal mucosa has occurred. The risk for perforation may be increased in patients who have had prior endoscopic therapy for achalasia, including pneumatic dilation and botulinum toxin injection. If the perforation is unrecognized, there is a high risk for subsequent peritonitis or abscess formation.

The best management option for a perforation that is recognized acutely is primary closure and reinforcement with well-vascularized tissue. The likelihood of healing the perforation with this approach is greater than 90%. Perforations that are recognized late, after the development of peritonitis or abscess formation, are much more challenging to treat. Options include primary closure, esophageal exclusion, T-tube drainage, and esophageal resection.

Recommendation

Primary closure buttressed with healthy tissue.

Case Continued

You close the perforation with several interrupted sutures placed using a laparoscopic technique. Repeat endoscopy with air insufflation demonstrates no further air bubbling from the region of the leak. A partial anterior fundoplication is performed that completely covers the area of repair.

The patient is not allowed oral intake in the first 24 hours. He is started on clear liquids on the second postoperative day, which he tolerates well. He is discharged on a full liquid diet on the third postoperative day in good condition and with relief of dysphagia.

Presentation

A 46-year-old woman is referred to you by an oncologist with complaints of left-sided back pain for the past several weeks. She has been followed by her oncologist for a history of lymphoma for which she has been previously treated. She denies any weight loss, fever, chills, or night sweats and is a nonsmoker. Her physical examination reveals tenderness over the region of the fourth and fifth ribs in the left paravertebral region. She presents with the following chest x-rays.

Chest X-rays

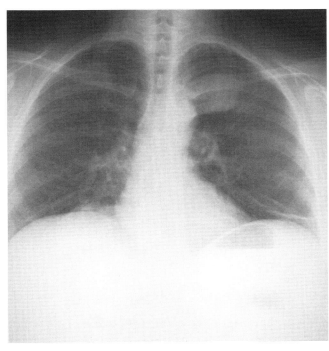

Figure 13-1

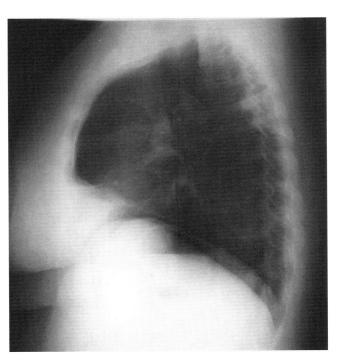

Figure 13-2

Chest X-ray Report

There is a posterior, paravertebral chest wall mass at the level of the fourth and fifth ribs. The lung fields are clear without evidence of other masses. The mediastinum appears unremarkable, without evidence of masses or adenopathy. There are no pleural effusions.

Computed tomography (CT) scans are performed to evaluate the chest x-ray finding. ▨

▨ CT Scans

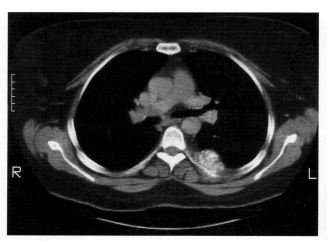

Figure 13-3

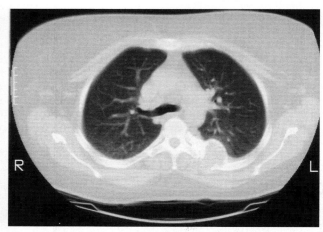

Figure 13-4

CT Scan Report

This study reveals a mass in the posterior paravertebral chest wall. The mass appears to be of bony origin with diffuse calcification within, and with adjacent rib destruction. There is underlying pleural thickening, with the mass protruding into the left hemithorax. There does not appear to be invasion into the lung parenchyma. There are no pleural effusions, lung nodules or masses, or mediastinal adenopathy. ▨

Differential Diagnosis

The patient has a new symptomatic chest wall mass. The differential diagnosis of a chest wall mass in the adult includes both benign and malignant pathology. Chest wall tumors include neoplasms of bone or soft tissues and may be primary or metastatic disease. The incidence of malignancy for all chest wall neoplasms is about 50%. The malignant processes may be primary tumors of the chest wall or metastatic to the chest wall. Primary chest wall malignancies make up about half of the malignant pathology. The other half is composed of metastatic disease to the chest wall. The four most common metastatic lesions to the chest wall are from breast, renal, colon, and salivary primaries. Soft tissue tumors are the most common primary neoplasms of the chest wall. Malignant fibrous histiocytoma, chondrosarcoma, and rhabdomyosarcoma are the most common malignant neoplasms of the chest wall. Cartilaginous tumors, desmoids, and fibrous dysplasia are the most common benign neoplasms of the chest wall. CT is needed to delineate the anatomy of the chest wall mass further and to plan subsequent therapy.

Discussion

This mass may be a benign or malignant primary tumor or a metastatic lesion to the bony skeleton from another primary. The mass appears to be a lesion of the bony skeleton. About 60% of all thoracic bony skeletal neoplasms are primary tumors of the chest wall; the rest are metastatic. The benign primary bone tumors are osteochondroma, chondroma, fibrous dysplasia, and histiocytosis X, with osteochondroma being most common (about 50%). The malignant primary bone neoplasms are myeloma, chondrosarcoma, Ewing's sarcoma, and osteogenic sarcoma, with myeloma being most common. The incidence of malignant bony skeleton tumors is 90%.

Recommendation

After a thorough history, physical examination, and evaluation to rule out other primary malignancies and other sites of metastatic disease, the lesion of the bony skeleton of the chest wall must be evaluated. Tissue diagnosis is required.

Discussion

The goal is to obtain a tissue diagnosis of the neoplasm in order to define the need for further treatment, surgical or medical. One needs to follow a general algorithm for the tissue identification of all chest wall neoplasms. If the lesion is suspected to be that of metastatic disease to the chest wall from a distant known primary, then a fine-needle aspiration biopsy is usually adequate to obtain a tissue diagnosis. In contrast, because most primary malignant neoplasms have a benign counterpart, adequate tissue examination is essential; thus, fine-needle aspiration is not a high-yielding technique. Biopsy of primary lesions therefore needs to be conducted by core biopsy or incisional biopsy of the neoplasm to obtain an adequate tissue sample. As stated previously, because the likelihood of a thoracic bony skeleton neoplasm being malignant is high, an excisional biopsy with a clear margin is the preferred option.

Small neoplasms of the chest wall (up to 4 or 5 cm in diameter) are diagnosed by complete excision. A margin of 1 to 2 cm should be obtained. Chest wall reconstruction and wound closure for small resections do not require complex reconstructive techniques. If the pathology of the specimen is benign, no further treatment is necessary. If the pathologic evaluation shows a malignant tumor that is better treated with adjuvant methods, further adjuvant therapy is offered. If, on final pathology, the surgical margin is involved, a wide resection is needed.

For a primary lesion greater than 5 cm in diameter, an incisional biopsy is performed. The skin incision is made such that it can be included within the margins of resection.

Case Continued

A CT-guided percutaneous core biopsy is performed through a posterior approach. Histology reveals osteogenic sarcoma.

Diagnosis and Recommendation

The diagnosis of osteogenic sarcoma is consistent with the patient's history of radiation. Osteogenic sarcoma commonly occurs in long bones of teenagers and young adults, with a second peak at about the age of 60 years. It is found less frequently in the ribs. Osteosarcoma affects more men than women and can present with rapidly enlarging tumors. Radiographically, it appears as bone destruction with indistinct borders that gradually merges into normal bone. The tumor is large and lobulated and usually extends through the bone into adjacent soft tissue. Microscopically, the predominant component may be bony, cartilaginous, or fibrous.

Osteogenic sarcoma is composed of three distinct disorders. *Primary high-grade osteogenic sarcoma* is the most common, arising from the medullary canal. It is a highly malignant tumor that metastasizes in 80% of patients treated by surgery alone. *Secondary osteogenic sarcoma* is associated with Paget's disease, bone infarct, fibrous dysplasia, and previously radiated bone. The most common tumors in patients after chest radiation are osteogenic sarcomas and soft tissue sarcomas. The most common history of chest radiation is for lymphoma or breast cancer. Secondary osteogenic sarcoma is rare in the young population. *Juxtacortical osteogenic sarcomas* are mostly low-grade lesions but may also occur as high grade. The grading of osteosarcoma is based on the number of mitosis and the degree of differentiation.

In the absence of metastasis, the treatment consists of wide resection of the tumor, including the entire involved bone and adjacent soft tissues (lung or muscle). Margins of resection include 3 cm of uninvolved tissue or uninvolved rib above and below the tumor with a 5-cm clear rib margin. Full-thickness chest wall resection including parietal pleura should be performed. Contiguous structures invaded by tumor should also be removed. Included with the specimen should be one normal myofascial plane below the skin. Overlying skin should always be resected if involved by tumor or if it was part of a previous biopsy incision. Positive margin of tumor has an impact on local recurrence and survival.

Postoperative X-ray and Resected Specimen

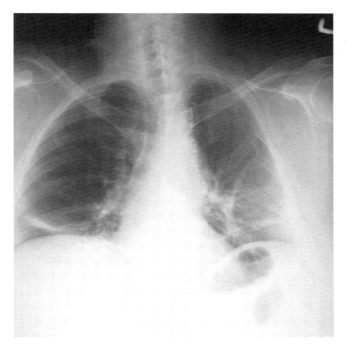

Figure 13-5

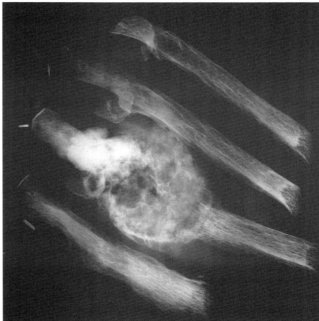

Figure 13-6

Case Continued

Discuss the role of adjuvant therapy or neoadjuvant therapy.

Discussion

Low-grade osteogenic sarcomas, intramedullary or juxtacortical, are associated with a greater than 90% overall survival rate with wide surgical excision alone. Adjuvant chemotherapy is not indicated in these cases. For high-grade osteogenic sarcoma, wide surgical excision must be combined with adjuvant chemotherapy. Patients who present with metastatic disease have a poor prognosis with about a 10% 5-year survival rate.

When indicated, systemic adjuvant chemotherapy is required to eradicate metastatic deposits. High-dose methotrexate is a major component of current multiagent regimens, most often with doxorubicin and cisplatin. Neoadjuvant chemotherapy has not had a clear survival benefit. Postoperative chemotherapy is indicated even if the neoplasms have not responded to the neoadjuvant regimen. Osteogenic sarcomas are resistant to radiation therapy.

Case Continued

After resection of the bony chest wall and soft tissue, a large defect is present. What are the options for reconstruction?

Discussion

Upper and posterior chest wall defects that are covered by the scapula may not need reconstruction. For the bony thorax, small defects (less than 5 cm) may not need prosthetic reconstruction. With larger defects, a reconstruction is necessary; Marlex mesh (Bard Inc., Murray Hill, NJ) or Gore-Tex patch (W. L. Gore & Associates, Flagstaff, AZ) may be used. In addition, a methyl methacrylate and Marlex mesh "sandwich" contoured to the bony thorax can be used as an alternative. For soft tissue reconstruction, the graft types include myocutaneous rotational flaps and myocutaneous free flaps. The greater omentum is used for an infected recipient site and is covered by a split-thickness skin graft. The three myocutaneous flaps used in chest wall reconstruction are the latissimus dorsi (based on the thoracodorsal artery), pectoralis major (based on the lateral thoracic, thoracoacromial, and internal mammary arteries), and rectus abdominis (based on the superior and inferior epigastric arteries).

Presentation

A 62-year-old woman presented to her primary care doctor because of a persistent cough for the past 4 weeks. The primary care physician noted some wheezing and treated her for a presumptive diagnosis of asthma. She was referred to a thoracic surgeon after she expectorated blood-tinged mucus.

The patient denies fever, occupational exposures, or any travel history. Her past medical history includes diabetes. She is a former smoker and has a 20-pack-per-year smoking history.

The physical examination reveals a moderately obese woman who is in no respiratory distress. There is no cervical adenopathy. Her cardiac tones are normal. Inspiratory wheezing is present on auscultation of her chest. She presents with the following chest x-rays.

■ Chest X-rays

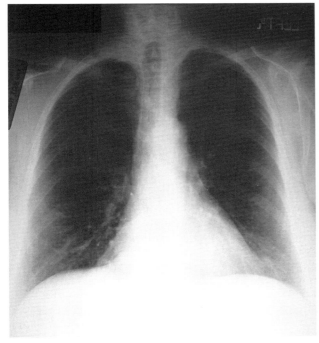

Figure 14-1

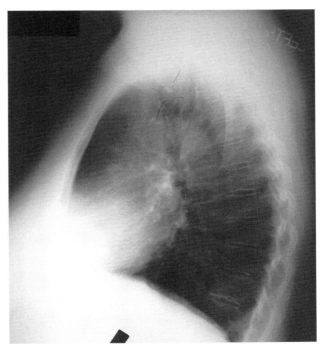

Figure 14-2

Chest X-ray Report

This study demonstrates a 1.5-cm rounded density within the trachea. The heart and great vessels are normal. The lung fields are clear. ▪

Discussion

Adult-onset asthma is unusual. A tracheal tumor should be considered in the differential diagnosis of patients with a persistent cough and wheezing, especially with associated hemoptysis.

Primary tracheal tumors are rare; they may be benign or malignant. One third of tracheal tumors are squamous cell carcinoma; one third are adenoid cystic carcinoma; and one third have a variety of benign and malignant causes. Squamous cell carcinoma tends to occur posteriorly in the distal one third of the trachea. Adenoid cystic carcinoma, formerly known as *cylindroma*, is more common in the upper one third of the trachea. Other malignant tumors of the trachea include carcinoid tumors, which include typical and atypical histologic types, adenocarcinoma, and small cell carcinoma.

Benign tumors tend to be round and smooth. Calcification within the tumor usually indicates a benign process. This is seen in hamartomas and chondromas. The exception is chondrosarcoma, which is malignant and may have calcifications. Other benign tumors of the trachea include papillomas, fibromas, and hemangiomas. Malignant tumors are irregular and may be ulcerated. Hoarseness usually signifies malignancy with involvement of the recurrent laryngeal nerve. Secondary malignant tracheal tumors include tumor extension from the larynx or thyroid, lung cancer, esophageal cancer, and metastatic disease from a distant primary cancer.

Cough is a common symptom associated with tracheal tumors. Wheezing and stridor are caused when the airway narrowing becomes more profound. This wheeze is more prominent during inspiration and is different from that of asthma, which occurs in expiration. Dyspnea and shortness of breath are common presenting features and occur when the tracheal cross-sectional area is reduced to one-third its original size. Hemoptysis occurs in 25% of patients and is most commonly seen with squamous cell carcinoma. Benign tumors are usually not associated with hemoptysis.

Many patients with tracheal tumors have a delayed diagnosis because of seemingly normal appearance of their chest x-ray. Careful inspection of the tracheal air column on plain chest x-rays is essential and may demonstrate the presence of a tracheal neoplasm, as it does in this patient. Tomograms and oblique and lateral views of the trachea using soft tissue technique visualize most tumors. Maneuvers such as swallowing and neck hyperextension may be used to demonstrate disease located in the upper trachea. These imaging techniques have largely been replaced by thin-cut computed tomography (CT) scans and magnetic resonance imaging (MRI) studies.

CT scans can be used to generate high-resolution images of the trachea, especially if thin (3-mm) cuts are obtained. The presence and degree of obstruction and invasion of the trachea, as well as lymph node involvement, can be assessed using high-resolution CT scanning. MRI, although not absolutely necessary, may provide enhanced images that aid in preoperative determination of the degree of invasion into surrounding tissues and blood vessels. The coronal and sagittal views are useful in determining the length of the tracheal neoplasm. Barium esophagogram may demonstrate esophageal compression or invasion and should be obtained in cases in which dysphagia is also present. Pulmonary function tests show the classic obstructive pattern, with a decreased forced expiratory volume in 1 section (FEV_1) and peak flow rate. The expiratory flow–volume loop is flattened.

Case Continued

CT scans of the chest are obtained.

CT Scans

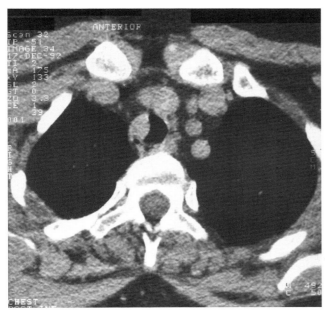

Figure 14-3

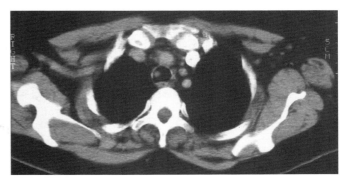

Figure 14-4

CT Scan Report

CT scans are performed that demonstrate an intratracheal tumor obstructing the lumen about 50%. Grossly, this tumor is not invading through the tracheal wall. There is no lymph node enlargement. The tumor extends for 1.5 cm along the length of the proximal trachea.

Discussion

Bronchoscopy with frozen section may be deferred until the time of operation if tracheal resection is clearly indicated. Preoperative bronchoscopy requires some sedation, which may lead to airway obstruction, in which case intubation may not be successful when there is significant tumor obstruction. In addition, emergent tracheostomy may limit options for surgical resection. If airway obstruction develops, coring away the tracheal tumor may be performed with a biopsy forceps through a rigid bronchoscope. The yttrium-aluminum-garnet (YAG) laser may also be useful to control bleeding with débridement of the tumor.

Bronchoscopy can provide important information on the exact location and extent of the tumor. This information is important in preoperative planning of a tumor resection. The degree of tracheal narrowing is noted because of its importance in anesthetic management during the resection. The vocal cords are inspected to assess preoperative function. The procedure must be performed in the operating room by an experienced endoscopist equipped with the appropriate instrumentation to control tumor hemorrhage and secure the airway. An assortment of rigid bronchoscopes, biopsy forceps, and instruments for emergency tracheostomy should be available. Appropriate anesthesia support is also mandatory as well as racemic epinephrine and steroids to treat airway edema.

Case Continued

A flexible fiberoptic bronchoscopy is performed with topical anesthesia and minimal sedation. The patient is spontaneously ventilating for the procedure. The tumor is found along the right side in the proximal one third of the trachea. The bronchoscope is easily passed beyond the tumor, demonstrating a normal distal airway. The length of the tumor is 2.0 cm (four tracheal rings). The tumor is not excessively vascular, and a biopsy is performed. There is no excessive bleeding.

Histologic Finding

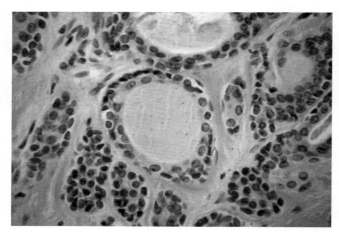

Figure 14-5   See Color Plate 6 following page 114.

Biopsy Report

Hematoxylin and eosin staining of the specimen cuboidal cells arranged in a cylinder or duct pattern consistent with adenoid cystic carcinoma. ▧

Discussion

Adenoid cystic carcinoma tends to occur in the upper one third of the trachea. This is a slow-growing malignancy that arises in the bronchial glands. It is histologically similar to salivary tumors and is not associated with smoking. These tumors extend along the submucosa and adjacent nerve sheaths and may invade through tracheal rings. They tend to displace, rather than invade, adjacent structures. The tumor may be present microscopically well beyond the gross region of the tumor. Local recurrence may occur long after primary resection. Microscopic disease at the surgical margin and positive regional lymph nodes do not affect prognosis; thus, a limited resection with a microscopically positive margin is favored over a resection that jeopardizes the anastomosis because of increased tension.

Squamous cell carcinoma of the trachea affects men more commonly than women and is associated with smoking. It locally invades and spreads to regional lymph nodes. Patients with squamous cell carcinoma should be screened for additional primary malignancies of the aerodigestive tract.

Case Continued

The patient is subsequently taken to the operating room. An arterial line is placed. The patient is fiberoptically intubated successfully, although the ventilating bronchoscope is immediately available. A shoulder roll is placed, and the neck and chest are prepped. An anterior cervical incision is made. Dissection is carried down to the trachea. The anterior pretracheal plane is entered, and dissection to the carina is performed. A sterile Tovell tube is passed through the operative field to the anesthesiologist; this tube is used to ventilate after the trachea is divided. Six tracheal rings are excised. The frozen-section analysis shows microscopic tumor at the distal margin. An additional 1 cm of trachea is excised, and frozen-section analysis is negative for tumor. The anastomosis is performed using interrupted 3-0 polyglactin sutures. A suprahyoid laryngeal release is performed to minimize anastomotic tension. The chin is sutured to the anterior chest. The patient is extubated and taken to the intensive care unit.

Discussion

The trachea is about 11 cm in length and has 18 to 22 rings. Each ring is about 0.5 cm. The blood supply to the trachea arises from the inferior thyroid artery superiorly and the bronchial arteries inferiorly. The blood vessels enter the trachea laterally, and the supply is segmental.

The operative approach to upper tracheal lesions is through an anterior cervical incision. This may be extended into an upper sternotomy to enhance exposure to the mediastinum. The lower trachea is best approached through a right posterolateral thoracotomy. The patient should be carefully evaluated preoperatively with bronchoscopy, and a surgical plan should be formulated.

The goals of the surgical resection are to remove the tracheal neoplasm with clear margins and to reconstruct the trachea with a tension-free anastomosis. About one half of the trachea may be resected safely. Several principles apply to successful tracheal resection. The trachea can be mobilized using several release maneuvers. Dissection of the anterior plane to the level of the carina should be done in all cases; avoiding lateral dissection preserves the segmental blood supply. A suprahyoid laryngeal release or a hilar release may be used to decrease suture line tension.

Flexing the neck and, at the end of the operation, suturing the chin to the anterior chest help remove tension for the suture line. Extubation should be performed at the end of the procedure to minimize anastomotic trauma. Tracheostomies are rarely necessary after resection. If one is required, it should not be placed through the anastomosis, but rather below the anastomosis if possible.

Case Continued

The final pathology report notes microscopic involvement at the resection margin in the perineural sheath.

Discussion

This patient should be managed with close, long-term follow-up and postoperative radiation therapy. Postoperative radiation (5,000 cGy) is recommended in patients with adenoid cystic and squamous cell carcinoma of the trachea.

Presentation

A 52-year-old man is admitted to the pulmonary service with complaints of recurrent hemoptysis of mild to moderate severity, ongoing for the past 6 to 8 months, with occasional expectoration of blood measuring about 200 mL. The patient also reports a chronic nonproductive cough without fever, chills, weight loss, or night sweats. Past medical history includes an emergency department admission at the age of 18 years for fever, cough, dark yellowish productive sputum, and pleuritic chest pain. Since then, the patient denies a history of asthma, bronchitis, or pneumonia. He is a nonsmoking farmer who has lived in Tennessee all his life. Physical examination is remarkable only for irregular heartbeat, egophony, and whispered pectoriloquy over the right upper lung fields. His only medication is amiodarone, 200 mg daily. In the emergency department, the following chest x-rays and computed tomography (CT) scans are obtained.

Chest X-rays

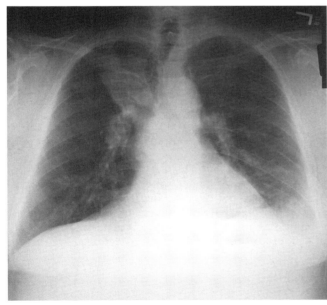

Figure 15-1

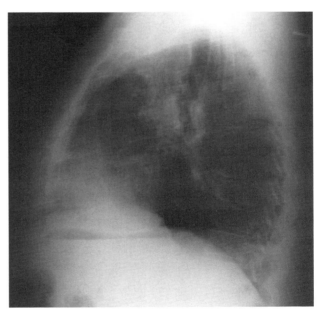

Figure 15-2

Chest X-ray Report

A posteroanterior and lateral chest x-ray of the chest demonstrates tracheal deviation to the right, suggesting ipsilateral volume loss. In addition, complete opacification of the right upper lobe consistent with collapse, multiple stations of calcified lymph nodes, obscured left hemidiaphragm, and costophrenic sulcus are also noted. The right heart border and the cardiophrenic angle are also not well visualized. ▦

▦ CT Scans

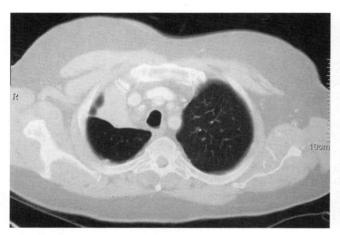

Figure 15-3

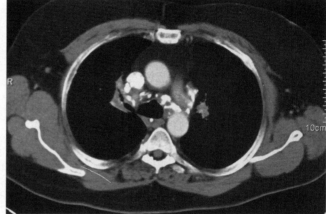

Figure 15-4

CT Scan Report

There is volume loss in the right upper lobe and an infiltrative pattern extending to the right hilum. The right upper lobe bronchus is encased. There are enlarged left hilar lymph nodes in addition to calcified lymph nodes at the right paratracheal, subcarinal, and aortopulmonary window regions. ▦

Differential Diagnosis

The differential diagnosis in a 52-year-old man with cough, hemoptysis, and radiographic findings as described above includes cancer, tuberculosis, bronchiectasis, broncholithiasis, and silicosis. Given the patient's occupation and the fact that the patient is a resident of an area of the Mississippi River endemic for histoplasmosis, broncholithiasis is a likely diagnosis. His emergency department visit 34 years ago may have been for a previous pulmonary fungal infection.

Diagnosis and Recommendation

Bronchoscopy should be performed in any patient who presents with hemoptysis and is hemodynamically stable. Bronchoscopy may aid in establishing a diagnosis localizing and quantifying the bleeding, and in selected patients, it may allow for therapeutic intervention. Furthermore, a Mantoux purified protein derivative (PPD) skin test should be performed to evaluate for exposure to tuberculosis.

Case Continued

The Mantoux PPD skin test is negative. At bronchoscopy, inflammation of the mucosal orifice of the right upper lobe bronchus is noted along with visible broncholiths, which are obstructing the airway. There is a trickle of fresh blood at the right upper lobe orifice and in the right main-stem bronchus. Although the carina is splayed, the left side of the airway, from the carina to the tertiary bifurcations, is bloodstained but otherwise normal. There are no endobronchial masses. It is concluded that the patient is bleeding from a broncholith in the right upper lobe, with associated inflammatory changes. Operative intervention is recommended.

Surgical Approach

The patient is taken to the operating room, where he undergoes a right posterolateral thoracotomy. On inspection, the right upper lobe is completely collapsed. There are bulky calcified nodes from the carina to the takeoff of the upper lobe bronchus and along the origins of the branches of the pulmonary artery to the upper lobe. Because a right upper lobectomy is contemplated, the dissection is commenced by dividing the posterior mediastinal pleura. The lymph nodes are carefully dissected. The dissection is especially tedious at the base of the apicoanterior trunk of the pulmonary artery, where sudden bleeding occurs. The bleeding appears to be from the main pulmonary artery. Manual compression is applied, which decreases but does not stop the bleeding.

Recommendation

The pericardium should be opened, and the main pulmonary artery should be controlled while an assistant maintains manual compression on the bleeding site.

Case Continued

The pericardium is opened and the main pulmonary artery is encircled and controlled with a tourniquet. During dissection and control of the main pulmonary artery, the patient loses about 2.5 to 3 L of blood, his mean arterial pressure decreases to 45 mm Hg, and his heart rate increases to 135 beats/min. The patient receives 6 units of packed red blood cells, at which time the pressure is temporarily stabilized, but the bleeding from the main pulmonary artery is not adequately controlled. Each attempt at repair seems only to enlarge the defect.

Recommendation

Salvage right pneumonectomy.

Case Continued

A salvage right pneumonectomy is performed. The carinal lymph nodes are removed by broncholithectomy and curettage. Postoperatively, the patient requires ventilator support for 4 days. The chest x-ray demonstrates fluffy infiltrates in the left lung. Although the patient's recovery is slow, he is transferred to a rehabilitation center on the tenth postoperative day.

Discussion

Broncholithiasis is a rare pulmonary pathology thought to result from the deposition of calcium salts in the lymph nodes in response to a healing granulomatous infection. Mucoid concretions of bronchiectasis may present in a similar way. Often, the presence of broncholithiasis is asymptomatic, and the diagnosis is made incidentally on a routine chest x-ray. The signs and symptoms range from cough, fever, chills, atelectasis, and expectoration of the broncholithic stones (lithoptosis) to life-threatening conditions such as massive hemoptysis, sepsis from obstructive pneumonia, and esophagorespiratory fistula.

A chest x-ray showing tracheobronchial, hilar, or subcarinal calcifications, especially in association with distorted airway or collapsed lung, should raise suspicion of this disease entity. Calcification and extent of nodal involvement can be assessed by a computed tomography (CT) scan of the chest. The presence of broncholiths alone is not an indication for intervention, but some form of intervention should be considered when debilitating signs or symptoms develop. These signs and symptoms include esophagorespiratory fistula, recurrent or massive hemoptysis, pulmonary infections, or intractable cough.

Whenever possible, the first line of treatment is endoscopic removal of the broncholiths. This modality is best suited for the stones that have extended well into the bronchial lumen. The use of excessive force or traction is discouraged for fear of inducing vascular disruption or airway perforation. Thoracotomy may be preferred in the presence of life-threatening complications. The actual procedure ranges from broncholithectomy to all forms of pulmonary resection. The goals of operation are two-fold: first, removal of all visible stones without complications, and second, removal of all diseased lung while preserving as much lung parenchyma as possible. As the above case clearly points out, it is important to obtain proximal control of the pulmonary artery before dissecting calcified lymph nodes that are adjacent to the pulmonary artery or its branches. These operations are technically challenging because the presence of densely calcified nodes is compounded by surrounding reactive inflammation and fibrosis.

Presentation

A 31-year-old man with a history of renal failure, joint pain, weakness, and persistently elevated serum calcium recently underwent a 3.5-gland parathyroidectomy followed by a neck reexploration and retrieval of the remaining parathyroid for persistent hypercalcemia.

Chest X-rays

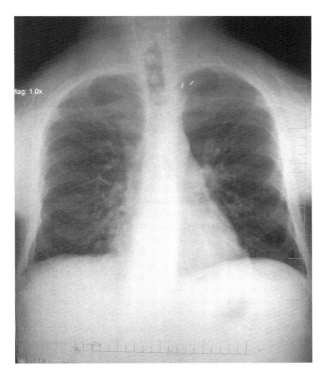

Figure 16-1

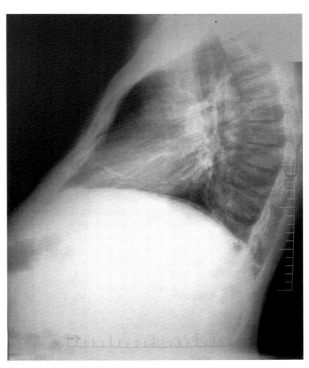

Figure 16-2

Chest X-ray Report

The trachea is midline; there are surgical clips in the left neck, consistent with the past surgical history. The lung fields are unremarkable. The heart is of normal size. There are no pleural effusions. On the lateral view, there is evidence of kyphosis. ▪

Differential Diagnosis

Ninety percent of patients with hypercalcemia have either primary hyperparathyroidism or malignancy. Primary hyperparathyroidism may be due to solitary adenomas or multiple endocrine neoplasia. In the case of malignancy, hypercalcemia is a serum abnormality found during the clinical evaluation for the patient's symptoms associated with the malignancy. These symptoms may include weight loss, fatigue, and night sweats. Malignancies that may cause hypercalcemia include metastatic breast cancer and solid tumors such as lung and renal cancers. Additionally, hematologic malignancies, such as lymphoma, leukemia, and multiple myeloma, may also cause hypercalcemia.

Less common causes for hypercalcemia include vitamin D intoxication, idiopathic hypercalcemia of infancy, hyperthyroidism, thiazide diuretics, and vitamin A intoxication. When associated with renal failure, etiologies for hypercalcemia include severe secondary hyperparathyroidism, aluminum intoxication, and milk-alkali syndrome.

Discussion

In this scenario, the patient undergoes two neck dissections and removal of all four parathyroid glands, which on histologic examination demonstrates parathyroid hyperplasia. Despite the removal of all parathyroid tissue in the neck, hypercalcemia (9.5 to 12.0 mg/dL) and severely elevated parathyroid hormone levels (1,200 to 1,700 mg/dL) persist.

Although all parathyroid tissue is removed from the neck, ectopic parathyroid tissue can still be present. Embryonically, the superior and inferior parathyroid glands develop separately. The superior parathyroid glands arise from the fourth branchial pouch along the posterolateral lobes of the thyroid gland. The inferior parathyroid glands develop from the third branchial pouch and migrate with the thymus; ectopic parathyroid may be found in the anterior mediastinum and, less commonly, in the middle and posterior mediastinum.

Technetium 99m (^{99m}Tc) sestamibi scintigraphy has been used to localize ectopic parathyroid adenomas because of its ability to concentrate in these structures. To concentrate sestamibi, tissues must be more metabolically active than surrounding tissue. Sestamibi is specific for mitochondrial membranes in direct correlation to the respiration rate of the cells. Large groups of cells with high concentrations of adenosine triphosphate (ATP) are detected as a hot spot on the film with a gamma camera. In cases of parathyroid adenoma, the normal parathyroids are metabolically inactive as an appropriate response to high concentrations of circulating calcium and do not appear on the gamma image. However, the parathyroid containing the adenoma continues to be metabolically active and concentrates the sestamibi. False-positive results can occur in certain situations in which surrounding tissue is also metabolically active, such as in thyroid adenomas, inflammatory lymph nodes, diffuse thyroid hyperplasia, and metastatic thyroid cancer. For this reason, sestamibi scans for first-time operations in the neck are controversial. In contrast, this test has been advocated for identifying ectopic parathyroid adenomas.

Other radiographic studies include angiography, chest computed tomography (CT), chest magnetic resonance imaging (MRI), and positron-emission tomography (PET). Angiography of internal mammary and thyrocervical arteries has a sensitivity of 84% for localizing a mediastinal parathyroid. Previously, chest CT was only 35% sensitive, but with spiral CT scan, the sensitivity approaches 50% to 75%. Sensitivity of MRI and PET scanning is about 70%.

Case Continued

A CT scan of the chest and ^{99m}Tc sestamibi scintigraphy study are performed.

CT Scan and Technetium 99m

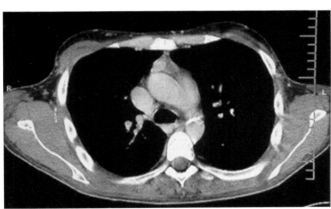

Figure 16-3

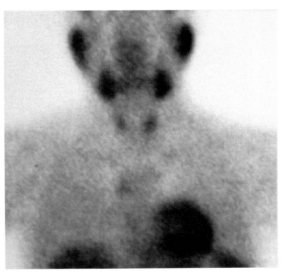

Figure 16-4

Radiographic Report

The mediastinal window of the chest CT reveals a discrete mass in the anterior mediastinum overlying the proximal arch of the aorta. This finding is correlated with uptake of ^{99m}Tc in the mediastinum.

Discussion

This finding is highly suggestive of an ectopic mediastinal parathyroid adenoma. As shown in this case study, ^{99m}Tc sestamibi scintigraphy and CT scan are effective in localizing ectopic parathyroid adenomas. Some centers claim 100% specificity for finding adenomas when applied to the proper patient population with sporadic primary hyperparathyroidism.

The mediastinal parathyroid adenoma should be resected. Surgical approach through a median sternotomy can be considered. Alternatively, a right thoracotomy can be performed, with the mass localized and excised from the anterior mediastinum. If the surgeon anticipates difficulty in localizing the mass, 20 to 25 mCu of ^{99m}Tc sestamibi can be injected 1.5 to 2.5 hours before incision. Using a gamma probe, the mass can be localized. Furthermore, using video-assisted thoracic surgery (VATS), the gamma probe can be introduced through a small skin incision, and the mass can be localized and excised endoscopically.

Preoperative serum parathyroid hormone, ionized calcium, and phosphorous levels should be obtained. The same serum assays should be drawn intraoperatively, immediately after excision of the mass and every 5 minutes until documentation of reduction of the parathyroid hormone levels is confirmed. Ionized calcium and phosphorous levels should also be obtained. Care should be taken when manipulating the mass. Fragmentation of the mass could lead to seeding of the parathyroid adenoma in the chest. If the VATS approach is used, the specimen should be removed from the hemithorax using an endoscopic bag. After the specimen is removed, it should be examined with the gamma probe to document the high concentration of uptake of ^{99m}Tc. A frozen section of the specimen confirms the finding.

Intraoperative Photographs

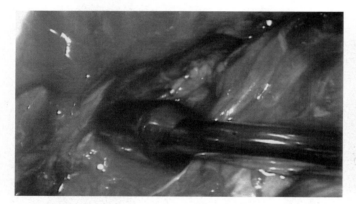

Figure 16-5 See Color Plate 7 following page 114.

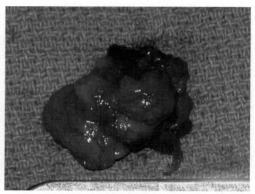

Figure 16-6 See Color Plate 8 following page 114.

Postoperative Management

Postoperative management should parallel the postoperative management of total parathyroidectomy, including aggressive management of calcium levels. Calcium should be supplemented both orally and intravenously until a steady state is obtained.

Presentation

A 50-year-old man is admitted to the hospital with fever and a headache. The patient has a medical history of human immunodeficiency virus (HIV) and hepatitis C. The patient reports a 20-pack-per-year smoking history and that he stopped smoking 5 years ago. During his last physician visit 3 months earlier, he was treated for a fever and cough. Chest x-rays are obtained on his present admission.

Chest X-rays

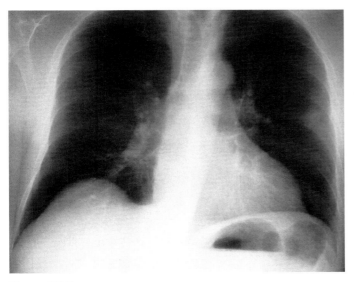

Figure 17-1

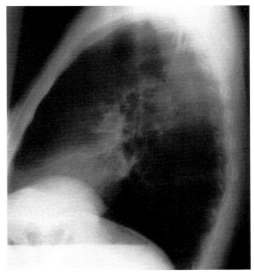

Figure 17-2

Chest X-ray Report

A round nodule is demonstrated in the left lung field. There are no pleural effusions. The mediastinum is not enlarged, and the heart size is normal.

Case Continued

Computed tomography (CT) scans of the chest are recommended to delineate the mass and examine the mediastinum for enlarged lymph nodes.

CT Scans

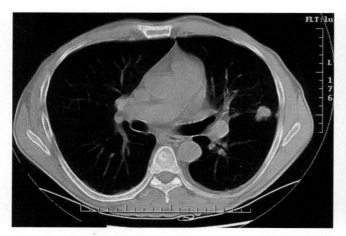

Figure 17-3

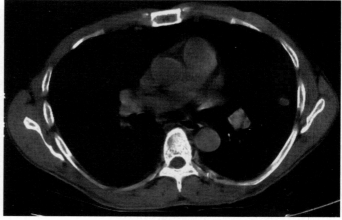

Figure 17-4

CT Scan Report

The CT scans demonstrate a solitary pulmonary nodule in the left upper lobe. The lesion is noncavitary and noncalcified. There are no enlarged lymph nodes in the hilar or mediastinal regions. ■

Recommendation

Sputum cultures and Mantoux purified protein derivative (PPD) skin test.

Case Continued

The Mantoux PPD skin test is negative, and the sputum cultures demonstrate no growth. Because of continuing febrile episodes and no source of infection, a recommendation is made by the infectious disease service to obtain a percutaneous needle biopsy for histology and culture. The biopsy is performed under CT guidance, but histologic evaluation is not diagnostic. After the procedure, the patient is short of breath, with decreased breath sounds over the left lung field. Chest x-ray shows a 30% pneumothorax on the left side. The patient undergoes a pigtail catheter placement.

Chest X-ray

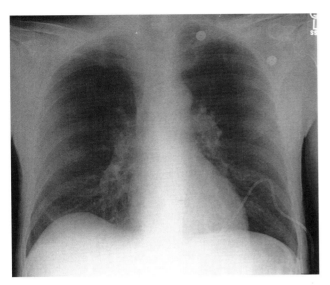

Figure 17-5

Chest X-ray Report

The left lung nodule is present. There is no pneumothorax. A pigtail catheter is present in the left chest.

Case Continued

The patient's cough and fever respond to antibiotics, and the patient is discharged home. Over the next few months, the patient continues to feel weak. Laboratory examination reveals decreasing CD4 cell counts. The patient's medical regimen is adjusted, but he is readmitted with cough and fever. A follow-up chest x-ray shows the nodule to have increased in size. A repeat CT scan of the chest is obtained, which demonstrates an interval increase in the size of the nodule. The lesion again is noncavitary and noncalcified with no significant adenopathy. The differential diagnosis includes infectious causes such as atypical mycobacterial infections; histoplasmosis; *Nocardia*, *Candida*, and *Aspergillus* species infection; and malignancy. Malignancy in this patient includes HIV-defining malignancies such as Kaposi's sarcoma and non-Hodgkin's lymphoma. Other non–HIV-defining tumors seen in HIV patients are Hodgkin's disease, squamous cell cancers, lung cancer, gastric cancer, testicular cancer, melanoma, and leiomyosarcoma.

Given the patient's poor medical condition, a second percutaneous needle biopsy is performed and is positive for non–small cell carcinoma, possibly an adenocarcinoma. Options for treatment are discussed with the patient and include no treatment and supportive care, radiation therapy, and surgical resection. The patient elects surgical resection. Pulmonary function tests showed a forced expiratory volume in 1 second (FEV_1) of 3.34 L (89% of predicted) and a diffusing capacity of lung for carbon monoxide (D_{LCO}) 78% of predicted.

■ Surgical Approach

Flexible bronchoscopy reveals no evidence of endobronchial disease. The patient is then intubated with a double-lumen endotracheal tube. The patient is placed in the right lateral decubitus position, and a diagnostic thoracoscopy is performed through a port in the mid-axillary line and the seventh intercostal space. No evidence of metastatic disease is identified within the chest. In the left upper lobe, a 2-cm mass is observed dimpling the visceral pleural surface. After placement of two additional thoracoscopy ports in the fifth intercostal space, one anterior and one posterior, the remainder of the chest is examined. Using an L-hook cautery, the fissure between the upper and lower lobes is completed. In this case, the fissure is complete, but in cases of an incomplete fissure, the endo GIA stapler is used to divide the lung parenchyma after identifying the branches of the pulmonary artery. After the fissure is completed and the pulmonary artery clearly identified, the individual branches to the upper lobe segments are gently dissected out using a standard right-angle clamp and an endoscopic dissecting sponge. The pulmonary artery anatomy to the left upper lobe is variable, and there may be four to seven individual branches that require ligation. The branches to the lingula segments are divided first using the reticulating endo GIA vascular stapling device. Dissection then continues proximally to divide the branches to the left upper lobe segments with the stapler inserted either anteriorly or posteriorly, depending on the angle. The most proximal branch of the pulmonary artery is above the left upper lobe bronchus and may be difficult to visualize with the camera in the inferior port site. Before dividing this branch, the superior pulmonary vein is fully dissected and divided with a vascular stapler introduced through the posterior port site. The camera is switched to the posterior port site to visualize the arterial branch. The stapler is then introduced through the inferior port site to divide the most proximal branch of the pulmonary artery. The GIA stapler is then placed across the bronchus and closed. The left lung is ventilated to ensure that the lower lobe bronchus is not included in the device, and the bronchus is then stapled and divided. The anterior port site is slightly enlarged to accommodate a large specimen bag, and the lobe is removed. A mediastinal lymph node dissection is performed and the bronchus checked for air leaks before a single chest tube is placed and the incisions are closed.

Case Continued

The chest tube is removed on the second postoperative day. The patient recovers uneventfully and is discharged on the fourth postoperative day.

Discussion

Lung cancer has been reported with increasing frequency in the HIV population. Although the association remains uncommon, the observed-to-expected ratio for primary lung cancer in the HIV population compared with the general population is 6:5. As with other HIV-defining malignancies, lung cancer may be more aggressive and present at a more advanced stage. The median age in the HIV group with lung cancer is about 50 years, which is 13 years younger than in the general population. Tobacco use is equal in both groups and is not considered a confounding factor, which may explain the earlier age in which patients with HIV presents with lung cancer. No correlation is present between CD4 cell counts and stage of lung cancer at presentation. Pulmonary complications remain a cause of considerable morbidity in this immunocompromised group. The video-assisted thoracic surgery (VATS) approach to minimize postoperative recovery may be advantageous in this group of patients.

Presentation

A 55-year-old white man presents to your office having been referred by a gastroenterologist. The patient has a long-standing history of acid reflux symptoms. He was diagnosed with Barrett's esophagus 5 years before his clinic visit and had undergone periodic endoscopic surveillance. He was not taking any acid suppression medications because his reflux symptoms were adequately controlled with antacids. Recent endoscopic biopsies demonstrated possible high-grade dysplasia. He has had no previous surgery. His examination is normal.

Case Continued

The gastroenterologist provides you with the results of a barium swallow, which demonstrate a normal esophagus with a small hiatal hernia. The stomach is normal. There was mild reflux of contrast into the esophagus during the examination. Previous endoscopy identified Barrett's esophagus beginning 30 cm from the incisors and extending to the gastroesophageal junction 35 cm from the incisors. No masses or ulcerations are evident. There is moderate esophagitis proximal to the squamocolumnar junction. There is a small axial hiatal hernia. The stomach and first portion of the duodenum are normal. During the past 3 years, the patient has had periodic endoscopic evaluations with surveillance biopsies. Histologic report is provided as follows.

Report of Endoscopy 3 Years before the Current Clinic Visit

Esophagitis. Barrett's metaplasia without evidence of dysplasia.

Report of Endoscopy 1 Year before the Current Clinic Visit

Esophagitis. Barrett's metaplasia with a single focus of low-grade dysplasia.

▇ Endoscopy 1 Month before the Current Clinic Visit

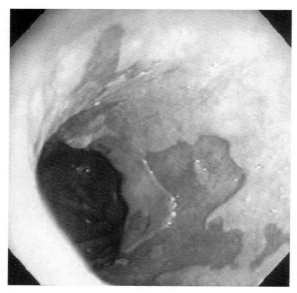

Figure 18-1

Endoscopic Report

Esophagitis. Barrett's esophagus with a single focus of high-grade dysplasia. ▇

Differential Diagnosis

This patient has a prolonged history of acid reflux symptoms and has had Barrett's esophagus confirmed on multiple endoscopies. The patient has not taken acid suppression medications regularly and has had esophagitis in each of his biopsies. The finding of a single focus of high-grade dysplasia is suggestive for the possible presence of invasive cancer. It is necessary at this point to reconfirm the diagnosis of high-grade dysplasia. The initial diagnosis of high-grade dysplasia may be erroneous, particularly when it is made in the presence of esophagitis. Other possible diagnoses are Barrett's esophagus with low-grade dysplasia, Barrett's esophagus without dysplasia, and invasive adenocarcinoma. The pathology slides should be reviewed by a specialist.

Case Continued

The pathology slides are reviewed by a gastrointestinal pathologist, who confirms the findings of Barrett's esophagus and esophagitis, but reports no evidence of high-grade dysplasia.

Recommendation

Intensive acid suppression medication followed by endoscopy and repeat biopsy in 2 months.

Case Continued

Repeat upper endoscopy demonstrates Barrett's esophagus with no esophagitis and no dysplasia.

Recommendation

In the absence of dysplasia, you recommend that the patient continue acid suppression medication and have surveillance endoscopy in 6 months.

Discussion

Surveillance endoscopy and intensive acid suppression make up the standard of care for this patient. There is no indication for antireflux surgery in patients with Barrett's esophagus in the absence of important reflux symptoms. Antireflux surgery does not decrease the likelihood of developing dysplasia, nor does it reduce the risk for dysplasia progressing to invasive cancer.

Case Continued

Surveillance endoscopy is performed at 6 months and demonstrates low-grade dysplasia. Repeat endoscopy 1 year later demonstrates multifocal high-grade dysplasia without evidence of a mass or ulceration. The presence of multifocal high-grade dysplasia is confirmed by an expert pathologist. The patient is again referred to you.

Recommendation

Computed tomography (CT) scans of the chest and abdomen and endoscopic ultrasonography (EUS).

CT Scans

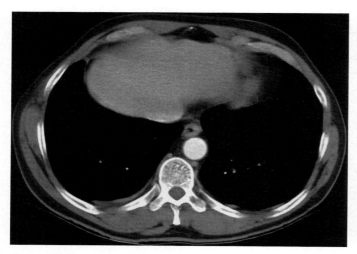

Figure 18-2

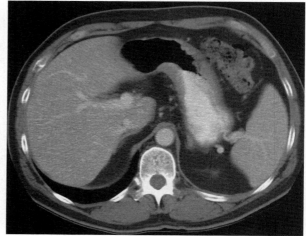

Figure 18-3

CT Scan Report

The lung fields are clear, there is no evidence of an esophageal mass, there is no adenopathy, and the liver and adrenal glands are normal. ▪

EUS

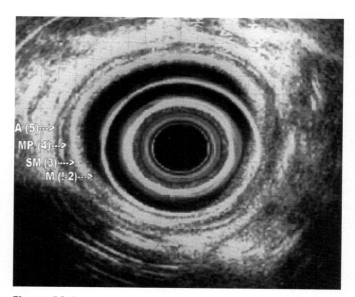

Figure 18-4

EUS Report

There is mild concentric thickening of the distal esophagus corresponding to the Barrett's segment. No tumor mass is evident. The lymph nodes are normal in size and appearance. ▪

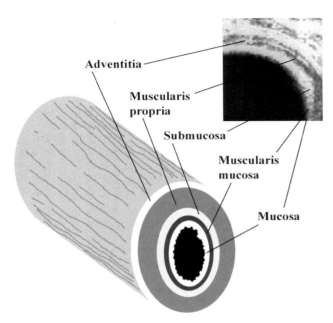

Figure 18-5 Appearance of different layers of the esophagus on endoscopic ultrasound.

Discussion

This patient has documented multifocal high-grade dysplasia in Barrett's esophagus and is otherwise healthy. The risk for progression from high-grade dysplasia to invasive cancer is up to 40% within 4 years. More than 40% of patients who undergo esophagectomy for a preoperative diagnosis of high-grade dysplasia have invasive cancer in the resected specimen. Of those patients ultimately diagnosed with invasive cancer, 25% have stage II disease or worse. Based on these data, surgical treatment of high-grade dysplasia is appropriate in patients who can tolerate the procedure.

Standard therapy for Barrett's esophagus high-grade dysplasia is esophagectomy. This procedure removes most of the esophagus, making surveillance unnecessary in the future. It is also an appropriate treatment for cancer, should it exist unknowingly. The risk for operative mortality after esophagectomy is less than 3%, and long-term quality of life in these patients is good.

The optimal operative approach for esophagectomy is controversial. There is no apparent advantage to more extensive operations compared with standard operations, and transthoracic, transhiatal, and minimally invasive techniques share similar risks for complications and durations of hospital stay. Long-term function after reconstruction with stomach appears to be similar to function after more complicated reconstruction procedures such as colon interposition.

A variety of alternative therapies for Barrett's esophagus with high-grade dysplasia that destroy the affected region of mucosa are being developed. These procedures include endoscopic mucosal resection and ablative techniques using cautery, laser therapy, and photodynamic therapy. The immediate risk associated with these procedures is low, although many patients develop benign strictures, which are sometimes difficult to manage. Most procedures are not successful in eliminating the Barrett's segment, and often there is residual high-grade dysplasia. These patients therefore continue to require close surveillance. The long-term outcomes after these treatments are unknown.

Recommendation

Transhiatal esophagectomy and gastric pull-up.

Case Continued

The operation proceeds uneventfully, and the postoperative course is unremarkable. The patient is discharged on the eighth postoperative day tolerating a soft solid diet.

Pathology Report

Barrett's adenocarcinoma with invasion into the muscularis propria. No lymphatic invasion. The lymph nodes are not involved.

Discussion

The patient has a stage IIA Barrett's adenocarcinoma. Prospective studies have demonstrated no survival advantage for postoperative adjuvant chemotherapy, radiotherapy, or combined therapy. Routine follow-up usually includes periodic examination, chest x-ray, and possibly CT scan of the chest and abdomen. The benefit of surveillance endoscopy is not known.

Presentation

You are called by the emergency department to evaluate a 45-year-old Vietnamese man with hemoptysis. He reports having streaks of blood in his sputum for the past few weeks but has now coughed up about 30 mL of blood. He is hemodynamically stable without respiratory distress.

Past medical history is significant for tuberculosis diagnosed 2 years ago and treated with isoniazid, rifampin, pyrazinamide, and ethambutol for a period of 6 months.

Review of systems is significant for recent fevers and cough.

■ Chest X-rays

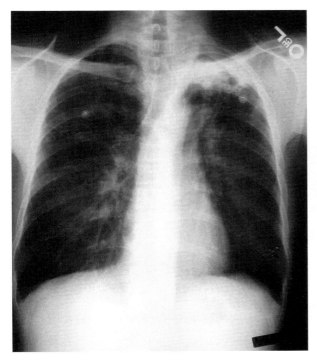

Figure 19-1

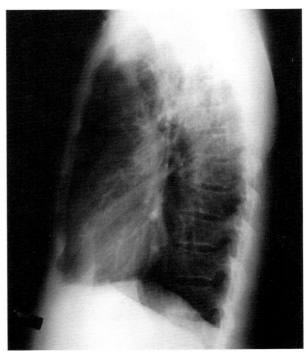

Figure 19-2

Chest X-ray Report

The left upper lung field contains an ill-defined opacity. The left hilum is elevated, which indicates left upper lobe involvement. There is no evidence of a mediastinal shift or effusion.

Differential Diagnosis

The opacity seen on the chest x-rays could represent an infectious or neoplastic process. This patient's complaints of fever, cough, and hemoptysis are consistent with either diagnosis. However, given the history of previous treatment for tuberculosis, a superinfection or reactivation tuberculosis is the more likely diagnosis.

Discussion

Patients with chronic lung diseases are prone to developing fungal infections. In the case of tuberculosis, aspergillus is the most common organism. Hemoptysis is frequently present and can occur as life-threatening hemorrhage. The underlying tuberculosis is typically active in 20% to 50% of cases.

Recommendation

Computed tomography (CT) scans of the chest to delineate the left upper lung field process.

CT Scans

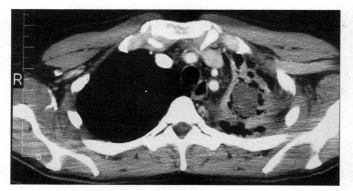

Figure 19-3

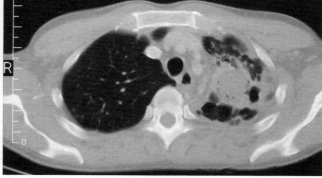

Figure 19-4

CT Scan Report

The left upper lobe contains an ovoid mass with surrounding consolidation.

Discussion

The CT scan finding is consistent with the suspected diagnosis of aspergilloma. The typical radiographic finding is of a mobile mass, which moves in a cavity as the patient changes position. There is often a lucent, crescent-shaped area over the opaque mass (Monad's sign).

Recommendation

Bronchoscopy is performed to assess inflammatory changes in the tracheobronchial tree and to obtain bronchial washings for culture and smears for tuberculosis, fungi, and other organisms.

Discussion

Positive sputum cultures by themselves are not sufficient to make a diagnosis of aspergilloma. Clinical and radiographic findings are sufficient for diagnosis of aspergilloma. However, sputum culture and smears are necessary to determine the possible reactivation of tuberculosis.

Case Continued

The patient undergoes flexible bronchoscopy, which reveals blood in the left upper lobe bronchus. Washings contain aspergillus hyphae. The patient subsequently has a second episode of 800 mL of hemoptysis.

Discussion

Aspergillus is a fungus transmitted as airborne spores found in soil, decaying vegetable matter, water, and ventilation systems. *Aspergillus fumigatus* and *Aspergillus flavus* are the species most commonly isolated. Clinical presentation can occur as hypersensitivity lung disease, aspergilloma, or invasive pulmonary infection, depending on the immune status of the patient. The presenting symptoms are usually fever, cough, pleuritic pain, and dyspnea. Hemoptysis ranges from blood-tinged sputum to exsanguinating hemorrhage. Usually, cavitary lesions occur in patients with previous chronic lung disease, such as tuberculosis, histoplasmosis, bronchiectasis, sarcoidosis, and lung abscess. The disease needs to be treated promptly because it progresses quickly. Amphotericin B is the treatment of choice, although nystatin, itraconazole, and iodides can also be used.

The approach to the patient with hemoptysis is controversial. A patient with massive hemoptysis, more than 600 mL per 24 hours, requires urgent surgical resection. In a patient who has had massive hemoptysis but is not actively bleeding, percutaneous Gelfoam embolization with subsequent resection is indicated. Gelfoam embolization offers immediate control of bleeding in 77% of cases. The indication for bronchial artery embolization includes stabilizing the patient with massive hemoptysis and controlling bleeding in the patient who is not a candidate for surgery owing to advanced pulmonary disease.

The decision to proceed with surgery must factor the extent of pulmonary disease and the severity of hemoptysis. Simple lesions can be resected with low risk. However, the more complex masses with extensive parenchymal involvement often result in a complicated postoperative course. Mild or moderate hemoptysis in a stable patient should be resected if the lung disease permits resection.

Recommendation

In this case, the underlying lung disease involves a significant portion of the left upper lobe as demonstrated by the elevated left hilum on the chest x-ray. In addition, the disease process has already resulted in hemoptysis. In this case, a surgical resection should be undertaken.

Discussion

Resection should incorporate the entire lesion, and parenchymal margins should be free of disease. Examination of the specimen typically reveals a smooth, cavitated lesion containing a mass of necrotic hyphae, fibrin, and inflammatory cells. There is often surrounding consolidation or areas of infarcted tissue. Methenamine silver staining demonstrates septate hyphae, blood vessel invasion, and thrombosis.

Case Continued

The patient undergoes left thoracotomy. Extrapleural dissection is required to free the lung from the apex owing to inflammation from old tuberculosis infection. Significant parenchymal disease necessitates left upper lobectomy. There is no evidence of pleural or chest wall involvement. The patient has an uncomplicated postoperative course.

▮ Histologic Slides

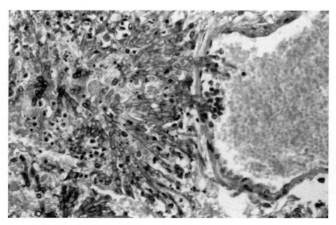

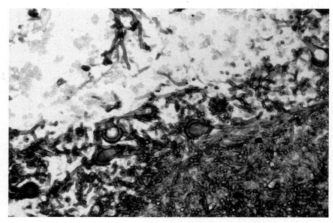

Figure 19-5   See Color Plate 9 following page 114.   **Figure 19-6**   See Color Plate 10 following page 114.

Report of Histologic Findings

The image on the left demonstrates dichotomous branching of aspergillus hyphae invading a blood vessel wall. The image on the right is a methenamine silver stain demonstrating hyphae, conidophores, and spores of *Aspergillus* species.

Recommendation

Because the fungal ball has been completely resected, no further treatment is indicated.

Discussion

Immunocompromised patients typically present with complex forms of the disease and should be maintained on antifungal drugs for a period of time after surgery to ensure eradication of the organism.

Presentation

A 57-year-old woman presents with increasing shortness of breath during the past 3 months. Her medical history includes breast cancer, for which she underwent a left modified radical mastectomy, a prophylactic right mastectomy, and first-stage breast reconstruction. The patient received chemotherapy and radiation initially and is currently receiving tamoxifen. The patient is hemodynamically stable. Respiratory rate is 12 breaths/min. Breath sounds are diminished on the right.

■ Chest X-rays

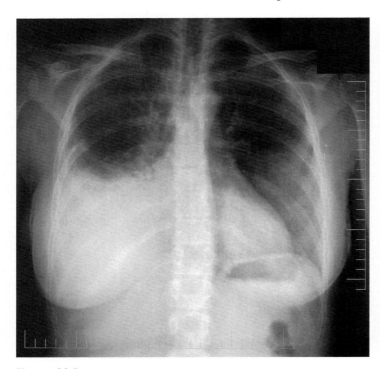

Figure 20-1

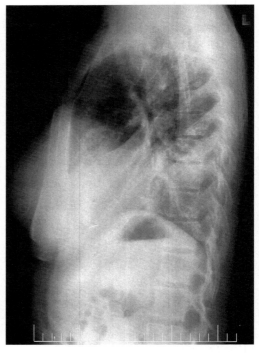

Figure 20-2

▦ Chest X-ray Report

There is a large right pleural effusion. There is also linear atelectasis at the base of the right lung consistent with compression atelectasis.

The left lung field is clear. There are surgical clips in the left axilla and bilateral breast implants.

CT Scan Report

Right pleural effusion consistent with the findings on the chest x-ray. The lung fields are clear of masses and infiltrates; however, compressive atelectasis is present in the right lower lobe. ▦

Differential Diagnosis

The diagnosis of pleural effusions should be divided into two categories: transudative and exudative effusions. Based on the type of effusion and the clinical history, a differential diagnosis is formulated. The distinction between transudates and exudates can be made based on the criteria proposed by Light and colleagues in 1972. Using Light's criteria, a pleural effusion is considered an exudate when:

1. Pleural fluid lactate dehydrogenase (LDH) is greater than two thirds of the upper limit of normal for serum LDH.
2. The pleural fluid LDH–to–serum LDH ratio is greater than 0.6.
3. The pleural fluid protein–to–serum protein ratio is greater than 0.5.

Forty-three percent of patients with an exudate have a malignancy, and 83% of patients with a transudate have congestive heart failure. Other causes of transudative effusion include cirrhosis, nephrotic syndrome, myxedema, peritoneal dialysis, hypoproteinemia, Meigs' syndrome, and sarcoidosis. Exudative effusions are caused by neoplastic disease, infectious disease, pulmonary infarction, collagen vascular diseases (rheumatoid arthritis, systemic lupus erythematosus), gastrointestinal diseases (pancreatitis, pancreatic pseudocyst, esophageal rupture, subphrenic abscess, hepatic abscess), trauma (hemothorax, chylothorax), and other causes (after radiation therapy and after myocardial infarction).

Other laboratory tests can be performed on the pleural fluid to help narrow the differential diagnosis. White blood cell counts greater than $10,000/mm^3$ suggest an empyema, whereas red blood cell counts greater than $100,000/mm^3$ suggest trauma, pulmonary infarction, or malignancy. Elevated amylase levels are often found with esophageal perforations, acute pancreatitis, and a ruptured pancreatic pseudocyst. The diagnosis of chylothorax can be made by demonstrating elevated levels of cholesterol, triglycerides, and chylomicrons in the pleural effusion. If the glucose in the pleural fluid is lower than in the serum, the diagnoses of tuberculosis, rheumatoid arthritis, empyema, and malignancy should be entertained. A low pleural fluid (pH less than 7.2) suggests contamination with bacteria. A parapneumonic effusion containing glucose greater than 40g/dL, pH greater than 7.2, and LDH greater than 1,000 units/L would likely resolve with treatment of the pneumonia. However, if the glucose is less than 40g/dL or the pH is less than 7.2, a thoracostomy tube is generally necessary to treat the effusion. Some exceptions include rheumatoid arthritis, tuberculosis, and malignant effusions, in which the pH is regularly less than 7.2 and a thoracostomy tube is not necessary.

Cytologic examination should be routinely performed on pleural fluid specimen. In patients with malignant pleural effusions, the initial specimen reveals a diagnosis of malignancy 60% of the time. Accuracy increases to 90% when three separate specimens are obtained.

Case Continued

A thoracentesis is performed, and 500 mL of bloody effusion is obtained. The results are shown in Table 20-1.

Using Light's criteria, the pleural fluid fulfills all three criteria for an exudate: the pleural fluid LDH–to–serum LDH ratio is 0.67, the pleural fluid protein–to–serum protein is 0.59, and the pleural fluid LDH high reference range is 0.71. Given the patient's history of breast cancer and the fact that pleural white blood cell count, pH, and glucose do not suggest infection, it is likely the fluid is a malignant effusion. Pleural fluid is sent for cytologic examination, which demonstrates malignant cells.

Recommendations

There are several approaches to the management of a malignant pleural effusion. Considerations should be made as to whether the patient is experiencing symptoms from the effusion (such as shortness of breath, chest pain, and cough). If the patient is not experiencing symptoms, and the effusion is small to moderate, a decision may be made to observe the progression of effusion. A thoracentesis should be performed to establish the diagnosis, and serial chest x-rays can be obtained for comparison. When the pleural effusion is moderate to large, the effusion should be drained because the fluid will cause compressive atelectasis and can also create a fibrinous peel, preventing full lung expansion.

Table 20-1: Results of Thoracentesis

Test	Pleural Fluid	Blood	Reference
LDH	521	781	340–670 U/L
Protein	4.2	7.1	6.3–8.6 g/dL
WBC	1,000		$4.3–10.8 \times 10^3/mm^3$
RBC	80,000		
PH	7.17		
Glucose	51	101	

LDH, lactate dehydrogenase level; WBC, white blood cell count; RBC, red blood cell count.

The goals of treating malignant pleural effusions are (a) evacuate the effusion from the pleural space, (b) appose the visceral and pleural surfaces of the lung, and (c) create pleurodesis to prevent recurrence of the effusion.

Three options are available to evacuate the effusions and provide appropriate apposition of visceral and pleural surfaces. First, serial thoracentesis can be performed when the patient develops symptoms. This is less than optimal because repeat procedures are uncomfortable and leave the patient at a higher risk for pneumothorax. Also, thoracentesis will evacuate fluid only. It does not provide an effective means of pleurodesis and therefore is associated with a high incidence of recurrent pleural effusions. For these reasons, thoracentesis should be used for diagnosis and, in some patients, for the initial recurrence. If the effusion continues to recur, an alternative method should be considered.

Various methods are available to achieve pleurodesis. Thoracotomy and pulmonary decortication for malignant pleural effusion is usually not recommended because of significant morbidity and high mortality. Alternatively, video-assisted thoracic surgery (VATS) insufflation of talc is an effective treatment of malignant effusions. Although VATS insufflation of talc is highly effective, this modality requires hospital admission, general anesthesia, and chest tube management. Alternatively, the effusion can be drained by a thoracostomy tube (28 French), followed by chemical pleurodesis when the drainage subsides. Chemical pleurodesis through a tube thoracostomy is less invasive and can be performed by instilling a sclerosing agent into the thoracic cavity. Several sclerosing agents are available, including bleomycin, doxycycline, and iodized talc. Bleomycin is expensive and may cause leukopenia. Iodized talc is mixed with sterile saline to form slurry, which is injected through a thoracostomy tube. Talc causes severe pleuritis and is an excellent sclerosing agent. Success rates of up to 96% have been reported; however, there are several associated disadvantages. Talc pleurodesis through a tube thoracostomy is often not uniform and can cause loculations of fluid within the thoracic cavity. Additionally, talc microemboli, pneumonitis, and acute respiratory distress syndrome have been reported. Doxycycline, a derivative of tetracycline, has been used successfully with response rates of more than 80%. Doxycycline is mixed with 1% lidocaine and 0.9% saline and delivered through a thoracostomy tube. It is more uniformly distributed throughout the hemithorax and may cause a more uniform pleurodesis.

Chemical pleurodesis is administered through a thoracostomy tube. The tube is then clamped for 4 hours, unclamped, and placed at 20 cm of suction. The tube is left in place until about 100 mL per day are drained. Hospitalization for chemical pleurodesis averages more than 6 days. Because chemical pleurodesis is painful, patients may require narcotics before the procedure.

Another option for pleurodesis is placement of a chronic indwelling thoracic catheter, such as the Pleurx catheter (Denver Biomedical, Golden, CO). The patient or a family member drains the fluid on a daily or every-other-day basis. By keeping the fluid from accumulating within the thoracic cavity, the visceral and parietal surfaces can adhere. Additionally, the presence of an indwelling Silastic catheter may cause irritation and inflammation of the two surfaces, resulting in a spontaneous pleurodesis. Placement of this catheter involves a minor outpatient procedure under local anesthesia, and patients can easily drain their effusions at home. When fluid drainage is less than 50 mL per day, the catheter is removed in the clinic with local anesthesia. In comparison with chemical pleurodesis, this procedure is less painful and requires no hospital stay.

In this case, the patient chooses the Pleurx catheter and home drainage.

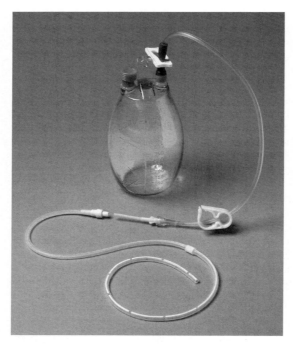

Figure 20-3 Pleurx catheter system (Denver Biomedical, Golden, CO).

Chest X-rays

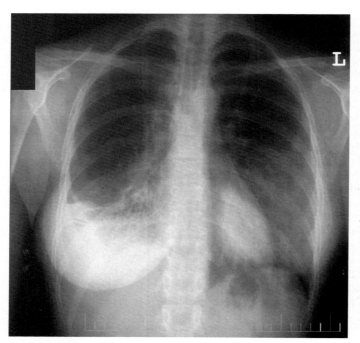

Figure 20-4

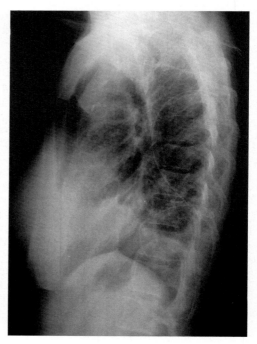

Figure 20-5

Chest X-ray Report

Right pleural effusion has decreased in size; reticular opacities are seen involving the right lower lung zone. The remaining lung fields are clear. The right-sided catheter is noted. There is a small right apical pneumothorax.

Case Continued

The patient continues to self-drain for 3 months, after which time minimal daily effusion is evacuated. The patient is seen in the office, and the catheter is removed under local anesthesia.

case 21

A 36-year-old man is referred to your office by his primary medical doctor for evaluation of difficulty swallowing. He presents with the following chest x-rays.

Chest X-rays

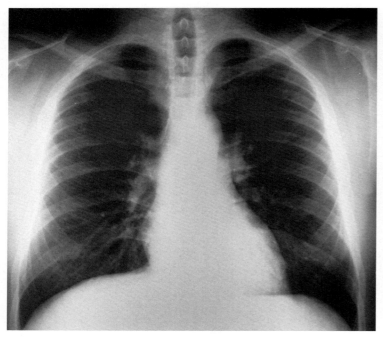

Figure 21-1

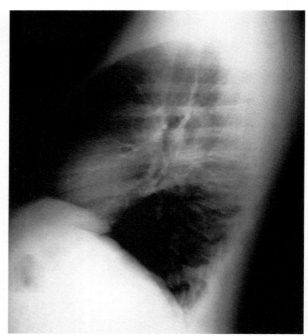

Figure 21-2

Chest X-ray Report

The lung fields are clear. The heart size is normal. The mediastinum is clear without any evidence of masses. █

Differential Diagnosis

In addressing symptoms of dysphagia (difficulty swallowing), the physician needs to conduct a thorough history to differentiate it from the symptoms of odynophagia (pain with swallowing) and globus (sensation of lump in the throat). Furthermore, symptoms of dysphagia can be divided into oropharyngeal dysphagia and esophageal dysphagia. Oropharyngeal dysphagia is the dysfunctional transfer of food bolus past the pharynx and upper esophageal sphincter and is more common in elderly patients, with stroke being the primary causative pathologic process. Esophageal dysphagia is caused by disordered peristaltic motility or conditions that obstruct flow of food or liquid bolus through the esophagus. Achalasia and scleroderma are the leading causes of esophageal motility disorders, with cancer, stricture, and Schatzki's ring being the most common causes of esophageal obstruction.

Recommendation

A detailed history and physical examination are necessary to distinguish the symptoms of dysphagia from odynophagia and globus. A thorough physical examination, including a neurologic examination, is necessary.

Case Continued

The patient complains that food is sticking in his chest after swallowing. He denies any difficulty with swallowing and does not experience coughing during swallowing. He reports symptoms only with swallowing solids; liquids do not produce any symptoms. The patient states he is otherwise healthy and rarely ever takes medications except over-the-counter pain medications for occasional musculoskeletal aches after intense workouts. The patient denies any weight loss. His symptoms have progressed in the past 2 to 3 years. The patient states that he has been evaluated for these symptoms within the past week and that he did not follow up with his prior physicians because of his extreme discomfort during an esophagoscopy. He further reports that a biopsy was performed at that time and was normal.

On examination, vital signs are stable. Full physical and neurologic evaluation is normal.

Recommendation

The history of this patient suggests an esophageal dysphagia. To confirm the diagnosis, a barium esophagogram is an appropriate initial test because previous esophagoscopy was normal.

Esophagograms

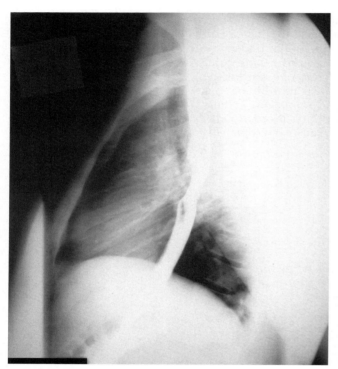

Figure 21-3

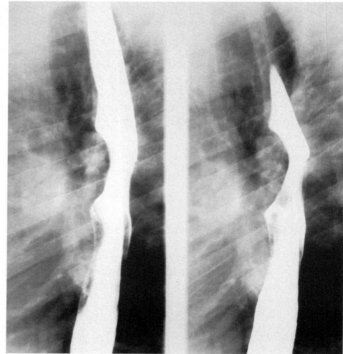

Figure 21-4

Esophagogram Report

The barium esophagograms demonstrate a concave mass in the mid-esophagus with a smooth surface and with no apparent mucosal abnormality. The rest of the esophagus appears normal with no pathology. ▪

Diagnosis

The appearance of the mass on esophagogram is most consistent with an esophageal leiomyoma.

Discussion

Esophageal leiomyomas are benign lesions of the muscular wall of the esophagus. The incidence of this lesion is very low, with all benign tumors of the esophagus composing less than 1% of all esophageal neoplasms. Leiomyomas, however, are the most common of all the benign esophageal masses of the esophagus, and intramural esophageal polyps are the second most common. Esophageal leiomyomas are rarely symptomatic unless the size approaches or exceeds 5 cm in diameter.

Leiomyomas that exhibit symptoms clinically are most commonly found in the middle (40%) and distal esophagus (50%). Only 10% are identified in the proximal third of the esophagus. They are twice as common in men, and only 2% are found in children. These tumors, as well as other benign tumors of the esophagus, can cause obstruction with aspiration and severe pulmonary complications.

Radiographically, plain chest x-ray is seldom diagnostic, but occasionally calcification within the leiomyoma is apparent. The most appropriate diagnostic test for esophageal leiomyomas is a barium contrast esophagogram. Schatzki described the appearance of a leiomyoma on barium study as a crescent-like filling defect. The junction of the lesion with the normal esophagus has a characteristic sharp angle of demarcation. The esophageal mucosa overlying the lesion is characteristically smooth, with regular mucosal folds apparent above and below the lesion as well as on the opposite esophageal wall. Patients with the characteristic barium esophagogram appearance for leiomyoma rarely need further diagnostic evaluation. Esophagoscopy is only necessary if other pathologic diagnoses are entertained or if the symptoms do not appear to correspond with the clinical presentation. Esophagoscopy demonstrates a mobile mass bulging into the esophageal lumen. The overlying mucosa appears without irregularities. The lumen of the esophagus is narrowed with minimal obstruction. Esophageal leiomyomas are round or ovoid smooth masses with occasional lobulations.

Recommendation

Right thoracotomy and excision of the leiomyoma. A thoracoscopic approach is also an option for leiomyoma resection.

Discussion

Tumors of the middle third of the esophagus are approached through the right chest. Tumors of the distal third of the esophagus are approached through the left chest. The upper third of the esophagus may be best approached through a right thoracotomy or a left cervical approach, depending on the level of the lesion. After exposure of the mediastinum, the mediastinal pleura is incised, and the esophagus is mobilized. The esophageal muscularis is incised longitudinally, and after the leiomyoma is identified in its entirety, it is bluntly dissected and enucleated. The mortality rate with enucleation approaches 0%.

Case Continued

A right thoracotomy is performed, and the esophagus is mobilized. During the blunt dissection and enucleation for the leiomyoma, a defect occurs in the esophageal mucosa.

Recommendation

Mobilization of the esophagus at the level of the defect should be performed. The mucosa is approximated with an absorbable interrupted suture. The muscularis layer is closed with interrupted nonabsorbable sutures. Drainage of the pleural cavity is performed, and a Gastrografin swallow is obtained on the fifth postoperative day to evaluate for an esophageal leak.

Discussion

The recent history of the esophagoscopy and biopsy may have contributed to the complication that occurred during resection of the leiomyoma. Biopsy of a suspected leiomyoma is contraindicated because the mucosa is not involved and surgical enucleation may result in perforation, as occurred in this scenario. Esophagoscopy, although not necessary in the diagnosis of leiomyoma, may be performed to assess other coexisting pathologies.

An asymptomatic patient with an incidental finding of a small leiomyoma may be followed as an outpatient with annual chest x-rays and a barium esophagography. This should be continued for any lesion that is less than 4 cm in diameter, without obstruction, bleeding, or suspected malignancy. Enucleation is performed if the mass enlarges, ulceration is present in the mass, the mass has central necrosis, or the mass appears heterogenous on ultrasonographic examination.

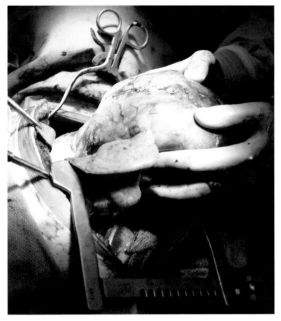

Color Plate 1 See Figure 1-5.

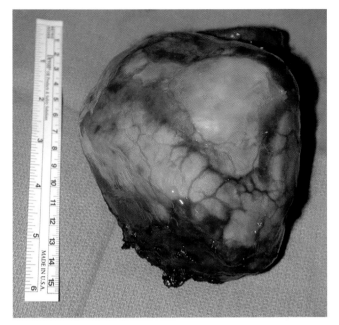

Color Plate 2 See Figure 4-5.

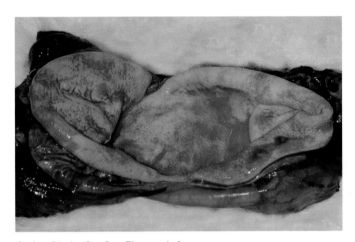

Color Plate 3 See Figure 4-6.

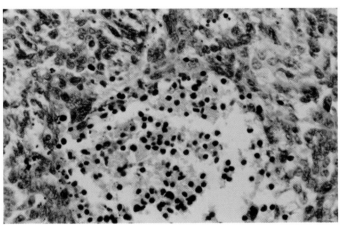

Color Plate 4 See Figure 6-6.

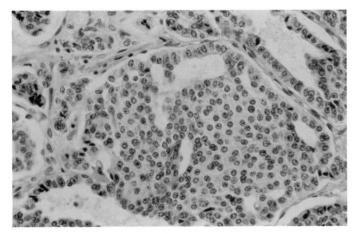

Color Plate 5 See Figure 6-9.

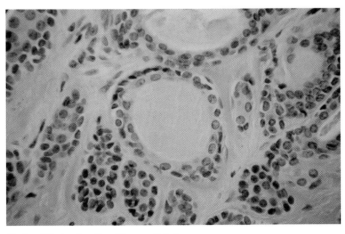

Color Plate 6 See Figure 14-5.

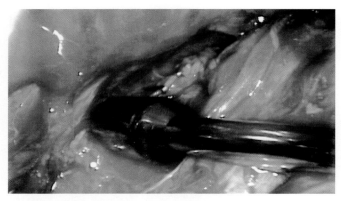

Color Plate 7 See Figure 16-5.

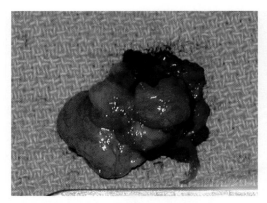

Color Plate 8 See Figure 16-6.

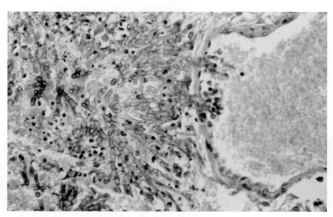

Color Plate 9 See Figure 19-5.

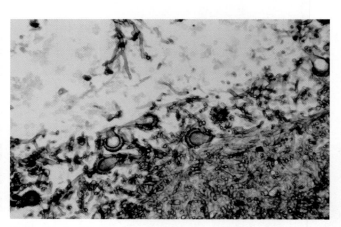

Color Plate 10 See Figure 19-6.

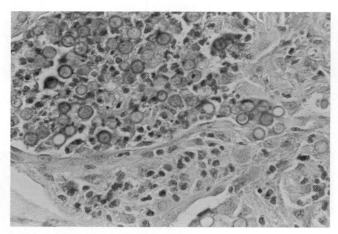

Color Plate 11 See Figure 26-3.

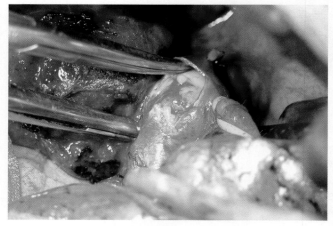

Color Plate 12 See Figure 28-7.

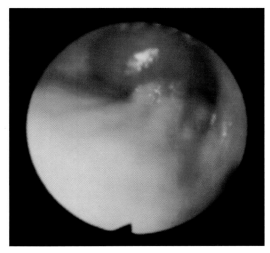

Color Plate 13 See Figure 31-5.

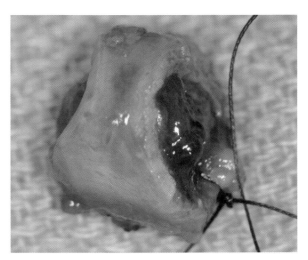

Color Plate 14 See Figure 31-6.

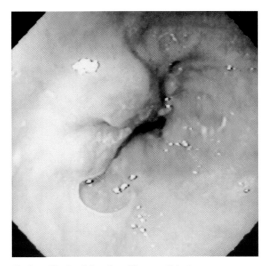

Color Plate 15 See Figure 34-4.

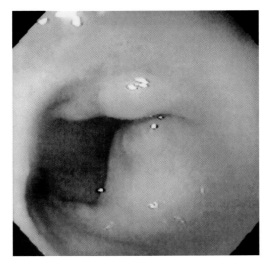

Color Plate 16 See Figure 34-5.

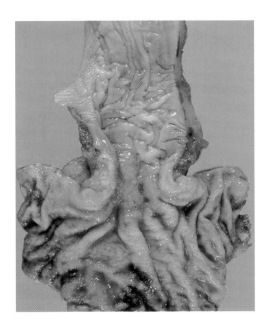

Color Plate 17 See Figure 34-6.

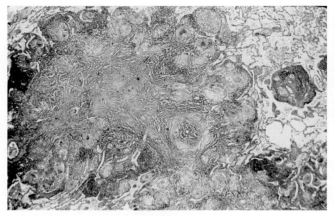

Color Plate 18 See Figure 42-5.

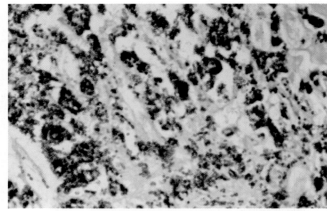

Color Plate 19 See Figure 42-6.

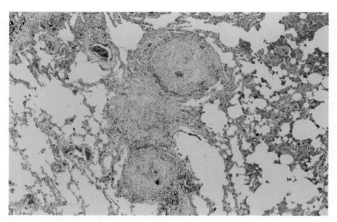

Color Plate 20 See Figure 46-5.

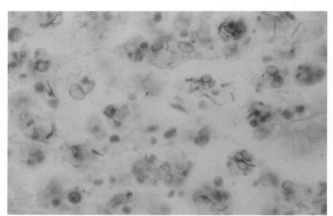

Color Plate 21 See Figure 46-6.

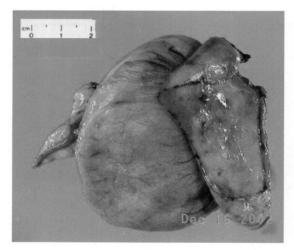

Color Plate 22 See Figure 47-6.

Presentation

A 51-year-old woman is referred to a thoracic surgeon because of an abnormal finding on chest x-rays that were obtained as part of a preoperative evaluation for an elective cholecystectomy.

■ Chest X-rays

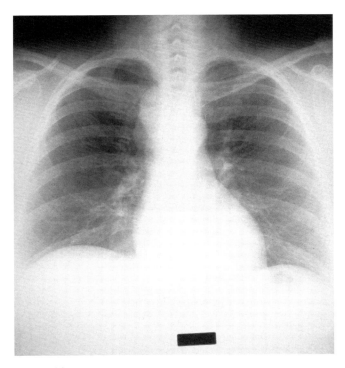

Figure 22-1

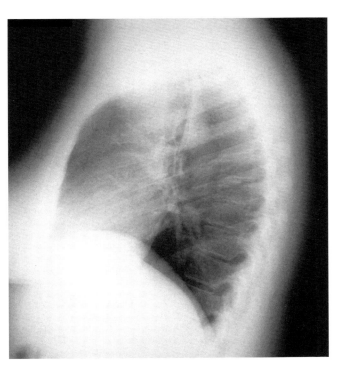

Figure 22-2

Chest X-ray Report

The chest x-rays demonstrate a mass in the right superior mediastinum. The heart is of normal size, and there are no lung masses or pleural effusions.

Discussion

The patient reports a 30-pack-per-year smoking history and coughing episodes almost every morning. She has no history of hemoptysis, fevers, night sweats, chills, pleuritic pain, or complaints suggesting heart disease. Physical examination shows no palpable masses in the neck or supraclavicular area.

Recommendation

Computed tomography (CT) scans.

■ CT Scans

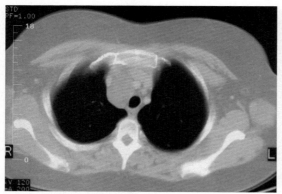 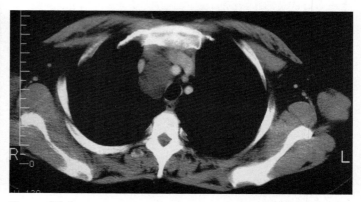

Figure 22-3   **Figure 22-4**

CT Scan Report

The CT scans demonstrate a homogeneous right superior mediastinal mass measuring 5 cm × 4 cm. The mass is adjacent to the trachea. There are no other lung nodules or infiltrates.

Discussion

The right paratracheal mass displaces the superior vena cava laterally and distorts the trachea medially. This mass may represent a primary mediastinal malignancy or a metastatic cancer. Likely tumors include lymphoma, non–small cell or small cell lung carcinoma, and thyroid carcinoma. The homogeneous appearance of the mass and lack of symptoms suggest the mass may be a mediastinal cyst. Enteric mediastinal cysts include bronchogenic cysts and duplication cysts of the bronchus or esophagus. Neuroenteric cysts are unlikely because they are usually found in the posterior mediastinum. Mesothelial cysts are also unlikely in this scenario because these cysts are usually adjacent to pericardium and communicate with the pericardial space (pericardial or "springwater" cyst). Chest x-rays may provide the diagnosis in 90% of the cases. However, a CT scan is a more sensitive study. Given the clinical scenario of this patient and the radiographic findings, the most likely diagnosis of this mass is a bronchogenic cyst.

Bronchogenic cysts appear on CT scan as a uniloculate or occasionally multiloculate mass with Hounsfield unit density from nearly water (0 to 20) to 90. Bronchoscopy may show extrinsic compression of the trachea by the cyst. Rarely, a fistulous communication to the cyst is found on bronchoscopic examination, with drainage of mucopurulent debris into the airway. If the diagnosis of bronchogenic cyst is suspected but other diagnoses are also considered, biopsy of the mass can be performed by mediastinoscopy, mediastinotomy, or thoracotomy. If the mass is small and asymptomatic, it may be observed with routine follow-up. Any symptoms of infection, airway compression, or enlargement of the cyst should prompt consideration for operative resection. Generally, symptomatic or poorly characterized masses should be removed. Mediastinal cysts are excised through a muscle-sparing thoracotomy. The goal of the operation is complete excision of the cyst. Occasionally, there are dense adhesions between the cyst and vital mediastinal structures rendering complete excision dangerous. In such instances, the cyst may be opened and the remaining mucosa ablated with argon plasma, laser, or cautery energy. Alternative approaches include drainage of the cyst through a mediastinoscopy, video-assisted thoracic surgery (VATS) excision, cyst aspiration, and injection of the cyst with a sclerosing agent. However, when a bronchogenic cyst is aspirated, it frequently recurs.

Case Continued

A muscle-sparing posterolateral thoracotomy is performed, and the cyst is completely excised from the upper mediastinum.

Discussion

Bronchogenic cysts originate from the primitive foregut and may either be mediastinal or peripheral (parenchymal) in location, depending on the timing of the formation of the cyst from the ventral foregut. Early budding leads to mediastinal cysts and later gestational events lead to peripheral or parenchymal cysts. Because the origin of the cyst is the primitive foregut, it may be lined with ciliated columnar or squamous epithelium. Mucous glands are present in both types of cysts, causing the cysts to fill often under pressure. This causes compression of the adjacent structures, especially the neonatal airways. Bronchogenic cysts may cause life-threatening respiratory distress in neonates, whereas older children and adults display milder symptoms or no symptoms. It has been estimated that one third of adults with bronchogenic cysts are asymptomatic. A residual communication of the cyst with the airway is possible. In such patients, spillage of mucus and contamination of the cyst contents occur with resultant pulmonary infection.

case 23

Presentation

A 35-week premature female neonate, weighing 3 kg, is initially discharged home. After 4 days, she is brought to the emergency department by her parents with dyspnea, nasal flaring, tachypnea, and mild cyanosis. She improves slightly with inhalers and humidified oxygen. Breath sounds are decreased on the right side. Endotracheal intubation is not necessary in the initial management.

Differential Diagnosis

The differential diagnosis for severe respiratory distress in a newborn includes congenital heart disease such as vascular rings or slings, mediastinal tumors, bronchogenic cysts, bronchopulmonary dysplasia, congenital lobar emphysema, pulmonary arteriovenous malformations, cystic adenoid malformation, pulmonary sequestration, tracheomalacia, congenital diaphragmatic hernia, and vocal cord malfunction.

Chest X-ray

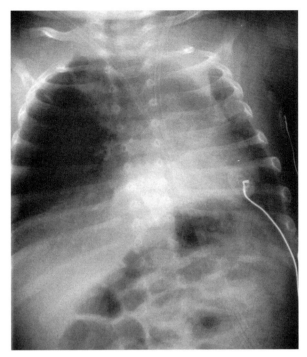

Figure 23-1

Chest X-ray Report

Hyperinflation of the left lung with mediastinal shift to the left side.

CT Scans

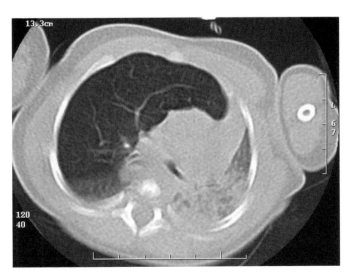

Figure 23-2

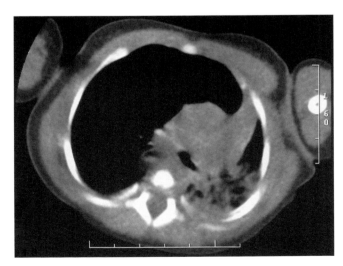

Figure 23-3

CT Scan Report

Hyperinflated right middle lobe with bronchovascular markings noted to the periphery of the lung. There is mediastinal shift to the left side with atelectasis of the left lung consistent with congenital lobar emphysema. ▪

Discussion

Congenital lobar emphysema is defined as a postnatal overdistention of a histologically normal lobe. The upper and middle lobes are most commonly affected, and the process is usually confined to a single lobe (left upper, right middle, right upper). The etiology of this entity is not identified in 50% of patients. In the remainder of patients, hyperinflation is caused by a ball-valve effect at the level of the lobar or segmental bronchus with distal air trapping due to bronchopulmonary dysplasia, hypertrophic mucus membrane, or mucus plug. Rarely, extrinsic bronchial compression from either an enlarged cardiac chamber or pulmonary arteries in congenital heart disease can cause distal air trapping and lobar emphysema. It is estimated that 15% to 20% of children with congenital lobar emphysema have a congenital heart defect. In these cases, correction of the cardiac defect may result in resolution of the emphysematous changes. Most patients present within the first week to first month of life, and the remainder present within the first 6 months of life. This diagnosis may be confused with tension pneumothorax. Placement of a chest tube may cause lung injury with persistent air leak and bronchopleural fistula.

Plain chest x-ray typically demonstrates overinflation of a lobe with mediastinal shift to the contralateral side. Computed tomography (CT) scan is useful in delineating extrinsic causes of congenital lobar emphysema.

Recommendation

Preoperatively, cardiac echocardiogram is necessary to exclude congenital heart disease. Intraoperatively, bronchoscopy, right posterolateral thoracotomy, and right middle lobectomy should be performed.

Case Continued

Cardiac echocardiogram shows the presence of a patent foramen ovale. No other anomalies are detected.

The patient is brought into the operating room and placed in the supine position. Flexible bronchoscopy reveals bronchomalacia in the right bronchus. Selective left main-stem intubation is attempted. However, the patient experiences significant hemodynamic instability and desaturation.

Approach

Small neonates are very sensitive to orotracheal manipulations. By intubating and inflating the giant right middle lobe, the heart chambers are likely to be compressed, resulting in hemodynamic compromise. Compression of normal lung parenchyma by the right middle lobe results in an acute increase in pulmonary vascular resistance, resulting in desaturation owing to right-to-left shunting across a patent foramen ovale.

Tidal volumes need to be minimized, and respiratory rate needs to be increased. High ventilatory pressures should be avoided. This is best achieved initially by an experienced anesthesiologist performing hand ventilation. The endotracheal tube is positioned in the mid-trachea. High-frequency ventilation can be used if these maneuvers are unsuccessful.

Case Continued

A right posterolateral incision is performed, the right middle lobe is found to be grossly overinflated, and the parenchyma is abnormally friable and poorly perfused. The middle lobe has herniated through the incision, precluding any maneuvers inside the chest. A stapling device is used to remove part of the middle lobe to identify the fissure and mediastinal structures. A standard middle lobectomy is completed. Two chest tubes are placed, one anteriorly and the second posteriorly. The thoracotomy is then closed in layers. There is immediate improvement in the neonate's saturation and hemodynamics.

Discussion

The only therapy for symptomatic congenital lobar emphysema is prompt resection of the involved lobe. Reported mortality rates for surgery are in the range of 10% to 30%. Survival depends heavily on associated defects, mainly heart defects. Children without associated cardiac defects have normal development. There is compensatory growth of the remaining lung tissue, with a residual pulmonary volume of about 90% predicted.

Chest X-ray, First Preoperative Day

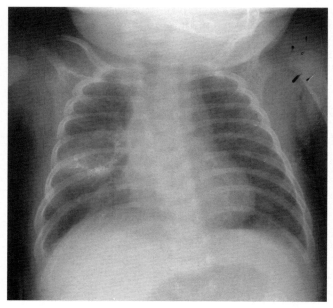

Figure 23-4

Case Continued

The patient remains intubated overnight. The chest tube is removed and the patient extubated. There are no further complications.

Presentation

An 87-year-old woman is referred to you with complaints of blood-streaked sputum for the past 3 weeks. The patient reports a productive cough for several
months. She also reports a two-pack-per-day smoking history for the past 15
years.

Past surgical history is pertinent for a previous hiatal hernia repair. On review
of systems, the patient denies any current heartburn or dysphagia but does admit
to a 5-pound weight loss and recent upper back pain.

On physical examination, the breath sounds are diminished at the bases, and
there is wheezing present over the right chest. In addition, there is focal chest wall
tenderness over the right lower ribs posteriorly.

The following x-rays are obtained.

Chest X-rays

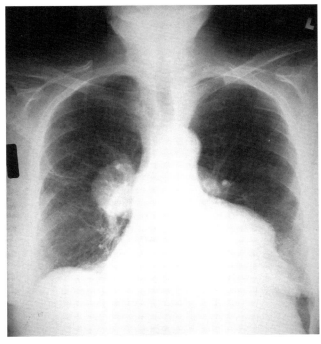

Figure 24-1

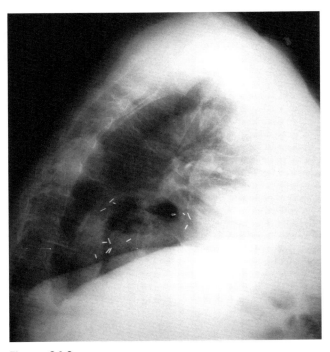

Figure 24-2

Chest X-ray Report

There is an irregular density in the right chest, possibly in the middle or right lower lobe. On the left side, there are postsurgical clips, and the left heart border is irregular, suggesting recurrence of the hiatal hernia. ▪

Differential Diagnosis

Hemoptysis usually indicates the presence of infectious or neoplastic lesions of the lung. Given this patient's strong smoking history and the presence of an irregular density on chest x-ray, a lung malignancy is the most likely diagnosis.

Recommendation

Computed tomography (CT) scans of the chest are needed to define the location and extent of the mass and to aid in staging.

▪ CT Scans

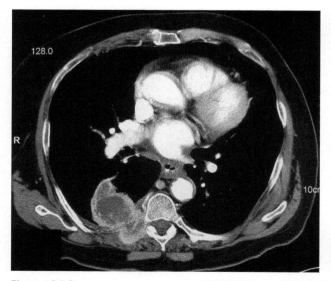

Figure 24-3

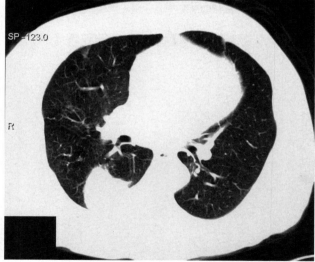

Figure 24-4

CT Scan Report

There is a large, necrotic, pleural-based mass in the right lower lung posteriorly. This mass, which measures 8 cm × 5 cm, invades the adjacent rib and extends into the paraspinous musculature. Nonspecific parenchymal opacification is present in the right upper lobe laterally. There are no pulmonary nodules and no enlarged lymph nodes in the hilum, mediastinum, or axillary region. There are no pleural or pericardial effusions. ▪

Recommendation

Further staging with positron-emission tomography (PET).

Discussion

The CT scan demonstrates a T3 N0 M0, stage IIB neoplasm. Accurate staging is necessary to determine resectability of this lesion. PET imaging adds metabolic information to the anatomic definition already provided by the CT scan. This information is important because physiologic changes precede anatomic changes. In PET imaging, a radiographic tracer accumulates in metabolically active tissues and then releases positrons, which are detected by the scanner. Lung cancers are known to have high glucose metabolism; thus, an appropriate glucose analogue tracer is used. In identifying malignant lung lesions, this method is 92% sensitive and 90% specific. It is important to remember that different types of tumors have different affinities for the tracer. False-negative results are more likely to occur with bronchioloalveolar cancers.

PET is also useful for assessing the mediastinum and distant sites for evidence of spread. The accuracy is variable based on a number of studies but appears to be superior to that achieved with CT scanning. In fact, PET is also more accurate than bone scanning in detecting metastases.

PET Scan

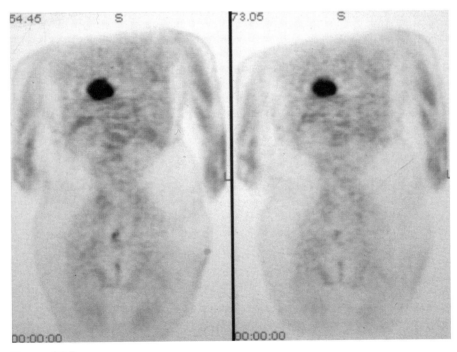

Figure 24-5

PET Scan Report

There is a single area of uptake in the right chest without evidence of mediastinal or distant disease. ▪

Recommendation

In high-risk procedures, especially in an elderly patient, it is appropriate to confirm the diagnosis using CT-guided needle biopsy before embarking on an operation.

Case Continued

A CT-guided biopsy was performed without complication. Final pathology demonstrates poorly differentiated non–small cell carcinoma.

Discussion

According to the clinical staging, this tumor represents a T3 lung cancer (chest wall involvement) without evidence of metastasis. If imaging suggests mediastinal lymph node enlargement or activity, mediastinoscopy should be performed. Involvement of mediastinal nodes, T3 N2, carry unfavorable prognosis, and alternative therapies can be considered.

Recommendation

Surgery to include right lower lobectomy with *en bloc* resection of any involved chest wall and mediastinal lymphadenectomy.

Discussion

A right posterolateral thoracotomy through the fifth intercostal space provides optimal exposure in this case. The first step would be to examine the lung tissue for the presence of other nodules and then to assess resectability of the lesion itself. If the tumor invades only the pleura, an extrapleural approach may suffice. However, if there is no clear plane present between the parietal pleura and the chest wall, the overlying ribs and intercostal muscles should be removed *en bloc* with the adherent lobe. The resection margin should be selected several centimeters beyond the gross tumor line to include a rib above and below the tumor. A complete mediastinal lymphadenectomy should then be performed.

Reconstruction of the chest wall defect is undertaken to provide stability and avoid respiratory compromise. Posterior defects, under the scapula, rarely require reconstruction. Other defects require prosthetic mesh fixation to the remaining rib margin and muscle flap with existing chest wall musculature. Prosthetic reconstruction materials include Gore-Tex patch (W. L. Gore & Associates, Flagstaff, AZ), Marlex mesh (Bard Inc., Murray Hill, NJ), and combination of Marlex and methylmethacrylate.

Case Continued

A right posterolateral thoracotomy is performed through the fifth intercostal space. The tumor in the right lower lobe is adherent to the seventh rib posteriorly and extends toward the sixth and eighth ribs on either side. A right lower lobectomy with *en bloc* resection of the posterior chest wall, including ribs six, seven, and eight, is performed, as well as a mediastinal lymphadenectomy. The chest wall defect is reconstructed with a 2-mm Gore-Tex patch. The patient is successfully extubated on the operating table and has an uneventful postoperative course.

Final pathology is a T3 N1 M0, stage IIIA, poorly differentiated non–small cell lung cancer.

Recommendation

The patient in this case has stage IIIA disease, and surgical margins are free of microscopic cancer. Postoperative radiation and chemotherapy in large clinical series has not proved to be of benefit. Postoperative radiation can decrease the incidence of local recurrence when regional nodes are involved.

Discussion

Numerous trials have been done to assess the applicability and efficacy of adjuvant chemotherapy. Alkylating agent trials have shown surgery alone to be more beneficial, whereas studies of cisplatin-based treatment show a favorable outcome with chemotherapy. No particular group of patients has been shown to obtain consistent benefit from chemotherapy, and its use should therefore be limited to protocol situations.

In patients with advanced disease, adjuvant radiation may be beneficial for local control; however, no long-term survival advantage has been demonstrated. Nevertheless, studies show that patients who receive adjuvant radiation with completely resected disease have better 5-year survival rates.

Overall, it appears that adjuvant therapies are safe, but their degree of efficacy has yet to be determined. Even with optimal treatment, median survival for stage IIIA disease is about 1 year, with a 5-year survival rate of 15% to 20%.

case 25

Presentation

A 44-year-old man presents to the emergency department after a night of binge drinking complaining of dysphagia and odynophagia. He admits to having vomited several times. Physical findings include tachycardia, fever (temperature 100.8°F), and decreased breath sounds at the left base.

Differential Diagnosis

In a patient who presents with esophageal symptoms after episodes of vomiting, esophageal perforation must be strongly considered. Other possible diagnoses include aspiration pneumonia, esophagitis, and peptic ulcer disease.

Discussion

Barogenic esophageal perforation due to emesis is a well-recognized cause of esophageal perforation. It typically occurs in younger men and is often related to an episode of alcohol abuse. The rupture usually occurs in the distal esophagus, permitting saliva and gastric contents to leak into the mediastinum and possibly the pleural spaces. The peristaltic activity of the esophagus and negative intrathoracic pressure facilitate rapid accumulation of these digestive fluids, leading to inflammation and the development of multisystem organ failure if the condition is left untreated.

A high index of suspicion is appropriate when esophageal perforation is part of the differential diagnosis. A contrast esophagram is useful and should be performed in patients who are able to cooperate with the procedure. Radiography permits accurate assessment of the site of the leakage and the cavity into which the leakage drains. In patients who are not able to cooperate with such an examination, upper endoscopy is performed.

The site of the leakage helps determine how to approach the patient surgically. Patients who have mid-esophageal leaks are best approached through a right thoracotomy because the aortic arch interferes with adequate access from the left chest. Most other patients are approached through a left thoracotomy because the lower esophagus is more readily accessible and because the left pleural space is more often involved in the process.

Recommendation

Chest x-ray. Contrast esophagram.

Chest X-ray

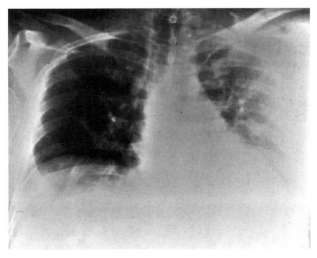

Figure 25-1

Chest X-ray Report

Small left pneumothorax, large left pleural effusion.

▧ Contrast Esophagram

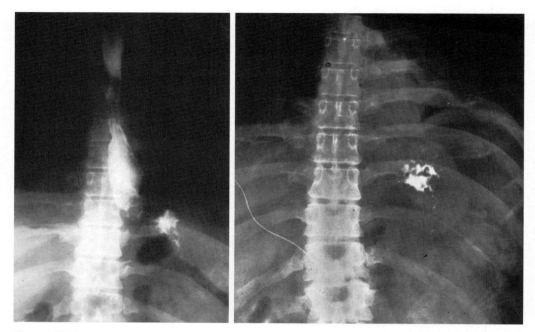

Figure 25-2

Contrast Esophagram Report

Contrast extravasates outside of the esophageal lumen just above the level of the esophagogastric junction. ▧

Diagnosis and Recommendation

Esophageal perforation with drainage into the left pleural space. You recommend primary closure of the perforation.

▧ Surgical Approach

You perform a left thoracotomy. Gastric contents and saliva are irrigated from the pleural space and mediastinum. A 3-cm perforation is identified 2 cm above the hiatus. The edges are trimmed, and the defect is closed in two layers. The closure is reinforced with a large pleural flap. Chest drains are placed, and a nasogastric tube is passed.

Case Continued

During the fifth postoperative day, the patient is hemodynamically stable but remains tachycardic with episodic temperature elevations to 101.2°F. The chest tube drainage decreases as expected, but the chest x-ray demonstrates accumulation of fluid in both pleural spaces.

Discussion

The physiologic response to reliable closure of an esophageal perforation is manifested by rapid clinical improvement, including reduction in fevers and tachycardia. Chest tubes should adequately evacuate serous pleural fluid that is generated in response to pleural and mediastinal inflammation. Patients who fail to follow this clinical course must be suspected of having a persistent leak or may be developing an empyema.

Evaluation of patients who remain ill after initial surgical therapy for perforation is aimed at determining the adequacy of drainage of the thorax and whether there is a persistent leak. Contrast esophagram and computed tomography (CT) scan are sufficient radiographic studies for these purposes.

The decision regarding proper management of a failed primary repair of an esophageal perforation is challenging. The basic principles include adequate drainage of the mediastinum and pleural spaces, preservation of the esophagus if its function can be maintained, and provision for gastric drainage and enteral nutritional support during what is likely to be a prolonged hospital stay.

Recommendation

CT scan and contrast esophagram.

Contrast Esophagram

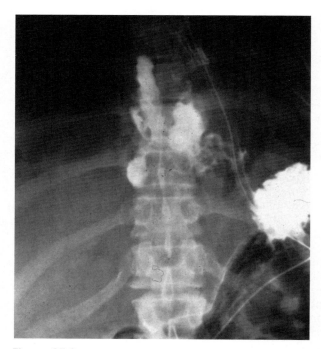

Figure 25-3

Contrast Esophagram Report

There is persistent drainage of contrast from the distal esophagus that collects in the right and left pleural spaces. Some of the contrast passes into the stomach. ▨

CT Scan

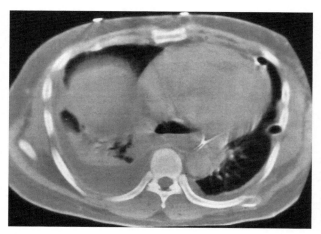

Figure 25-4

CT Scan Report

Bilateral pleural effusions are present; the right pleural effusion is larger. There is a large mediastinal fluid collection with an air–fluid level within it. Some consolidation is evident at the base of the right lower lobe.

Discussion

The radiographic findings indicate that there is a persistent defect in the esophagus leaking into both pleural spaces; furthermore, these images also indicate that both pleural spaces are inadequately drained. In view of these findings, it is unlikely that another attempt at repair of the esophagus is likely to succeed. Because the function of the esophagus was normal before the perforation, it is appropriate to attempt to preserve the esophagus rather than perform an esophagectomy at this point in time.

Control of the leak combined with preservation of the esophagus is most easily accomplished by excluding the esophagus, diverting saliva through a cervical esophagostomy. An alternative option might be placement of a T tube in the esophageal perforation.

Recommendation

Pleural drainage, cervical esophagostomy, gastrostomy, and jejunostomy feeding tube.

Surgical Approach

The left thoracotomy is reopened, and the pleural space is evacuated. A limited decortication is performed. Drains are placed to control the pleural space and the mediastinum, including the area of perforation. A right chest tube is placed. Through a cervical incision, an end-esophagostomy is performed. The closed distal end of the cervical esophagus is sewn to the side of the proximal esophagus so that it can be identified when the esophagostomy is taken down. Through a laparotomy, a draining gastrostomy is placed, and a feeding jejunostomy is created.

Case Continued

The patient recovers quickly from the drainage and diversion procedure and is discharged 2 weeks after his second operation. After 3 months, during which time he recovers his strength and his performance status improves, a contrast study is performed through the gastrostomy tube and demonstrates no leakage from the distal esophagus. The cervical esophagostomy is taken down, and an end-to-end esophagoesophagostomy is performed. The patient is advanced to a regular diet within 10 days and subsequently recovers uneventfully.

case 26

Presentation

A 24-year-old man is sent to your office by his primary medical physician for recommendations regarding an abnormal chest x-ray. The patient presents with a history of pneumonia, which was treated with several courses of antibiotics without any significant improvement in radiographic findings. The patient's physical examination is significant for rales over the right upper lung field. He denies any travel except for a camping trip 3 months ago in Mississippi. The patient's past medical, work, and social history are unremarkable, with no risk factors for human immunodeficiency virus (HIV).

Chest X-rays

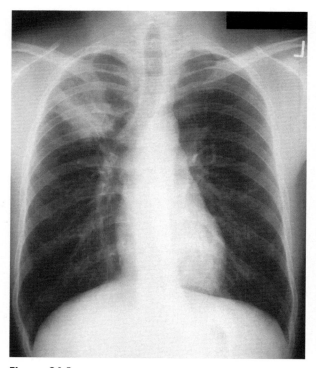

Figure 26-1

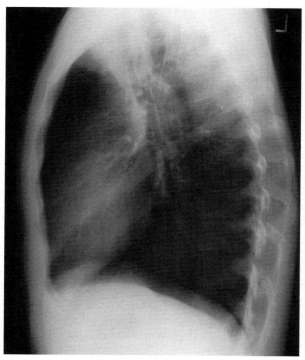

Figure 26-2

Chest X-ray Report

A right upper lobe infiltrate is present. A mass lesion with distal atelectasis cannot be excluded. There is no evidence of a pleural effusion. The heart size is normal.

Case Continued

A detailed history reveals that the patient has had a chronic cough, which has been productive of mucopurulent sputum with occasional chest discomfort and episodes of hemoptysis during the past 2 months. The patient also reports low-grade fevers, malaise, generalized fatigue, and a 10-pound weight loss over a 1-month period. Although the patient has received several antibiotic regimens, which have included tetracyclines and macrolides, his symptoms and radiographic findings have not improved. Sputum Gram stain and cultures did not reveal any organisms.

Discussion

The patient's history, physical findings, and radiographic changes are suggestive of a chronic pulmonary infection. Given the resistance to antibiotic therapy, the diagnosis of atypical pneumonias should be further investigated. The causative pathogens of atypical pneumonias may be bacterial, fungal, or viral. In general, viral pathogens do not cause lobar pathology or mass-like lesions in immunocompetent patients. Fungal infection, in addition to an atypical bacterial etiology, including tuberculosis, should be evaluated. The more common pathogens of the atypical bacterial pneumonias in immunocompetent patients are *Mycoplasma pneumonia*, *Legionella pneumophila*, *Chlamydia pneumonia*, oral anaerobes, *Chlamydia psittaci*, and *Coxiella burnetii*. The patient's symptoms, radiographic findings, and travel history suggest a high likelihood of an endemic fungal infection such as histoplasmosis, blastomycosis, or coccidioidomycosis. Although the diagnosis of malignancy is highly unlikely in a 24-year-old, it should be excluded in any patient with a persistent mass or infiltrate that does not respond to antibiotic treatment.

Recommendation

Because the patient has consistent production of mucopurulent sputum, repeat sputum studies should be obtained. Stains and culture mediums for fungal, as well as mycobacterial, strains should be requested. Although the patient's history is not suggestive of exposure to tuberculosis, a tuberculin skin test should be performed. A flexible fiberoptic bronchoscopy with bronchial washings, bronchoalveolar lavage, and possible transbronchial biopsy should also be considered. Empiric treatment for fungus or tuberculosis is not indicated unless an organism is identified.

Discussion

Fungal infection of the lung is best established by staining or culture of the infecting organism. Occasionally, it is not possible to recover organisms in the stained specimens. The two stains most commonly used for demonstration of fungi are periodic acid–Schiff (PAS) and methenamine silver stains. Other stains include a wet sputum preparation with immediate KOH staining and cytologic evaluation with Papanicolaou's (PAP) smear. For optimal fungal cultures, all specimens should be inoculated on different types of culture media. Sabouraud's dextrose agar is an excellent medium because it inhibits contaminating bacteria. Specimens should also be inoculated onto a second medium containing antibiotics and cycloheximide to suppress less fastidious bacteria and contaminating molds. Because this medium inhibits *Cryptococcus neoformans* and *Aspergillus fumigatus*, Sabouraud's agar should be used in conjunction.

As for mycobacteria, acid-fast stain or fluorochrome is necessary. Culture media should include an egg base (Lowenstein-Jensen) and an agar base (Middlebrook 7H11 agar). A third medium to suppress nonmycobacterial organisms is also recommended.

Case Continued

Before the scheduled bronchoscopy, the sputum culture indicates the following finding.

▧ Histology

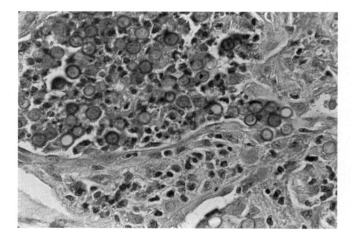

Figure 26-3   See Color Plate 11 following page 114.

Report of Histologic Finding

PAS staining demonstrates round, thick-walled organisms with broad base budding consistent with *Blastomycosis*. ▧

Discussion

North American blastomycosis is an endemic fungal infection that is caused by *Blastomyces dermatitidis*, a thermal dimorphic fungus. The spectrum of disease ranges from the asymptomatic acquisition to a rapidly progressive and life-threatening respiratory or disseminated illness. Blastomycosis is endemic to parts of the Midwestern and south-central United States and Canada with concentration along the Mississippi and Ohio Rivers and the Great Lakes. *B. dermatitidis* is acquired as an airborne spore. Some spores may escape the nonspecific defenses of the airway and reach the alveoli. It characteristically induces a granulomatous and pyogenic reaction with microabscesses and giant cells and occasionally caseation, cavitation, and fibrosis. The primary illness is therefore a lower respiratory infection. Symptomatic disease develops after an incubation period of 30 to 45 days. Some patients have an acute illness that resembles a bacterial pneumonia. The onset of symptoms is usually abrupt, with high fevers and chills followed by cough, which rapidly becomes productive of large amounts of mucopurulent sputum. These symptoms are more common in endemic outbreaks, whereas in sporadic cases, the onset of symptoms is more gradual. Some patients may present with a low-grade fever, productive cough, and weight loss. Extrapulmonary disease has been described in as many as 25% to 40% of patients with chronic blastomycosis. Skin lesions are highly variable in appearance, ranging from subcutaneous nodules and abscesses to papules and ulcers with heaped borders. Skin lesions may be single or multiple and may occur in crops of several new lesions daily. There is no characteristic chest x-ray pattern, and lesions may vary from single or multiple round densities throughout both lung fields to segmental or lobar infiltrates. Calcification in healed lesions is rare.

The skin and bony skeleton are the most common sites of symptomatic extrapulmonary spread. The prostate gland, meninges, oral pharynx, and abdominal viscera, including liver and adrenal glands, are involved less frequently.

Blastomycosis can present as a progressive infection in patients with T-cell defects, including organ transplant recipients and other patients being treated with high-dose glucocorticoid therapy for malignant and nonmalignant disorders. The disease can be cured in patients with intermediate degrees of immunosuppression. Blastomycosis in patients with acquired immunodeficiency syndrome (AIDS) is severe, and cure may be unlikely.

Recommendation

Itraconazole, 400 mg per day given orally for 6 months.

Discussion

The clinical spectrum of blastomycosis is variable. Infection may be asymptomatic or may present as an acute or chronic pneumonia. In addition, extrapulmonary disease may or may not be present. Spontaneous cures may occur in some immunocompetent individuals with acute pulmonary blastomycosis; nevertheless, most patients require therapy. In disease limited to the lung, cure may have occurred without treatment before the diagnosis was made. In contrast, all immunocompromised patients have progressive pulmonary disease or extrapulmonary disease and should be treated aggressively with amphotericin B. Other patients who should receive amphotericin B include patients with a life-threatening or central nervous system (CNS) disease and patients in whom azole treatment has failed. Amphotericin B is also the only drug approved for treating blastomycosis in pregnant women.

The azoles are an equally effective and less toxic alternative to amphotericin B for treating immunocompetent patients with mild to moderate pulmonary or extrapulmonary disease, excluding CNS disease. Ketoconazole has documented cure rates of 70% to 76% with doses of 400 mg per day and of 82% to 85% with doses of 800 mg per day. Relapse rates of 10% to 14% have been shown with ketoconazole, and follow-up is warranted for 1 to 2 years after treatment. Itraconazole is more readily absorbed, has enhanced antimycotic activity, and is better tolerated. It is effective in 90% to 95% of patients treated with 200 to 400 mg per day for 6 months. No therapeutic advantage is evident from the higher dose regimens. Fluconazole at doses of 400 to 800 mg per day shows 87% success in patients treated for a mean duration of 9 months. Itraconazole is the initial treatment of choice for non–life-threatening, non-CNS blastomycosis.

Case Continued

The patient is started on itraconazole, 400 mg per day, for a period of 6 months. His symptoms gradually improve and resolve. He returns for follow-up several times. The patient has several repeat chest x-rays. Toward the end of his antifungal therapy, the chest x-ray shows inadequate improvement with persistence of a right upper lung infiltrate.

Recommendation

Computed tomography (CT) scans of the chest are recommended. The study should be obtained to evaluate for an abscess and to undertake preoperative evaluation.

▪ CT Scans

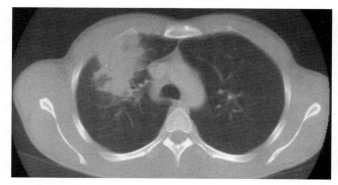

Figure 26-4

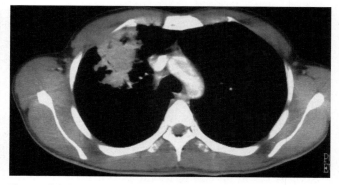

Figure 26-5

CT Scan Report

A 5 cm × 7 cm infiltrate in the right upper lobe with no evidence of an abscess is seen. There are no pleural effusions.

Recommendation

With the disease process confined to the right upper lobe, along with resistance to antifungal therapy, a right upper lobectomy is recommended.

Discussion

Most cases of pulmonary blastomycosis are managed medically. Surgical intervention is used in patients for whom medical management has failed and in those for whom no diagnosis has been confirmed using various diagnostic studies. In older patients in whom the diagnosis of cancer is more likely, thoracotomy is usually performed earlier in the diagnostic algorithm. Patients who undergo lung resection for blastomycosis should receive postoperative drug therapy with amphotericin B or itraconazole. Viable organisms are likely to persist in blastomycotic cavitary lesions; thus, resection of such lesions is indicated if they persist after adequate drug therapy.

case 27

Presentation

A 43-year-old woman comes to your office with a 4-week history of fever and night sweats accompanied by a 10-pound weight loss. She has no significant past medical or surgical history and is a nonsmoker.

■ Chest X-rays

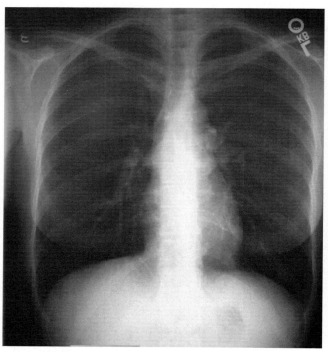

Figure 27-1

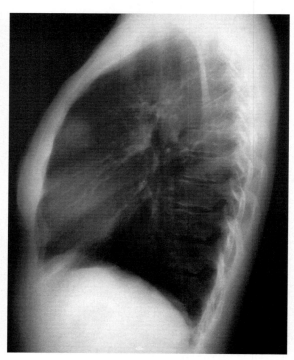

Figure 27-2

Chest X-ray Report

The lung fields are clear, and the cardiac silhouette is normal. There is a discrete density in the anterior mediastinum seen on the lateral view. ▪

Differential Diagnosis

The anterior mediastinum is bordered superiorly by the innominate vessels and inferiorly by the diaphragm. The anterosuperior aspect of the heart divides the anterior from the middle mediastinum. The contents of the anterior mediastinum include connective, lymphatic, and fatty tissues in addition to blood vessels, the thymus gland, and occasionally, parathyroid and thyroid tissue.

The most common anterior mediastinal tumor is a thymoma, which accounts for about half of all mediastinal tumors in adults. The next most prevalent mediastinal tumor is lymphoma, which includes Hodgkin's and non-Hodgkin's types, and is the most common of all mediastinal neoplasms. Germ cell tumors are also typically found in the anterior mediastinum and include teratoma, seminoma, choriocarcinoma, yolk sac tumor, and embryonal carcinoma. Thyroid masses, such as thyroid goiter or neoplasm, can also be present. Other tumors, such as thymic carcinoid, thymic cyst, thymolipoma, parathyroid adenoma, lymphangioma, hemangioma, fibroma, and fibrosarcoma, are less common histologic types of tumors that may be found in the anterior mediastinum.

Recommendation

Complete physical examination with careful attention to axillary and supraclavicular lymphadenopathy or other masses, and a testicular examination in men. Also, serologic tumor markers, such as a-fetoprotein, b-human chorionic gonadotropin, and lactate dehydrogenase, should be obtained. Computed tomography (CT) scans of the chest to delineate the mass and evaluate the status of intrathoracic lymphadenopathy are also necessary.

Test Results

The physical examination reveals no enlarged lymphadenopathy or masses. Serologic markers are negative. ▪

CT Scans

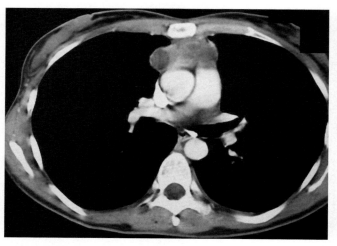

Figure 27-3

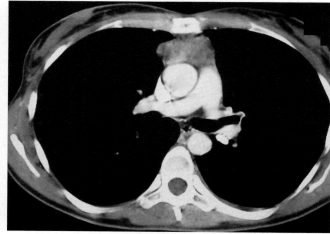

Figure 27-4

CT Scan Report

The CT scans of the chest show a heterogeneous mass, measuring 4 cm × 5 cm, in the anterior mediastinum. There are no enlarged mediastinal lymph nodes. There are no pleural effusions.

Discussion

Serologic markers are helpful in distinguishing among different anterior mediastinal masses. An acetylcholine receptor antibody level is diagnostic of thymoma. In young adults with suspicion of germ cell tumor, α-fetoprotein and β-human chorionic gonadotropin levels are suggestive of germ cell tumors. Although there are no specific markers for lymphoma, lactate dehydrogenase and alkaline phosphatase levels can be elevated.

Different imaging modalities aid in narrowing the differential for mediastinal masses. Plain chest x-rays, including a lateral view, are essential because mediastinal tumors are classified based on anatomic location. CT scanning is the next diagnostic modality of choice in most situations. If available, a spiral-type scan is better for reducing artifact, and intravenous contrast aids in assessing blood vessel involvement. The use of magnetic resonance imaging (MRI) is limited because of motion artifacts introduced by lung movement, but MRI can be used for soft tissue or vascular detailing. Gallium-67 scanning employs an iron analog to delineate both neoplastic and inflammatory lesions, and can be used to assess progress during treatment. Positron-emission tomography (PET) scanning can be used, although its role is still being investigated. If thyroid or parathyroid pathologies are suspected, ultrasound can be a good first imaging tool, followed by radionuclide thyroid scanning or parathyroid scintigraphy.

Recommendation

The history suggests lymphoma as the most likely diagnosis. This presumptive diagnosis needs to be confirmed with histologic evaluation.

Discussion

The diagnostic investigation of mediastinal masses is important because surgical intervention is not warranted for all cell types. It is often advisable to pursue tissue diagnosis before commencing treatment. However, there are instances in which immediate treatment is preferred, as in a case of large anterior mediastinal mass with α-fetoprotein or β-human chorionic gonadotropin levels above 500 ng/mL; these elevated levels of tumor markers are diagnostic for germ cell tumors.

There are several approaches to obtaining a tissue biopsy. The least invasive is percutaneous fine-needle aspirate with CT or ultrasound guidance, which is rarely associated with complications in the anterior mediastinum. The diagnostic accuracy of CT-guided core biopsy for lesions with suspected lymphoma ranges from 68% to 94%. Alternatively, extended cervical mediastinoscopy is a technically more demanding procedure that provides access to the superior mediastinum and upper portion of the anterior mediastinum. Anterior mediastinotomy, Chamberlain's procedure, is particularly well suited for evaluating mediastinal lymphadenopathy and large anterior tumors. Video-assisted thoracic surgery (VATS) is an excellent modality for obtaining biopsies of adequate size from multiple sites. When less invasive methods fail to provide adequate tissue for diagnosis, thoracotomy or sternotomy is performed, adequate tissue is obtained, and complete resection is considered based on histologic finding.

Case Continued

CT-guided needle biopsy is performed.

CT Scan (Needle Biopsy)

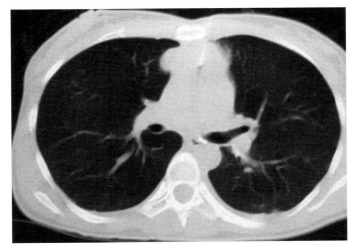

Figure 27-5

Histologic evaluation confirms the diagnosis of lymphoma. Immunophenotyping was performed for Reed-Sternberg cells and other lymphoid markers. Although larger tissue samples are often needed to classify lymphoma, in this case, the diagnosis of B-cell non-Hodgkin's lymphoma was made with needle biopsy.

Recommendation

Chemotherapy and radiation.

Discussion

Lymphomas represent about 15% of all mediastinal lesions. One third of mediastinal lymphomas are Hodgkin's lymphoma, and two thirds are non-Hodgkin's type. These lesions characteristically grow and displace surrounding tissues without eroding into them and only rarely have associated necrosis and cavitation.

Mediastinal disease is found in 60% of patients with Hodgkin's disease. There are four cell types, all with characteristic Reed-Sternberg cells: nodular sclerosing, lymphocyte predominant, mixed type, and lymphocyte depleted, which is most like non-Hodgkin's lymphoma. The disease can occur in any age group but peaks in the third decade as well as in patients older than 45 years of age. Younger patients usually have the more common nodular sclerosing type, whereas older patients have the mixed cell type, which is associated with more advanced stage. Although the actual cause is unknown, the disease may be caused by mycobacteria or Epstein-Barr virus and spreads from one lymph node station to adjacent ones.

Non-Hodgkin's lymphoma involves the mediastinum in 20% of patients, is of B- or T-cell type, and is of unknown cause. It usually affects patients in the first five decades of life and can be associated with pulmonary infiltrates and systemic adenopathy that skips lymph node stations.

Most patients are asymptomatic at the time of diagnosis. Any symptoms that are present are usually compressive in nature. There may be chest discomfort, hoarseness, or superior vena cava syndrome with large tumors. Less commonly, Horner's syndrome, stridor, or dysphagia may develop. Typically, patients present with palpable enlargement of axillary, supraclavicular, or cervical lymph nodes that is accompanied by mediastinal lymphadenopathy. Fever, night sweats, and weight loss, also called B-type symptoms, are more commonly seen with non-Hodgkin's type. More unusual complaints include pruritus or pain in lymph nodes after consuming alcohol.

Disease staging is based on lymph node involvement on CT scan and bone marrow biopsy. Staging laparotomy is no longer advised. Mediastinal disease is classified as stage I or II, whereas addition of abdominal disease or diffuse involvement is classified as stage III or IV.

Treatment of lymphoma is typically nonsurgical. The chemotherapy and radiation regimen is guided by cell type and stage. B-cell tumors are treated with both modalities, whereas T-cell tumors are best treated with chemotherapy alone. Combination chemotherapy is reserved for more advanced stages of disease.

Complete remission can be expected in 55% to 85% of patients, and late relapses are uncommon. Disease-free survival rate is better for Hodgkin's than non-Hodgkin's lymphoma.

Presentation

A 71-year-old woman presents to your office with complaints of a chronic dry cough. She has no significant past medical history. She walks every day for 30 minutes without symptoms of shortness of breath. She denies productive sputum, hemoptysis, weight loss, fever, chills, or night sweats. She is a lifetime nonsmoker and has not recently traveled outside the United States. She has an iodine allergy.

▨ Chest X-rays

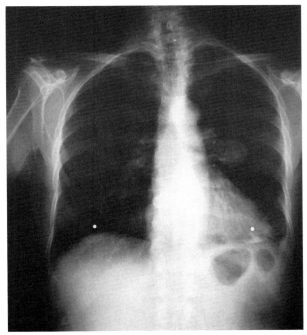

Figure 28-1

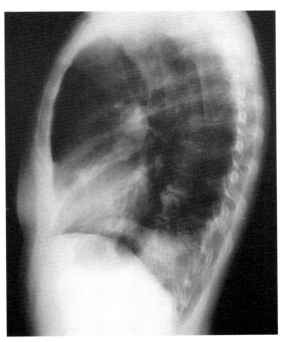

Figure 28-2

Chest X-ray Report

The trachea is midline. The heart size is normal. There is a small pleural effusion in the left chest. There is a round, smooth-edged, well-circumscribed mass located in the left mid-lung field. There is a clear line of demarcation between the border of the heart and the mass. ▨

Differential Diagnosis

Although this patient is a nonsmoker and only about 5% of patients with lung cancer are nonsmokers, the diagnosis of lung cancer should be considered. Passive smoking accounts for 25% of lung cancer in nonsmokers. Moreover, the risk for lung cancer increases 35% to 53% in nonsmokers who live with smokers. Because the anatomic location of the mass is central, other diagnoses that should be considered include mesodermal tumors such as angiosarcoma and hemangioma, arteriovenous fistulas, metastatic disease, and pulmonary artery aneurysms. Finally, hamartomas should also be included in the differential diagnosis. These tumors can appear round or lobulated but have a smooth border. Hamartomas are often calcified, and the finding of "popcorn" calcifications on chest x-rays is suggestive of this diagnosis.

Discussion

Further anatomic delineation of the mass in addition to evaluation of mediastinal structures is important in achieving a diagnosis and planning a therapeutic approach. For these reasons, a computed tomography (CT) scan of the chest and bronchoscopy is necessary. Aspiration of the left pleural effusion through a thoracentesis may also yield a diagnosis. Cytology from a pleural effusion yields a diagnosis of malignancy in 20% to 60% of patients with cancer. A positron-emission tomography (PET) scan may be considered, but it is more commonly used to assess metastases instead of diagnosing the primary lesion.

Recommendation

CT scan of the chest, bronchoscopy, and thoracentesis are recommended.

Case Continued

The bronchoscopy reveals no evidence of intrabronchial lesions or extraluminal compression. The bronchial mucosa in the left upper lobe bronchus appears hyperemic. Biopsies demonstrate macrophages and chronic inflammatory cells, but no neoplastic cells. A thoracentesis is performed at the time of bronchoscopy, and 100 mL of clear fluid is aspirated and reveals no malignant cells on cytologic examination.

CT Scans

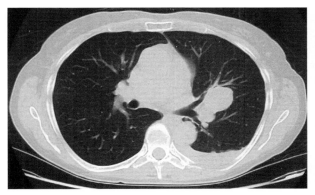

Figure 28-3

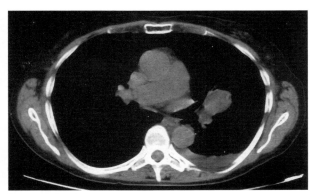

Figure 28-4

CT Scan Report

CT scans of the chest demonstrate a mass measuring 3 cm × 2 cm. The mass is slightly irregular in appearance. The bifurcation of the bronchus to the left upper and left lower lobe is visualized, and there is no impingement on these structures. Because no contrast was used in obtaining this study owing to the patient's allergy, comments on the proximity or involvement of the pulmonary artery cannot be made from this study. A small left pleural effusion is present. There are no enlarged lymph nodes.

Case Continued

Because this mass abuts the pulmonary artery and it is impossible to determine the involvement of the mass with the pulmonary artery owing to the lack of contrast, other radiologic examinations should be considered. A T2-weighted magnetic resonance imaging (MRI) study of the chest would show the relationship of the mass to the pulmonary artery. Additionally, a pulmonary artery angiogram might be considered in cases in which arteriovenous fistula or pulmonary artery aneurysm is suspected. An angiogram, however, is more invasive and requires a dye load, which should be avoided in patients with iodine allergies. To assess for metastatic disease, a PET scan is obtained.

▨ MRI Scan

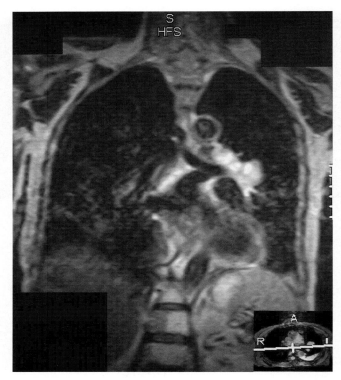

Figure 28-5

MRI Scan Report

The T2-weighted MRI depicts the mass as seen on the CT scan. Additionally, the mass extends into the left pulmonary artery and partially occludes it. Additional views (not shown) confirm that the pulmonary artery occlusion begins approximately 3 cm distal to the bifurcation of the main pulmonary artery. ▨

PET Scan

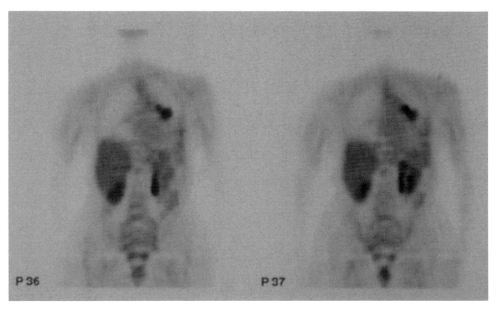

P 36   P 37

Figure 28-6

PET Scan Report

Radioisotope uptake is greatest in the region of the mass depicted on the CT scan. There is no evidence of other areas of uptake in the mediastinum.

Recommendations

Because the mass is centrally located and is close to or involves the pulmonary artery, a CT-guided biopsy cannot be performed safely. Nevertheless, the mass should be excised and the patient informed that a lobectomy or a pneumonectomy might be necessary given the proximity of the mass to the pulmonary artery. Pulmonary function testing should be performed in cases of marginal lung function and when pneumonectomy is considered. This patient had pulmonary function testing that revealed a forced expiratory volume in 1 second (FEV$_1$) of 1.74 L (96% of predicted), and the diffusing capacity of lung for carbon monoxide (D$_{LCO}$) was 72% of predicted. With these findings, the patient should tolerate a pneumonectomy.

Surgical Approach

A left posterolateral thoracotomy is performed through the fourth intercostal space. The thoracic cavity is explored, and there is no evidence of metastatic disease. The mass seen on the CT scan is palpated in the central part of the left upper lobe. Dissection is started in the hilum of the left lung, and the superior and inferior pulmonary veins are dissected. The major fissure is then dissected and the pulmonary artery visualized. The pulmonary artery is thick, full, and noncompressible, suggesting intraluminal occlusion. A core biopsy and frozen section of the mass are obtained and reveal malignant mesenchymal tumor. Because the tumor involves the pulmonary artery to the left upper lobe and left lower lobe, a pneumonectomy has to be performed. The pericardium is opened, and the pulmonary artery is dissected and excised. The proximal end is sutured with 4-0 polypropylene sutures. A lymph node dissection is performed.

Intraoperative Photograph

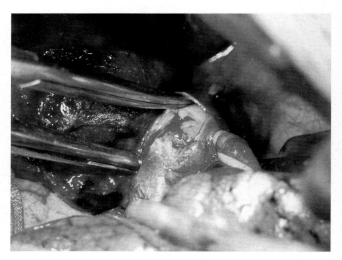

Figure 28-7   See Color Plate 12 following page 114.

Pathology Findings

Leiomyosarcoma filling the main pulmonary artery; upper lobe artery and branches; proximal left lower lobe artery, distal branches occluded by organizing thrombi; mass in middle to upper lobe, medial aspect; surgical margins of pulmonary artery and veins, and bronchus not involved. Lymph nodes were not involved with tumor.

Discussion

Pulmonary artery sarcomas are divided into three groups: fibroblastic or myofibroblastic sarcomas (50%), leiomyosarcomas (20%), and tumors requiring immunohistochemistry subclassification (30%). There are only 130 cases of primary pulmonary artery sarcoma published in the literature. Reports state a mean survival time of 1.5 months after diagnosis without surgical intervention. With surgery, mean survival time has been calculated at 10 to 19 months with an early mortality rate of 22%. Pulmonary artery sarcomas can be found along the pulmonary artery including the main pulmonary trunk and involving the pulmonary valve. Complete resection, along with prosthetic replacement of the valve, pulmonary trunk, or parts of the pulmonary artery, is recommended. At times, cardiopulmonary bypass and even hypothermic circulatory arrest has been implemented to complete the resection. In cases in which complete resection has not been feasible, endarterectomy of a pulmonary artery sarcoma has improved survival. Similarly to other sarcomas, survival benefit has been documented with successive resection of metastatic sarcoma to the lung. Because this tumor is rare, randomized trials for adjuvant therapy cannot be performed. In one small study, patients received postoperative chemotherapy with no documented tumor-free survival; however, the longest survivor without tumor recurrence received postoperative chemotherapy. Postoperative chemotherapy and radiation may play a role in the treatment of pulmonary artery sarcoma, but no study has proved this.

Presentation

A 65-year-old man is referred to you for management of esophageal cancer after being diagnosed 3 months before his appointment. Initially, the patient reported a 2-month history of progressive dysphagia to solids and a 15-pound weight loss. Evaluation at that time consisted of computed tomography (CT) scan, barium swallow, and endoscopic ultrasound (EUS). Diagnostic evaluation and histologic biopsy demonstrated a lower esophageal adenocarcinoma with transmural penetration of the primary tumor, and there was no involvement of adjacent structures; however, one enlarged lymph node adjacent to the lesser gastric curvature was identified. The past medical history was unremarkable.

The patient underwent multimodality therapy including chemotherapy (two cycles of cisplatin and 5-fluorouracil) and external-beam radiotherapy (50 Gy), which was completed 2 weeks before his appointment. There was only a modest radiographic response to this therapy. In addition, the patient has persistent dysphagia to soft solids and has lost another 10 pounds.

Chest X-ray

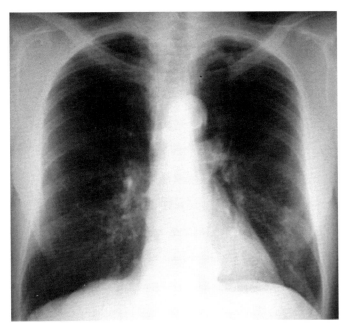

Figure 29-1

Chest X-ray Report

Findings consistent with diffuse emphysema. Mass effect in lower mediastinum adjacent to the left border of the spine. The heart is of normal size. There are no pleural effusions. ▨

▨ Barium Swallow

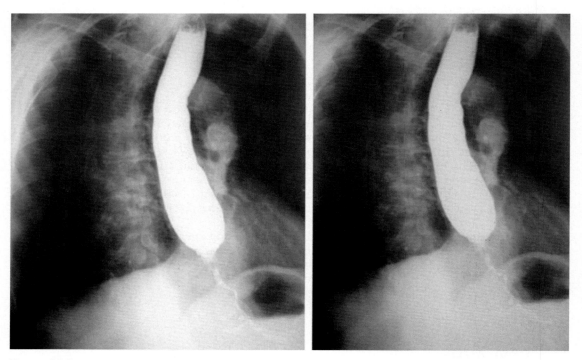

Figure 29-2

Barium Swallow Report

There is a mass in the lower thoracic esophagus with high-grade obstruction of the esophageal lumen. ▨

▉ CT Scan

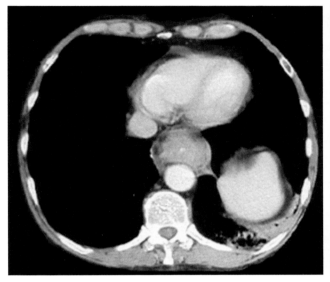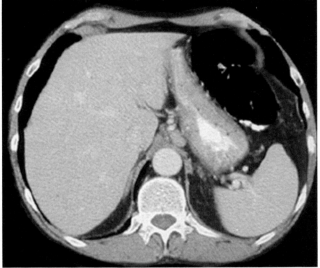

Figure 29-3

CT Scan Report

A mass is seen in the lower thoracic esophagus without obvious involvement of surrounding structures. Nonspecific infiltrate is seen at the base of the left lower lobe. An enlarged lymph node is seen adjacent to the lesser gastric curvature. Lungs are clear. Liver and adrenal glands are normal. ▉

Discussion

Despite the high frequency with which multimodality therapy for esophageal cancer is recommended, the benefit of multimodality treatment has not been proved. Most randomized studies demonstrate no apparent survival advantage for neoadjuvant chemotherapy, radiotherapy, or combined chemoradiotherapy. Studies suggest that there may be a survival advantage for neoadjuvant chemotherapy in patients with adenocarcinoma. Surgery remains an important component of potentially curative therapy for esophageal cancer.

Fortunately, there is no evidence that preoperative chemotherapy or radiation therapy has important adverse effects on intraoperative or postoperative complications. Neoadjuvant therapy does make the operation technically more difficult because normal tissue planes are sometimes obliterated after treatment. Transthoracic esophagectomy after radiation treatment allows dissection under direct vision, which is often a better technique than the so-called blind or blunt transhiatal esophagectomy technique.

The extent of resection and the choice of location are also influenced by the use of neoadjuvant therapy. When radiotherapy is administered preoperatively, every effort should be made to perform the anastomosis outside of the radiation field to minimize the risk for anastomotic complications.

Recommendation

Transthoracic near-total esophagectomy, gastric pull-up with cervical anastomosis, and a feeding jejunostomy.

Case Continued

You perform a modified Ivor Lewis esophagectomy, beginning with a right lateral thoracotomy incision and then repositioning the patient for an upper midline laparotomy and finally a cervical incision. A near-total esophagectomy is performed, a feeding jejunostomy is placed, and a pyloromyotomy is performed. The reconstruction is accomplished using tubularized stomach positioned in the bed of the resected esophagus. The anastomosis is created in the neck by stapling the back wall of the esophagus and the stomach using a linear cutting stapler and then suturing the front wall of the remaining defect. A nasoenteric tube is placed for gastric decompression.

The patient does well in the initial postoperative period. On the third postoperative day, he develops tachycardia and a low-grade fever. The following day, he has episodic atrial fibrillation, which is not associated with electrolyte abnormalities and responds appropriately to antiarrhythmic medications. On examination, the lungs are clear, and the chest and abdominal incisions are intact. The neck incision is swollen, but there is no discharge.

▢ Chest X-ray

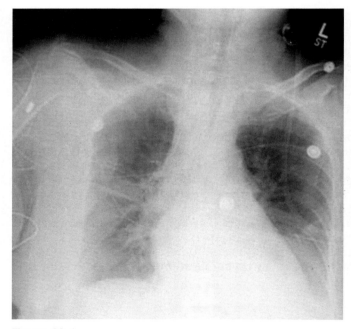

Figure 29-4

Chest X-ray Report

Small right pleural effusion. No pneumothorax. Chest tube in place. Widening of the mediastinum, presumably due to recent surgery and stomach pull-up. Nasogastric tube in place. ▪

Differential Diagnosis

The development of fever and tachycardia suggests an infection. The most common type of infection that develops after esophagectomy is anastomotic leak. Infections due to such leaks can sometimes propagate into the mediastinum, causing irritation of the pericardium with resultant supraventricular arrhythmias.

Fever and tachycardia may also be due to atelectasis, even in cases in which the atelectasis is not apparent on a chest x-ray. Arrhythmias may also result from manipulation of the pericardium at the time of the operation. The development of an empyema may also account for all of these findings, although the third postoperative day is early in the postoperative course for an empyema to be clinically apparent.

Important intraabdominal problems, such as leakage from the pyloromyotomy and mesenteric ischemia, are much less common but may also cause this clinical picture.

The physical examination is important in prioritizing the various possibilities. If the abdomen is benign and the chest is clear, attention is focused on the anastomosis. If there is any question about an intrathoracic process, a chest CT is obtained.

Recommendation

Because the neck incision is slightly swollen, you recommend drainage of the anastomosis as a diagnostic and therapeutic maneuver.

Discussion

Anastomotic leak may be due to breakdown of a segment of the anastomosis, dehiscence of a portion of the staple line used to create the gastric tube, or necrosis of the tip of the gastric tube. The latter complication may occur more frequently after a stapled anastomosis using the linear stapler technique than after a hand-sewn or end-to-end anastomosis.

Gastric tip necrosis results in a large volume leak and substantial loss of tissue. Healing of gastric tip necrosis by secondary intention is unlikely and increases the risk for catastrophic complications. Breakdown of the gastric tube can cause large mediastinal and pleural fluid collections, resulting in rapid clinical deterioration of the patient. Anastomotic leaks are usually relatively small and are successfully managed with drainage of the neck incision.

Differentiating among these causes is important in their management. If the neck wound is opened and only a small amount of drainage is evident, it is likely that a simple anastomotic leak exists. Larger volumes of drainage, unexplained potential spaces that have developed, and continued deterioration of the patient suggest a more ominous complication. Endoscopy and chest CT can help distinguish among these causes.

Case Continued

You open the incision at the bedside and probe the prevertebral region. A collection of saliva is released into the wound. The collection appears to track into the mediastinum. The wound is packed open. A CT scan of the chest is performed.

CT Scan

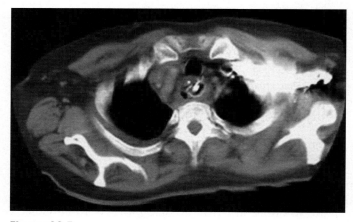

Figure 29-5

CT Scan Report

Small bilateral pleural effusions and right chest tube (not shown). Nasogastric tube in what appears to be a stomach pull-up in the posterior mediastinum. Small fluid collection adjacent to this structure in the upper mediastinum. ▨

Recommendation

Esophagoscopy and mediastinal drainage.

Case Continued

You perform flexible esophagoscopy in the operating room and identify the level of the anastomosis. The tissues appear viable. No anastomotic defect is evident, but a small amount of air bubbles appears out of the open neck incision. The neck incision is explored, and a collection of saliva is drained deep and inferior to the anastomosis. A flat suction drain is placed in the posterior mediastinum, and the wound is packed.

Chest X-ray

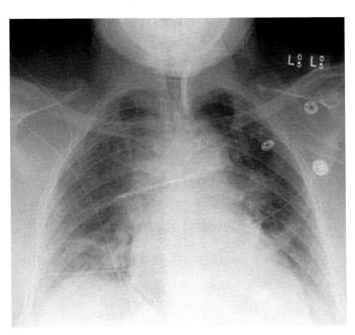

Figure 29-6

Chest X-ray Report

Indwelling mediastinal drain. The chest tube and nasogastric tube have been removed.

Case Continued

Drainage from the chest tube stops after 2 days and cultures of the fluid are negative. The chest tube is removed. Drainage from the cervical drain becomes negligible over a period of a week, after which the patient is started on sips of water, and no increase in drainage is noted. The drain is withdrawn, and the patient is discharged on a full liquid diet. After discharge, anastomotic dilation is necessary 4 weeks and 3 months after the operation.

Presentation

A 60-year-old woman presents to the emergency department and is admitted to the hospital with elevated temperature. She has been experiencing fatigue and myalgia for the past several days, but on the day of admission, she develops shaking chills and pleuritic chest pain.

Her past medical history is significant for a recent dental extraction of an abscessed tooth, hypertension, and diabetes. She is a long-time smoker of 40 pack-years. On physical examination, the patient appears toxic. Temperature is 104.3°F, pulse is 110 beats/min, and blood pressure is 100/60 mm Hg. She has no cervical adenopathy. Her extraction site appears to be healing, and there is no tenderness over this area. There are diminished breath sounds over the left hemithorax, and there is tenderness over her left chest.

Differential Diagnosis

The high temperature with chills this patient is experiencing is most likely of infectious etiology. Pneumonia, lung abscess, and empyema should be considered.

Case Continued

Blood cultures and laboratories are sent. The patient's white blood cell (WBC) count is 16,000/mm³. Broad-spectrum antibiotics and intravenous fluids are immediately begun. Chest x-rays are performed.

Chest X-rays

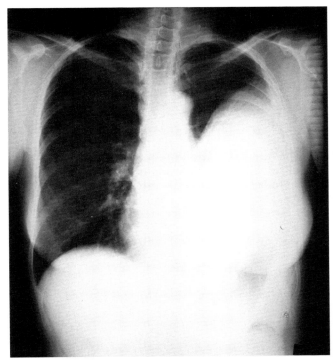

Figure 30-1

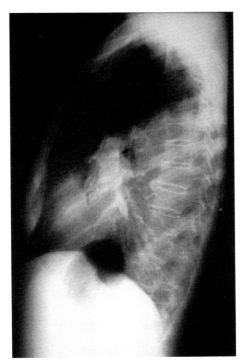

Figure 30-2

Chest X-ray Report

There is opacification of the lower two thirds of the left hemithorax. There are no masses or effusion in the left chest. The left heart border is not clearly defined.

CT Scans

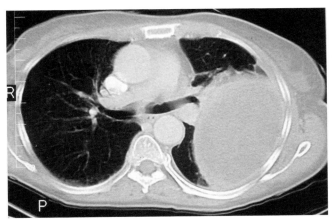

Figure 30-3

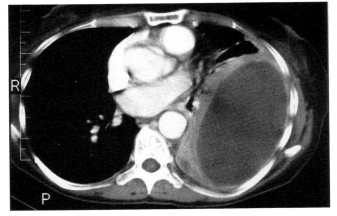

Figure 30-4

CT Scan Report

A homogenous fluid collection is noted compressing the left lower lobe. There is no air noted in the fluid or the soft tissues. There are no masses or effusion in the right thorax. ■

Case Continued

The patient had a chest tube placed into the collection on the left side at the bedside. More than 1,000 mL of foul-smelling, purulent material was removed. The Gram stain showed gram-positive rods, and the culture grew *Actinomyces meyeri*. The temperature returned to normal over the next 2 days.

Diagnosis

Empyema.

Discussion

An empyema is an infection within the pleural space. It most frequently results from a secondary infection of a reactive pleural fluid collection associated with a bacterial pneumonia (50%). Other causes of empyema include rupture of a lung abscess, generalized sepsis, posttraumatic, postsurgical, or resulting from extension of a subdiaphragmatic process. The infection here probably resulted from either a complicated pneumonic process associated with aspiration or direct hematogenous spread.

The development of a parapneumonic empyema is divided into the exudative, fibrinopurulent, and organizing phases. The exudative or acute phase is marked by the production of pleural fluid, which is reactive and initially noninfected. The pH is normal, and the lactate dehydrogenase (LDH) level is less than 1,000 IU/L. If the pneumonia is not appropriately treated, this fluid may become infected and progress to the fibrinopurulent or transitional phase. During this phase, there is accumulation of many WBCs and bacteria. Fibrin is deposited in an attempt to wall-off the process. Glucose and pH levels drop, and LDH level increases. Unless the process is interrupted, fibroblast proliferation and collagen deposition will become loculated, resulting in trapping of the underlying pulmonic tissue.

Clinical suspicion of an empyema should be considered when a patient's pneumonic symptoms fail to respond to appropriate antibiotic therapy. The symptoms of empyema vary from being asymptomatic to toxemic. Anaerobic infections tend to be slowly progressive, whereas aerobic infections worsen rapidly and may produce symptoms of fever, pain, and coughing. Suddenly, coughing up a large amount of purulent material signifies possible development of a bronchopleural fistula.

On physical examination, the patient will have decreased breath sounds over the fluid-filled space. There may be localized tenderness. In advanced stages, there may be crepitus in the soft tissues or drainage directly through the chest wall (empyema necessitatis). Initial evaluation is with chest x-rays but may also include decubitus views to determine whether the fluid is free flowing, indicating an earlier stage of empyema. Chest computed tomography (CT) is helpful in determining the presence of loculations and for placement of drainage catheters. Ultrasound provides similar information, but without much detail.

Thoracentesis can be used diagnostically and may be therapeutic if the empyema is in the exudative phase. An 18-gauge needle is placed into the cavity based on the location determined by CT or ultrasound. The specimen is sent for glucose, LDH, pH, protein, Gram stain, and culture. Antibiotics are adjusted based on sensitivities of the cultures. As many as 50% of the cultures will be negative if antibiotic therapy was initiated before the time that specimen cultures were obtained. Antibiotics should be continued until there is clinical resolution of the infection. Treatment of empyema must include adequate and dependent drainage. Repeat thoracentesis may be required to remove all of the fluid.

Chest tube drainage is required if the fluid is viscous or grossly purulent. The tube should be placed in the most dependent area of the cavity, and the tube is placed to suction. The chest tube is removed when there is minimal drainage and the lung has fully expanded without any remaining space. If a small space remains, the tube may be cut and converted to open drainage. After about 2 weeks of drainage, if a small space persists, the tube may then be converted to open drainage. Chest x-rays ensure that the lungs remain expanded, and the tube is slowly removed in weekly intervals.

Video-assisted thoracic surgery (VATS) is extremely useful and may be used as first-line therapy if there are multiple collections or loculations within the empyema. This requires that the patient is stable and can tolerate single-lung ventilation. Large fibrinous particles may be extracted through the port sites, and chest tubes can be positioned precisely. Limited débridement and decortication may also be performed.

With some success, fibrinolytic agents, such as streptokinase and urokinase, may be instilled through a chest tube to dissolve the fibrinous loculations. This therapy is conducted over a period of days by placing the fibrinolytic agent directly into the tube and allowing it to dwell for 8 hours while the tube is clamped.

Case Continued

A repeat chest x-ray and subsequent CT scan are obtained several days after chest tube placement.

Chest X-ray

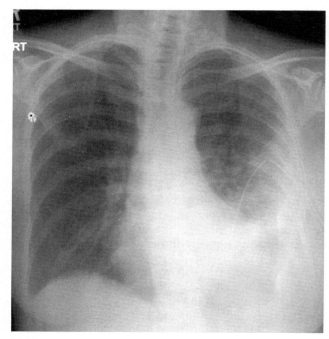

Figure 30-5

Chest X-ray Report

A left chest tube is noted. Compared with previous chest x-rays, there is less opacification in the left thorax, and the left heart border is more clearly delineated; however, the left lower lobe is not completely expanded. ■

CT Scans

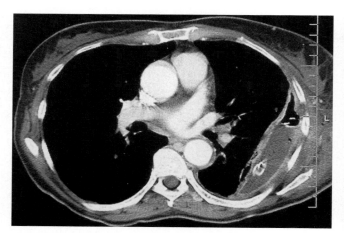

Figure 30-6

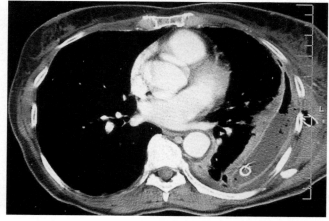

Figure 30-7

CT Scan Report

A focal, crescent-shaped fluid collection with an enhancing rind and pocket of gas is identified within the posterior lateral left chest, which extends from the level of the aortic arch through the dome of the diaphragm. A left thoracostomy tube is identified within this fluid collection, and the distal tip is located within the inferior portion of the fluid collection. Consolidation or atelectasis is noted within the adjacent left lung parenchyma. ■

Case Continued

Based on the incomplete resolution of infectious process in the left chest, the patient is taken to the operating room for a surgical intervention. Intraoperatively, a double-lumen endotracheal tube is positioned and an arterial line placed. The patient is placed in the right lateral decubitus position. The left chest is prepped, and a left posterolateral thoracotomy is performed through the sixth intercostal space. Dense fibrinous adhesions are encountered. The peel is decorticated from the visceral pleura, and large amounts of fibrinous debris are removed from the chest cavity. A partial pleurectomy of thickened and edematous pleura is performed as well. The lung is reexpanded, two chest tubes are positioned, and the chest is closed.

Discussion

Several therapeutic options are available for treatment of an infected fibrinous collection. Decortication is performed through a posterolateral thoracotomy. This offers the advantage of removing the infected, fibrinous material as well as freeing the trapped, defunctionalized lung. This, however, may be associated with significant morbidity and mortality in a debilitated patient. To be effective, the lung must be freed sufficiently to fill the thoracic cavity, with no space remaining. An empyemectomy is the *en bloc* removal of a mature empyema without opening the contaminated center. Thoracoplasty and muscle flap transposition are reserved for cases in which there is residual intrathoracic space remaining after more conservative treatments.

Alternatively, after allowing time for pleural fusion, the chest tube can be cut several centimeters from the skin surface. The open-tube drainage system can then be irrigated and slowly advanced over a period of several weeks while the inside of the cavity is allowed to granulate.

case 3

Presentation

A 51-year-old woman is referred to your office for cough and hemoptysis. Upon questioning, she admits to having noted blood in the sputum for the past 6 months. She denies any weight loss but notes progressive weakness. The patient denies any history of smoking.

She had no other medical problems until 2 years ago when she was found to have asthma, recurrent bronchitis, and hypertension. Past medical history includes a cholecystectomy. Her medications include ipratropium bromide (Atrovent), enalapril maleate (Vasotec), and potassium supplements.

Vital signs include a systolic blood pressure of 140/90 mm Hg, normal sinus rhythm at 70 beats/min, and a respiratory rate of 20 breaths/min. On physical examination, you note wheezing on inspiration. The heart sounds are normal, and there are no murmurs. Abdominal examination demonstrates a soft, nontender, nondistended abdomen with a thick scar. The patient reports having had healing problems after undergoing a cholecystectomy.

■ Chest X-rays

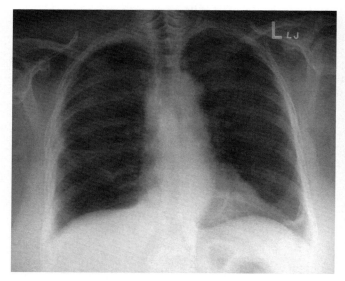

Figure 31-1

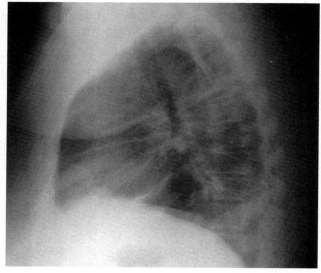

Figure 31-2

Chest X-ray Report

Normal chest x-rays. ▦

Differential Diagnosis

The main causes of hemoptysis in a patient with a normal coagulation profile include inflammatory, pulmonary, and cardiac etiologies. Inflammatory causes include bronchitis, which is the most common cause of hemoptysis. Other causes include bronchiectasis, lung abscess, and infectious etiologies, such as tuberculosis and histoplasmosis. Pulmonary causes include primary lung cancer, bronchial neoplasms, lung contusion, and trauma by a foreign body. Finally, cardiac causes of hemoptysis include mitral stenosis and acute mitral regurgitation.

Discussion

In this patient, who is a nonsmoker, a primary lung cancer is less likely. However, the weakness, hypertension, hypokalemia, and physical examination findings are suggestive of a paraneoplastic syndrome. Given the recent diagnosis of asthma and bronchitis, the diagnosis of an endoluminal neoplasm should be strongly considered.

Recommendation

Laboratory evaluation of electrolytes and computed tomography (CT) scans of the chest.

Test Results

Sodium, 152; potassium, 3.2; chloride, 92; bicarbonate, 28. ▦

▦ CT Scans

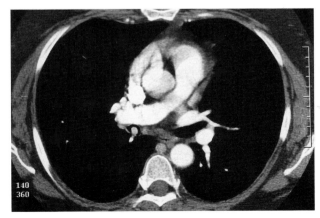

Figure 31-3

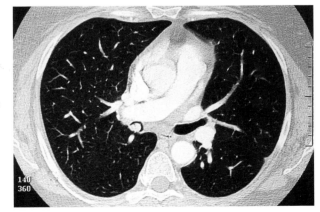

Figure 31-4

CT Scan Report

An endoluminal lesion with contrast enhancement is noted in the bronchus intermedius. There is no significant distal bronchiectasis or other postobstructive change. ■

Discussion

The electrolyte levels are suggestive of hypercortisolism. The sources include pituitary or adrenal pathology as well as steroid secretion as part of a paraneoplastic syndrome. In this case, in which an abnormal mass is demonstrated on the CT scans, paraneoplastic syndrome is highly probable.

With regard to the radiologic evaluation, chest x-rays often fail to detect an intraluminal abnormality, especially when there are minimal or no distal airway obstructive changes. However, CT scanning is more sensitive at demonstrating the neoplasm as well as defining the extent of parenchymal involvement. Presence of calcifications suggests the diagnosis of carcinoid tumor in 30% of cases, and evidence of contrast enhancement further implicates carcinoid. In addition, CT scan aids in assessing distal bronchiectasis and mediastinal lymph nodes.

Recommendation

Bronchoscopy should be performed to evaluate the location and extent of the tumor, as well as to obtain tissue diagnosis of the endobronchial lesion, which was demonstrated on the CT scan.

▨ Flexible Bronchoscopy

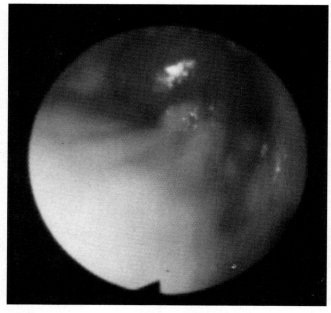

Figure 31-5   See Color Plate 13 on page 114.

Flexible Bronchoscopy Report

Bronchoscopic evaluation of the trachea and left tracheobronchial tree reveals no abnormalities. The carina is sharp and in the midline. The right upper lobe orifice is normal. Immediately beyond it, however, a polypoid tumor is noted. It is attached by a stalk to the lateral wall of the bronchus intermedius and is freely mobile in the lumen. The bronchoscope was passed beyond the tumor to the right middle and lower lobe segmental bronchi, which are found to be normal.

Biopsies of the tumor are obtained, which reveal typical carcinoid.

Discussion

Carcinoids represent 0.5% to 1.0% of all tracheobronchial tumors and are of typical and atypical varieties. They affect men and women in a wide range of ages, with a median age of 55 years.

The presenting symptoms depend on the location of the lesion. The more peripheral tumors are usually asymptomatic, whereas more centrally located lesions produce luminal obstruction leading to cough, wheezing, infection, and hemoptysis. Because these tumors are slow growing, symptoms may be present for extended periods of time before diagnosis is made.

Paraneoplastic syndromes are seen in 1% to 2% of patients with carcinoid tumors. Carcinoid syndrome, which includes bronchospasm, flushing, and chronic diarrhea, is the most common paraneoplastic syndrome and is usually associated with large lesions or liver metastases. Cardiac valvular problems may occur but affect the left-sided valves, unlike the right-sided abnormalities seen in patients with hepatic and gastrointestinal carcinoid disease. Cushing's syndrome can also be seen in these patients and is associated with lymph node metastases in 50%.

The diagnosis is generally made with a combination of radiographic studies and flexible bronchoscopy. Biopsies taken during bronchoscopy can lead to bleeding because deep samples are needed to assess these submucosal lesions accurately. Dilute epinephrine solution is generally sufficient to achieve hemostasis if bleeding is present after bronchoscopic biopsy. Fine-needle aspirate for peripheral lesions can be employed, but is not usually accurate, because carcinoid can appear pathologically similar to small cell cancer. Serum or urine studies tend to be helpful only when the carcinoid syndrome is present.

Typical carcinoids are usually central in location and tend to be single lesions that look soft and reddish-pink on bronchoscopy. They are occasionally pedunculated, and their site of origin can be from a stalk distal to the location of the tumor. Atypical carcinoids are located peripherally in half the cases and can be difficult to distinguish from small cell histology. They present in older patients and often spread to lymph nodes or distant sites. Oncocytic, clear cell, and melanocytic carcinoid variants can also be seen.

Recommendation

Because there is no radiographic evidence of metastatic disease, resection should be undertaken.

Discussion

Because these tumors usually invade locally, a conservative resection with preservation of lung tissue should always be considered.

Endoscopic resection was historically performed but should now be reserved for patients who are not operative candidates and patients who refuse open resection. The role of photodynamic therapy and other laser therapies in this situation is still being investigated.

The surgical approach should employ standard double-lumen intubation and should include octreotide if the patient had carcinoid syndrome, thereby avoiding intraoperative crisis during manipulation of the tumor. An assessment of the regional lymph nodes should be done first and biopsy samples sent for frozen-section analysis. If nodal disease is present, a formal cancer operation with mediastinal lymphadenectomy is indicated. If there is no spread to regional lymph nodes, a variety of local resections can be performed, depending on the location, extent, and size of the primary tumor. Options include bronchotomy and full-thickness excision of the mass, although this is rarely applicable. Anatomic segmentectomy is preferred for peripheral lesions. Lobectomy is done frequently because lesions are often near the origin of a lobar bronchus. Sleeve bronchial resection is an excellent option for preserving lung parenchyma. Pneumonectomy is rarely required.

Case Continued

The patient undergoes a right thoracotomy and sleeve resection of the lesion in the bronchus intermedius. A complete mediastinal lymphadenectomy is performed. The procedure is uncomplicated. Final pathology (see figure) reveals a completely resected typical carcinoid without any lymph node metastasis.

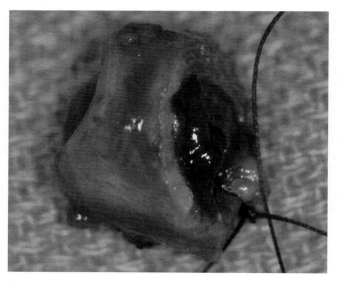

Figure 31-6   See Color Plate 14 on page 114.

The patient remains stable overnight, but the next day, a new and significant air leak is present.

Recommendation

Chest x-ray and bronchoscopy.

Discussion

A new postoperative air leak after a sleeve resection raises concerns of anastomotic complications, such as superficial necrosis, fistula, or complete dehiscence. The overall condition of the patient provides some clue to the extent of the problem. Bronchoscopy should be performed to assess the degree of necrosis or dehiscence. Superficial mucosal sloughing or small fistulas may heal with time; however, more extensive involvement or frank disruption should be treated with immediate salvage reoperation.

In this case, there was no evidence of pneumothorax on the chest x-ray. Bronchoscopy demonstrates some superficial sloughing with a small fistula.

Recommendation

Continued nonsurgical management with periodic bronchoscopic evaluation is sufficient.

Because on final pathology there was no evidence of metastatic disease, adjunctive therapy is not required.

Discussion

Carcinoids are not sensitive to radiation. However, some patients with incompletely resected lesions may benefit from radiation treatment. Chemotherapy (cisplatin and etoposide) can be considered for metastatic disease.

The prognosis depends on the aggressiveness of the primary tumor. For typical carcinoids, resection is curative, and prognosis is excellent, with a 5-year survival rate of 95%; if lymph node involvement is present, the 5-year survival rate is reduced to 70%. Patients with atypical carcinoids have a 5-year survival rate of about 60%; these tumors usually recur with distant metastases.

case ◼ 32

Presentation

A 25-year-old man is referred to you after an employment-screening chest x-ray reveals an abnormal finding. He is a recent college graduate previously employed as a waiter. He has no past medical or surgical history, has not traveled outside the United States, and denies any history of smoking. He does not have symptoms of weight loss, fever, chills, or night sweats. His vital signs are normal, and his physical examination is unremarkable.

◼ Chest X-rays

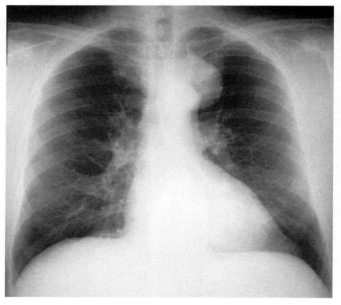

Figure 32-1

Figure 32-2

Chest X-ray Report

There is a posterior, paravertebral, round mass. The anterior mediastinum is not enlarged, and there are no other masses or pleural effusions.

Discussion

The patient has a recently discovered, asymptomatic, isolated, posterior mediastinal mass. Tumors most commonly found in the posterior mediastinum are those of neurogenic origin. Benign neurogenic tumors include schwannoma (neurilemmoma), neurofibroma, ganglioneuroma, chemodectoma, and pheochromocytoma. Neurofibrosarcoma, ganglioneuroblastoma, neuroblastoma, malignant chemodectoma, and malignant pheochromocytoma are the most common malignant neurogenic tumors. The neuroblastomas are very aggressive malignant tumors that usually present in early childhood and infancy; adult cases are rare. Most extraadrenal pheochromocytomas arise from the aortic body and are found in the retroperitoneum. Both chemodectomas and pheochromocytomas arise from paraganglionic tissue; however, chemodectomas are hormonally inactive. Hypertension associated with increased catecholamine metabolites in the urine is helpful in establishing the diagnosis of pheochromocytomas. Posterior mediastinal tumors may extend intraspinally or invade adjacent structures. Computed tomography (CT) is crucial in anatomic localization of the tumor and also in planning a diagnostic and therapeutic approach.

▨ CT Scans

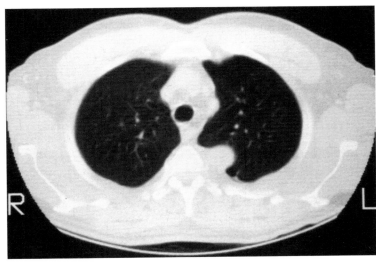

Figure 32-3

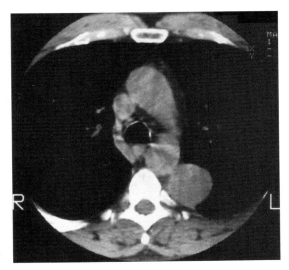

Figure 32-4

CT Scan Report

The CT scans of the chest demonstrate a 4-cm homogeneous mass in the left paravertebral sulcus. It approximates, but does not invade, the head of the rib or the transverse process of the vertebral body and does not extend to the intervertebral foramen. There is no mediastinal adenopathy, pleural effusions, or other masses. ▨

Discussion

Posterior mediastinal masses may be malignant or benign. The presence of pain may indicate tumor invasion of the chest wall or neural foramina. Benign tumors may arise from the nerve sheath (schwannoma and neurofibroma), sympathetic ganglia (ganglioneuroma), and paraganglion system (pheochromocytoma and chemodectoma). Pheochromocytomas have chromaffin-secreting cells, whereas paragangliomas have non–chromaffin-secreting cells. Tumor extension into the intervertebral foramen (dumbbell tumor) occurs in about 10% of neurogenic tumors. Although CT scan is the initial investigative test, magnetic resonance imaging (MRI) provides more accurate assessment of tumor extension to the intervertebral foramen. MRI should be obtained in patients with posterior mediastinal masses along the costovertebral sulcus and in patients with neurologic symptoms and CT scan findings suggestive of possible extension of the tumor to the intervertebral foramina.

Schwannomas and neurofibromas share common sites of origin, but neurofibromas tend to occur in younger patients (20 to 40 years of age), are often multiple, and may be associated with von Recklinghausen's disease. Von Recklinghausen's disease is an autosomal dominant disease with skin manifestation (café au lait spots) and multiple tumors. However, brain and spinal cord tumors are more common than thoracic tumors. Although most thoracic tumors in patients with von Recklinghausen's disease are neurofibromas, some may be schwannomas or a mixture of neurofibromas and schwannomas.

Vertebral sulcus tumors may be divided into two groups on the basis of CT and MRI findings: those that are purely intrathoracic (90%), as in this case, and those that invade the intervertebral foramina (10%). Patients in the latter group present with neurologic signs or symptoms in 60% of cases.

Percutaneous core biopsy is more useful than fine-needle aspiration biopsy in establishing the diagnosis, but because surgical resection is usually indicated, neither fine-needle aspiration biopsy nor core biopsy is usually recommended.

Recommendation

This is a single lesion of uncomplicated nature in the paravertebral sulcus of a healthy young man. The need for percutaneous biopsy has been excluded, and preoperative workup is in order. Surgical resection is recommended.

Case Continued

The patient is taken to the operating room. Under general anesthesia with double-lumen endotracheal intubation, a left posterolateral thoracotomy is performed. The chest is entered through the fourth intercostal space, and the tumor is found to be in close proximity to the nerve sheath. After careful dissection, the tumor is completely resected. A single 28-French chest tube is placed, and the patient is transferred to the recovery room extubated. The tumor measured 4 cm × 6 cm × 3.5 cm. The final histopathology is neurofibroma.

On the first postoperative day, the patient complains of a severe headache. The chest tube is draining 300 mL of clear fluid per shift. A chest x-ray demonstrates a small right-sided pleural effusion.

Recommendation

CT myelogram and neurosurgical consultation.

Discussion

Cerebrospinal fluid (CSF) leak to the pleural space is a rare complication of thoracic procedures. Patients usually complain of headaches but may have other neurologic symptoms, such as lethargy and mental status changes. The chest tube output is clear and cannot be differentiated from transudate based on chemical analysis. When clinical symptoms suggest a CSF leak, a CT myelogram should be obtained to confirm the diagnosis. Initial management of CSF leak is nonoperative. The patient is maintained on bed rest, and the chest tube is placed on water seal rather than on suction. The normal intrathoracic pressure is about -5 cm H_2O, whereas the pressure of the CSF is +10 cm H_2O. This pressure differential can be further exacerbated by the chest tube suction. The neurosurgical team may suggest placement of a lumbar drain. If nonoperative management fails, surgical treatment includes nerve root ligation or laminectomy and placement of an intradural or extradural patch.

Case Continued

The patient is maintained on bed rest, and the chest tube is placed to water seal. The CSF drainage decreases on the second and third postoperative days and stops on the fourth postoperative day. The chest tube is removed, and the patient recovers uneventfully.

Discussion

Neurofibromas, unlike schwannomas, which are almost entirely made up of Schwann's cells, have equal proportions of Schwann's cells and perineural cells. Single lesions tend to be asymptomatic and have a very favorable prognosis because recurrence after excision is rare. Patients with multiple lesions and those with lesions in association with von Recklinghausen's disease have a higher chance of developing malignant degeneration. Five-year survival rates with resection of neurofibrosarcoma are significantly lower in patients with neurofibromatosis than in patients without neurofibromatosis. Local recurrence or distant metastases may be seen 5 to 10 years after treatment.

Posterior mediastinal tumors may also be resected thoracoscopically. In this approach, three ports are used. One port is placed in the anterior axillary line at the fourth to fifth intercostal space; this port is used to retract the lung. Another port is placed posteriorly at the fourth intercostal space; and finally, the thoracoscope is introduced through a port in the seventh intercostal space, at the midaxillary line. With the lung deflated and retracted inferiorly, the adhesions are taken down, the mediastinal pleura is incised, and the mass is gently dissected away. The involved intercostal nerve is clipped and ligated and resected with the specimen. Care must be taken in dissecting the mass in the vicinity of the stellate ganglion because traction on this may result in a transient postoperative ptosis. The mass is placed in a pouch and removed through one of the enlarged intercostal space ports.

For intrathoracic tumors with intervertebral extension, the spinal component should be exposed first through a separate paravertebral incision, followed by laminectomy and an intraspinal dissection. A lateral thoracotomy to excise the remaining tumor is then performed. Alternatively, a combined approach can be undertaken in which a posterior thoracotomy with a vertical paravertebral extension is performed; this approach allows both operations to be completed through a single incision. The spinal laminectomy should be performed before intrathoracic manipulation of the tumor.

case ■ 33

Presentation

A 62-year-old Vietnam War veteran presents to the emergency department with complaints of acute shortness of breath. Over several months, he has had a productive cough, occasionally blood streaked, and left-sided pleuritic chest pain. He reports a decrease in his exercise tolerance as well as a 15-pound weight loss. He has a 36-pack-per-year history of smoking and drinks two or three cans of beer daily. On physical examination, vital signs are stable, temperature is 98.8°F, and oxygen saturation is 91%. Breath sounds are diminished in the left lower chest. The rest of the examination is unremarkable. In the emergency department, the following chest x-ray is obtained.

■ Chest X-ray

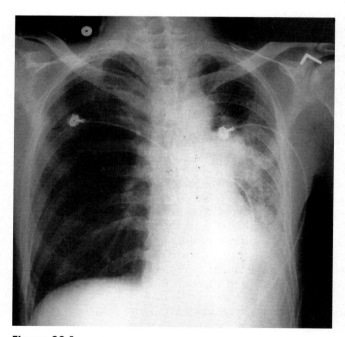

Figure 33-1

Chest X-ray Report

There is loss of volume of the left lung with compensatory shift of the mediastinum toward the left. The left hilum is enlarged, and there is an infiltrate at the left lung base. The right lung is hyperinflated. A fracture is present in the axillary portion of the third rib in the right chest.

Case Continued

The patient was admitted for antibiotic treatment, nutritional support, and further clinical assessment. During the hospital course, the patient was more dyspneic and hypoxic (saturation 83% on room air) requiring supplemental oxygen. The following chest x-ray was obtained on the second hospital day.

Chest X-ray

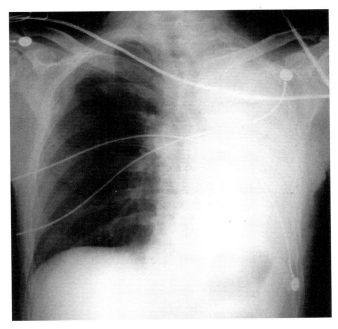

Figure 33-2

Chest X-ray Report

There is now total opacification of the left lung. This finding is compatible with atelectasis of the left lung, with a mediastinal shift to the left. The right lung is hyperinflated but clear of infiltrates.

Recommendation

A bronchoscopy to evaluate for endobronchial lesions as well as to obtain a tissue sample for diagnosis. In addition, computed tomography (CT) scans may identify an endobronchial lesion and other disease processes that may cause bronchial obstruction.

CT Scans

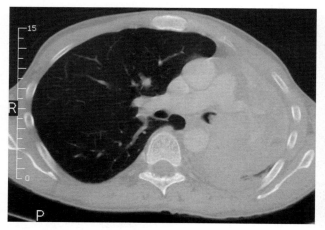

Figure 33-3

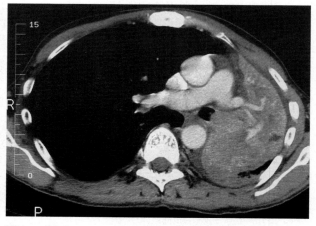

Figure 33-4

CT Scan Report

Most of the left lung is atelectatic, which is consistent with obstructive pneumonitis. An endobronchial mass obstructing the distal left main-stem bronchus is demonstrated. There is no mediastinal adenopathy. There is a small left pleural effusion. The right hilum and lung are unremarkable.

Differential Diagnosis

Bronchogenic carcinoma is highly considered in a smoker with blood-streaked sputum and an endobronchial lesion. Other possibilities include small cell carcinoma and bronchial carcinoid with parenchymal involvement. Obstructive pneumonitis is an indicator of advanced disease.

Case Continued

Bronchoscopy was performed, and a large polypoid mass was encountered more than 2 cm distal to the carina. This tumor obstructed the left main-stem bronchus. A biopsy demonstrated a squamous cell carcinoma. A metastatic workup was performed to determine resectability of this lesion. An MRI of the brain was negative. Liver function tests were normal. Bone scan was performed that showed an area of focal increased uptake of isotope in the axillary portion of the right third rib.

Bone Scan

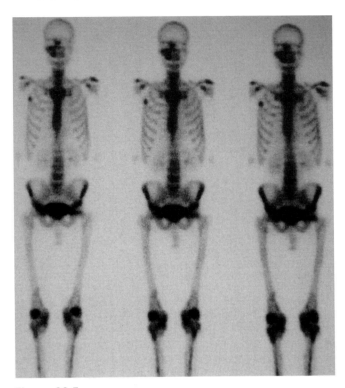

Figure 33-5

Discussion

The central location of this tumor suggests that this patient may require a pneumonectomy. Morbidity and mortality with pneumonectomy is of concern; therefore, one must carefully assess for distant metastatic disease as well as the patient's ability to withstand the operation. The surgeon must assess, based on bronchoscopic findings and radiologic evaluation, whether the lesion can be technically resected and whether the patient can tolerate surgery without major cardiac or pulmonary insult.

Case Continued

Evaluation of additional CT scan images shows the mass impinging on the inferior pulmonary veins, and pneumonectomy may require ligating the pulmonary veins intrapericardially. Cytologic examination of the pleural fluid is negative for malignancy and is most likely the result of obstructive pneumonitis. Pulmonary function tests show a forced expiratory volume in 1 second (FEV_1) of 1.82 L (58% predicted), forced vital capacity (FVC) of 2.53 L (64% predicted), maximum voluntary ventilation (MVV) of 61 L/min (40% predicted), and diffusing capacity of lung for carbon monoxide (D_{LCO}) of 14.8 mL per minute per mm Hg (70% predicted).

Split functions are not performed because the patient is physiologically using only the right lung, and despite blood shunting through the left pulmonary artery, the patient is comfortable with 2 L per minute of supplementary oxygen through nasal cannula. A stress test is negative, and the patient does not require coronary angiography in the preoperative assessment.

Recommendation

This patient requires a pneumonectomy if the right third rib lesion is benign. If the rib lesion is a metastatic implant, the disease will be categorized as stage IV lung cancer, and the patient will be offered palliative chemotherapy and radiation therapy without surgery. Although the rib lesion may be an area of a healing fracture, to determine resectability, a rib biopsy should be performed before embarking on a pneumonectomy.

Case Continued

A bone scan–guided localization of the rib lesion is obtained. A needle is inserted into the rib under scanning guidance, and the lesion is injected with a small amount of methylene blue dye. Intraoperatively, the patient is placed in a supine position with a sandbag under the right shoulder. The arms are suspended over the head to expose the axilla. Using the methylene blue stain as a guide, a small incision is made, and the abnormal segment of the third rib is clearly identified by the dye stain. Subperiosteal excision of the lesion is carried out, and the specimen is sent to pathology for decalcification. The microscopic diagnosis is osteoclastic callus formation with no evidence of malignancy.

The patient is prepared for a thoracotomy. He has a histologic diagnosis of malignancy based on the bronchoscopic biopsy of the endobronchial mass. Clinical staging shows no evidence of metastatic disease, and preoperative physiologic evaluation demonstrates that the patient was a candidate for pneumonectomy. Intraoperatively, an epidural catheter is placed for postoperative pain control. An arterial line is inserted for intraoperative and postoperative blood gas monitoring, and venous access lines are properly positioned. A right-sided double-lumen endobronchial tube is used for intubation, and placement is confirmed bronchoscopically. After positioning in a right lateral decubitus position, the patient is prepped and draped, and a lateral thoracotomy is performed. The latissimus dorsi muscle is dissected sufficiently to enable posterior retraction, the serratus anterior muscle is separated, and the chest is entered through the fifth intercostal space. The left lung is atelectatic, and a central mass is palpated. There is no evidence of intrapleural metastatic disease or other masses identified in either lobe. Palpation of the hilar structures reveals the tumor mass to involve the inferior pulmonary vein and extend to the pericardium at this level. This finding indicates that an intrapericardial pneumonectomy will be required. The inferior pulmonary ligament is then transected, and the posterior mediastinal pleura is opened along the esophagus and posterior hilum. The pericardium is then opened anteriorly between the phrenic nerve and the hilum, and palpation of the atrium reveals that the tumor mass does not extend into the atrium and that resection will be possible. The pericardium is then opened to the origin of the left main pulmonary artery, and it is freed by sharp scissor dissection. The distal main pulmonary artery is ligated with a large silk tie, and the proximal artery is stapled with a vascular stapler and transected. The superior pulmonary vein is then stapled proximally and distally inside the pericardium and transected. It is necessary to staple a small portion of the atrium to achieve a satisfactory margin of resection of the inferior pulmonary vein. There is no back bleeding because the vein is totally obstructed by tumor. The left main-stem bronchus is dissected to the level of the tracheo-bronchial angle and the carina, and level 7 lymphadenectomy is accomplished. The bronchus is then stapled and transected with a 4.8-mm leg-length stapler, and the lung is removed. The bronchial margin is free of microscopic disease on frozen-section study. Level 5 and 6 lymph nodes are removed for pathologic analysis with careful and meticulous preservation of the recurrent laryngeal nerve. The chest cavity is filled with saline, and the bronchial stump is tested for air leak at 30 cm of inflation pressure by the anesthesiologist. The bronchial stump is then covered with a pericardial patch, and the pericardial edges are reapproximated to close the defect partially. A single chest tube is left in place for proper mediastinal positioning.

The patient is extubated in the operating room, and the chest tube is connected to a water-seal chamber with the suction tubing removed. A postoperative chest x-ray shows the mediastinum to be in the midline, and the chest tube is clamped. Recovery is facilitated by control of thoracotomy incisional pain, careful fluid management, pulmonary supportive care, and early mobilization. The chest tube is removed in 24 hours, and the patient is ambulating. The patient requires supplemental oxygen by nasal cannula for several weeks postoperatively, but this is eventually weaned off.

▌Chest X-rays

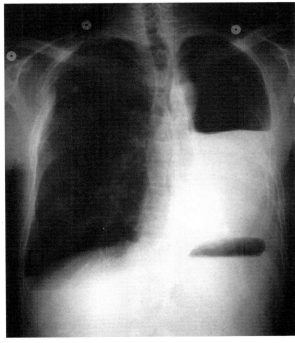

Figure 33-6

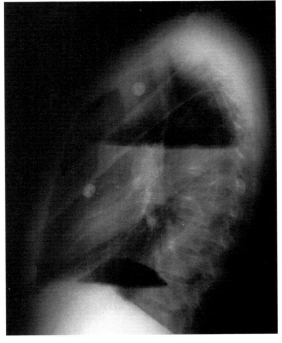

Figure 33-7

Chest X-ray Report

Post left pneumonectomy x-ray shows accumulation of fluid within the left thoracic cavity. There is shift of the mediastinum to the left and elevation of the left hemidiaphragm. ▓

Final Pathology

The final pathologic report is squamous cell carcinoma arising in the main-stem bronchus and extending into the upper lobe bronchus. The surgical-pathologic staging is stage IIIA (T3 N1 M0). The tumor is T3 because of extension to the mediastinal pleura. All resection margins are free of microscopic cancer. Postoperative adjuvant therapy is not administered to this patient.

Presentation

A 51-year-old man is admitted to the emergency department with a 2-month history of worsening episodes of dysphagia. He complains of retrosternal discomfort soon after ingesting solid food that lasts about 10 minutes. He has lost 10 pounds in the past 2 months. He is a nonsmoker but drinks one or two bottles of beer per day. On physical examination, the patient is somewhat cachectic, and his vital signs are stable. He has the following admission chest x-rays and esophagogram.

▨ Chest X-rays

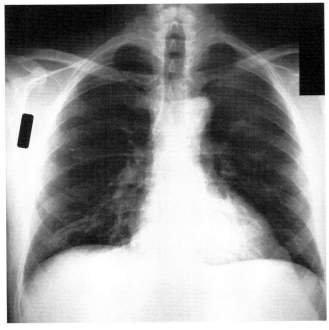

Figure 34-1

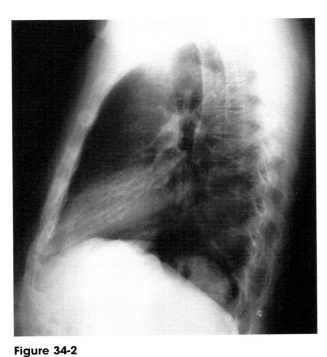

Figure 34-2

Chest X-ray Report

There are no lung masses. The heart is normal in size. There are no pleural effusions. ▨

Esophagogram

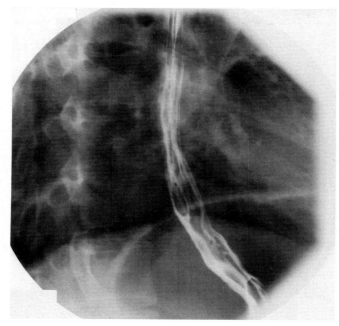

Figure 34-3

Esophagogram Report

There is free flow of contrast material through the esophagus to the stomach without evidence of a stricture, extrinsic compression, mass lesion, or mucosal irregularities.

Case Continued

The patient is discharged from the emergency department with instructions to follow up with his primary physician. After several weeks, the patient continues to complain of dysphagia. Based on the clinical symptoms, his physician suspects a motility abnormality and refers the patient to a gastroenterologist for an esophagoscopic study.

Esophagoscopies

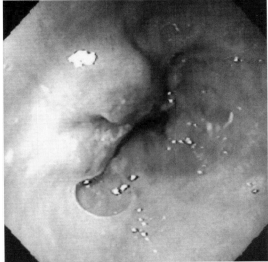
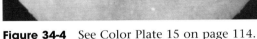
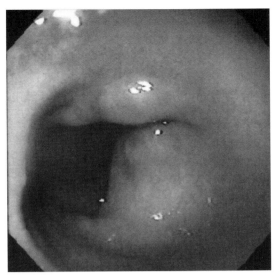

Figure 34-4 See Color Plate 15 on page 114.   **Figure 34-5** See Color Plate 16 on page 114.

Esophagoscopy Results

The gastroenterologist identifies a mucosal mass with an ulcerated surface, which starts at 36 cm and extends to 39 cm. Biopsy results reveal a moderately differentiated adenocarcinoma at the squamocardiac junction.

Discussion

The incidence of adenocarcinoma of the esophagus has been rising in the United States in the past two decades. It now surpasses squamous cell carcinoma, constituting 48% to 70% of all esophageal cancers. Most patients are males (male-to-female ratio of 6:1) in their seventh decade of life. Moreover, patients with Barrett's esophagus have a 40-fold increased risk for developing adenocarcinoma compared with the general population, and the risk persists even after corrective surgery for reflux disease. The incidence of adenocarcinoma is higher in whites than in blacks, which is the opposite relation from squamous carcinoma of the esophagus. Smoking and alcohol are other major risk factors in the development of adenocarcinoma of the esophagus. In comparison with squamous carcinoma, adenocarcinoma typically occurs in the lower one third of the esophagus. Exposure of the lower third of the esophagus to acidic gastric content may be a reason for the propensity of the lower third of the esophagus to be more susceptible to adenocarcinoma than to squamous carcinoma.

After the diagnosis is established by endoscopic biopsy, the next step is staging. Stage I (T1 N0 M0) is tumor limited to the mucosa and submucosa. Stage IIA (T2-3 N0 M0) denotes invasion of muscular wall and adventitia, and stage IIB (T1-2 N1 M0) indicates locoregional lymph node involvement. Regional lymph node metastasis, combined with invasion through the esophageal wall with or without involvement of local structures, is stage III (T3 N1 or T4 N0-1). Stage IV is distant metastasis (stage IVA indicates celiac lymph node metastasis in lower esophageal tumors and cervical lymph node involvement in upper thoracic esophageal tumors; IVB is any distant disease).

As in this case, an esophagogram is not sensitive in diagnosing early tumors. A high index of suspicion based on clinical symptoms and risk factors should prompt further evaluation. Although computed tomography (CT) scan is accurate in determining the size of the tumor and extension of the disease to the liver and adrenal glands, it is less reliable in identifying local invasion. Endoscopic ultrasonography is more sensitive than CT scan in evaluating the depth of invasion and lymph node extension. Although PET scanning may be useful in evaluating for metastatic disease, this test is not as sensitive for lymph node involvement. Sensitive and specific preoperative staging is important when the benefit of induction therapy becomes clear. Several studies are evaluating the benefit of cisplatin-based neoadjuvant chemotherapy in patients with esophageal cancer.

Recommendation

A thorough physical examination with careful evaluation of the supraclavicular lymph nodes. Also, to evaluate further the size of the tumor and lymph node involvement, a CT scan of the chest and an endoscopic ultrasound (EUS) study should be obtained.

Chest CT and EUS Report

There is prominence at the gastroesophageal junction measuring 2.1 cm. The esophagus proximal to the lesion is not distended. There is no hilar or mediastinal adenopathy. EUS shows the tumor extending through all layers of the esophagus, and regional lymph node enlargement is not detected. ▪

Surgical Approach

Based on the CT scan and EUS studies, this patient has clinical stage IIA disease. The treatment of choice is a surgical resection. Although several approaches may be appropriate for esophageal resection, for distal third tumors, a transhiatal esophagectomy can be performed with a mortality rate of 5%. The short gastric arteries are ligated, and the stomach is mobilized into the neck where an anastomosis (stapled or hand-sewn) is performed. Small mid-esophageal tumors are also amenable to a transhiatal approach, but large, bulky tumors may require thoracotomy, laparotomy, and cervical anastomosis. For mid-esophageal tumors, a left thoracotomy is performed, and the anastomosis is performed in the chest. For upper third esophageal tumors, a right thoracotomy and an abdominal incision are performed (Ivor Lewis procedure), and the anastomosis can be performed in the chest or in the neck with additional cervical exposure.

Case Continued

A midline abdominal incision is used to access the pathology. A 2-cm mass is palpable at the gastroesophageal junction. There is no gross invasion of the surrounding tissues. After a pyloroplasty is performed, the stomach is mobilized and brought up to the neck through a transhiatal approach. A stapled anastomosis is performed in the neck, the skin is closed, and the wound is drained with a Penrose drain. A nasogastric tube is placed in the stomach. A jejunostomy feeding tube is placed for postoperative nutritional support.

■ Specimen

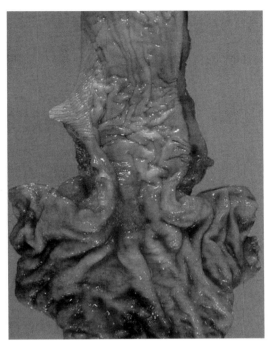

Figure 34-6   See Color Plate 17 on page 114.

Pathology Findings

Moderately differentiated adenocarcinoma of the gastroesophageal junction extending through the entire wall with no extension of the disease to regional lymph nodes. Surgical margins are free of tumor. ■

Final Pathologic Diagnosis

Esophageal adenocarcinoma stage IIA (T3 N0).

Case Continued

Enteral feeding is started on the second postoperative day through the jejunostomy tube. On the fourth postoperative day, the patient is noted to have serous drainage from the neck incision. A contrast swallow is performed.

▨ Postoperative Esophagogram

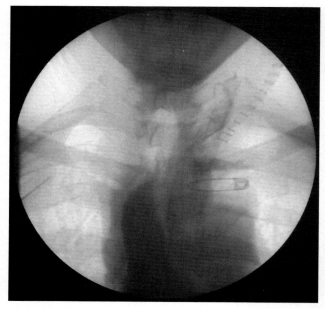

Figure 34-7

Esophagogram Report

There is flow of contrast to the stomach, and a small amount of contrast is extravasating and exiting the wound. ▨

▨ Approach

The patient has an anastomotic leak. Adequate drainage of the wound is maintained, and the patient is not allowed oral feeding. Enteral feeding is provided through the jejunostomy tube. Oral alimentation is begun when the drainage is minimal, which usually occurs after 5 to 10 days.

Discussion

Anastomotic leak occurs in about 5% to 10% of cases, usually between the second and seventh postoperative day. Surgical technique and diminished blood supply are factors attributed to anastomotic leaks. Most patients with cervical anastomosis can be treated conservatively with local wound care and cessation of oral intake. Healing may result in anastomotic stricture, which may necessitate future dilation. In contrast, intrathoracic anastomotic leak is much more devastating and often requires reoperation for anastomotic takedown and cervical esophagectomy. The mortality rate from intrathoracic leak may be as high as 50%. Prompt diagnosis and reoperation are necessary to prevent extension of mediastinitis.

Presentation

A 65-year-old man presents to the emergency department in moderate distress. The patient reports dyspnea on exertion and blood-streaked sputum for past 4 months. He now presents with an acute exacerbation, which began several hours before the emergency department admission. The patient was diagnosed with advanced non–small cell lung cancer 8 months ago, for which he received two cycles of chemotherapy. On physical examination, vital signs are stable, but room air saturations are 78%. On auscultation, there are decreased breath sounds over the left chest. The trachea is midline. The patient is treated initially with 100% oxygen, and full panel laboratory tests, an electrocardiogram, and the following chest x-rays are obtained.

Chest X-rays

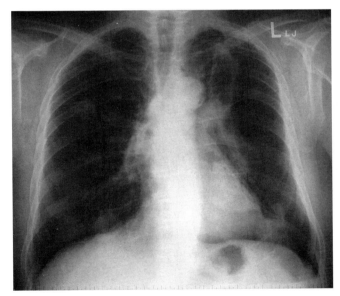

Figure 35-1

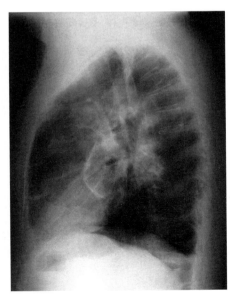

Figure 35-2

Chest X-ray Report

A large, left-sided pneumothorax is present with partial atelectasis of the left lung. There are several nodules in the right lung field. The left costophrenic angle is blunted. The heart size is not enlarged. ▨

Case Continued

A left-sided tube thoracostomy is placed in the emergency department with marked clinical improvement; however, repeat chest x-ray demonstrates a partially expanded left lung. The patient is admitted to the hospital, and the tube thoracostomy is placed on suction. Chest x-ray on the second hospital day shows nonexpansion of the lung and no air leak.

Recommendation

Failure of the lung to expand may be from either a large bronchopleural fistula with persistent air leak or airway obstruction by tumor, leading to atelectasis of a lobe or segment of the left lung. Computed tomography (CT) scans and bronchoscopy are necessary for further diagnosis and treatment planning.

▨ CT Scans

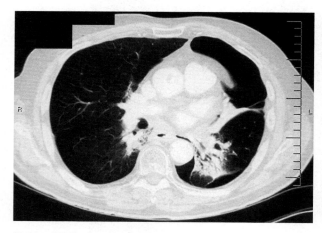 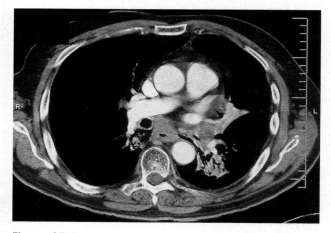

Figure 35-3   **Figure 35-4**

CT Scan Report

CT scans demonstrate collapse of the left upper lobe, partial consolidation of the left lower lobe, and nonvisualization of the left bronchi. In addition, there is a large left pneumothorax with mediastinal adenopathy. ▨

Case Continued

The patient is taken to the operating room for flexible and rigid bronchoscopy under general anesthesia. On examination with the flexible bronchoscope, the distal left main-stem bronchus is almost totally obstructed by tumor.

Recommendation

Laser coagulation of the tumor and placement of a stent after achieving adequate patency of the left main-stem bronchus.

Discussion

Several palliative treatment modalities are available to treat patients with advanced lung cancer and tracheobronchial airway obstruction. This obstruction can be from extrinsic compression of the airway by tumor, by enlarged lymph nodes, or by endobronchial disease. Treatments of endobronchial airway obstruction include debulking the tumor with forceps through a rigid bronchoscope, laser coagulation, photodynamic therapy, electrocoagulation, cryocoagulation, and brachytherapy. These treatments provide a mechanical means of reestablishing a patent airway and are usually followed by placement of a stent to maintain airway patency. External compression of a main-stem bronchus is treated by dilation and stent placement.

Although the potassium-titanyl-phosphate (KTP) laser and the carbon dioxide (CO_2) laser are available for use in the airway, the neodymium:yttrium-aluminum-garnet (Nd:YAG) laser is the most commonly used. The Nd:YAG laser has several advantages over the CO_2 laser. First, the laser can be delivered through a flexible quartz fiber and therefore can be applied through a flexible bronchoscope. Furthermore, the Nd:YAG laser produces coagulation necrosis with a 5-mm zone of necrosis, which allows débridement of lesions immediately after treatment with decreased risk for bleeding from the tumor. Although earlier use required high levels of power with increased risk for endobronchial fire, current applications are performed with low-power levels (less than 40 watts) and short pulses (less than 3 seconds). The maximum inspiratory oxygen should be less than 50% to minimize the risk for endobronchial fire. The major complication of the laser is the potential for perforation of major vascular structures, perforation of bronchial wall, and endobronchial fire.

Other palliative modalities have several disadvantages when compared with laser treatments. Photodynamic therapy requires administration of porfimer sodium (Photofrin) intravenously 48 to 72 hours before activation by light energy source. Several bronchoscopic procedures are necessary to remove the necrotic tumor. This modality is used for carcinoma *in situ* or carcinomas with only several millimeters of invasion and is not used in symptomatic patients with endobronchial occlusion requiring urgent treatment. Cryotherapy uses nitric oxide, CO_2, or liquid nitrogen to cause cell necrosis and death. As in photodynamic therapy, repeat bronchoscopies are necessary to remove the necrotic tissue; thus, their use in urgent airway management is limited.

After the patency of the airway is achieved, several stents are available to aid in maintaining patency of the airway. Two types of stents available are metal stents and Silastic stents. The most commonly used stent in the tracheobronchial tree is the Silastic stent, such as the Dumon stent (Novatech, Plan de Gras, France). Other Silastic stents include the Montgomery T tube (Hood Laboratories, Pembroke, MA), Hood stent (Hood Laboratories, Decatur, GA), and a Rusch Y stent (Rusch Inc., Duluth, GA). Advantages of the Silastic stent are that it can be easily removed and that the tumor cannot penetrate the lumen of the stent. These stents require precise positioning and are placed through a rigid bronchoscope under general anesthesia. The major disadvantage is that these stents can easily migrate. Metal stents include stents such as the Wallstent (Schneider Inc., Minneapolis, MN), Ultraflex (Boston Scientific, Natick, MA), Gianturco (Cook Inc., Bloomington IN), and Palmaz stent (Johnson & Johnson Interventional Systems, Warren, NJ). These stents are placed through a flexible bronchoscope under fluoroscopic guidance. Metal stents are composed of stainless steel wire (Gianturco) and cobalt-based alloy (Wallstent), which allows tumor growth into the lumen of the stent. Some metal stents such as the Ultraflex and the Wallstent are also available as covered stents and are designed to prevent tumor growth into the lumen of the stent. Metal stents form an epithelial growth over the wire mesh and usually cannot be removed. Other disadvantages of these stents include granuloma formation at the edges of the stent, hemorrhage from erosion of a vessel, and tracheoesophageal or tracheopharyngeal fistula.

Case Continued

A rigid bronchoscope is introduced, and the tumor is débrided from the left mainstem bronchus as well as from the left upper lobe bronchus with the aid of Nd:YAG laser. After achieving satisfactory airway patency and hemostasis, a silicone-covered Wallstent is placed in the left main-stem bronchus. The patient tolerates the procedure well and is extubated at the conclusion of the procedure. On the postoperative chest x-ray, the left lung is expanded. The chest tube is removed on the second postoperative day, and the patient recovers uneventfully and is discharged on the fourth postoperative day.

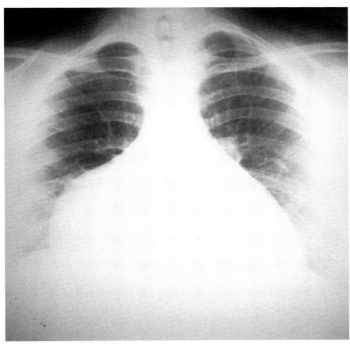

Presentation

A 22-year-old obese man with no significant medical problems presents to his primary care physician with right upper quadrant abdominal pain for the past 2 weeks. The patient has no complaints of nausea or vomiting but has a history of constipation for several years. Examination of the abdomen reveals mild tenderness over the medial right costal arch.

Chest X-rays

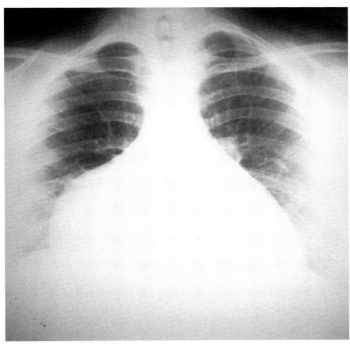

Figure 36-1

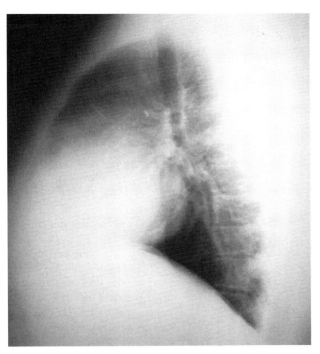

Figure 36-2

Chest X-ray Report

Posteroanterior and lateral chest x-rays demonstrate an abnormally large silhouette at the right cardiophrenic angle. This finding is consistent with a density behind the sternum as seen on the lateral x-ray.

Discussion

The differential diagnosis for the x-rays shown includes a pericardial cyst, lipoma of the epicardial fat, and diaphragmatic herniation. Computed tomography (CT) scans will aid in further diagnosis and planning treatment. Oral contrast should be administered to patients in whom the diagnosis of diaphragmatic hernia is highly suspicious.

■ CT Scans

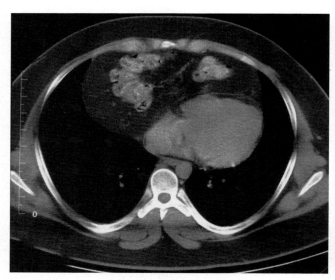

Figure 36-3

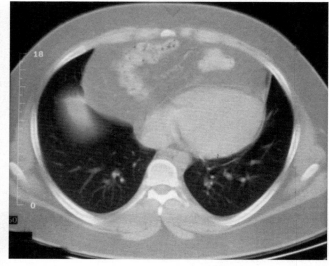

Figure 36-4

CT Scan Report

CT scans of the chest demonstrate the presence of contrast-filled bowel in the anterior mediastinum. There are no lung nodules or pleural effusions. The heart size is normal. ■

Discussion

The four types of diaphragmatic herniation are hiatal hernia, traumatic hernia, hernia of Bochdalek, and hernia of Morgagni. Diaphragmatic hernias of Bochdalek and Morgagni are congenital hernias. Bochdalek hernia is more common and is a posterolateral pleuroperitoneal defect more commonly found on the left side (85%). Hernia of Morgagni is a less common diaphragmatic hernia and is an anterior defect of the diaphragmatic insertion into the chest wall. This hernia is present mostly on the right side but has been reported on the left side or bilaterally. In the newborn, congenital diaphragmatic hernias can cause severe pulmonary hypoplasia and pulmonary hypertension, necessitating extracorporeal membrane oxygenation (ECMO). Hiatal hernias penetrate through the esophageal hiatus in the diaphragm. Traumatic hernias can result from penetrating or blunt trauma and can occur anywhere on the diaphragm. Initial diaphragmatic injury can be easily missed if bowel herniation is not present.

In evaluating the CT scan, the anterior and right-sided locations of the hernia substantiate the diagnosis of a foramen of Morgagni hernia. Although CT scan is usually diagnostic, other tests that may be useful in confirming the diagnosis include contrast upper gastrointestinal (GI) study and magnetic resonance imaging (MRI).

The herniation of abdominal viscera into the chest results in discomfort for the patient and the potential for bowel strangulation or obstruction. Although partial obstruction may be present in a foramen of Morgagni hernia, complete bowel obstruction is rare. Surgical repair is always indicated unless there are strong contraindications to an operative undertaking.

In children, foramen of Bochdalek hernia can be associated with chromosomal abnormalities, congenital heart defects, and intestinal malrotation.

Surgical Approach

An upper midline incision is used to repair a foramen of Morgagni hernia. The incision depends on surgeon preference, body habitus, and past surgical history. Subcostal, paramedian, and midline incisions have all been successfully used. Occasionally, the hernia is discovered incidentally during a thoracotomy. Closure can also be performed through the chest.

The principles of operative repair include reduction of the abdominal viscera into the abdomen, excision of the hernia sac, and tension-free closure of the diaphragmatic defect using primary suture repair or patch repair. Various types of nonabsorbable sutures have been used, and different patch materials, including polypropylene mesh and polytetrafluoroethylene (PTFE), have been used to close the defect. Currently, the PTFE patch is preferable because of its characteristic strength and resistance to adhesion formation. There is no evidence to support the use of one material over another. Some have reported successful closure of a foramen of Morgagni hernia laparoscopically.

Discussion

The retrosternal anterior diaphragmatic hernia, or foramen of Morgagni hernia, is an unusual clinical problem with an incidence of only 1% to 6% of all diaphragmatic hernias. It is less frequently encountered than the posterolateral hernia through the foramen of Bochdalek. The hernia occurs between the xiphoid and the costochondral attachments of the diaphragmatic muscle. It presents more frequently on the right side because the potential defect is obturated by the pericardium on the left. The ligamentum teres forms the medial border of the hernia. Foramen of Morgagni hernia is usually associated with a true sac, which is resected during surgical repair.

This entity is seldom encountered in childhood. Obese patients appear to present with this type of hernia more often than nonobese patients. This entity occurs more frequently in women than in men.

Although colicky pain is an unusual presentation in patients with this entity, dull and aching discomfort is more common. In patients with severe pain, one must suspect either bowel strangulation or obstruction. Urgent repair is indicated in cases in which volvulus or strangulation of bowel may be present. In general, foramen of Morgagni hernia is most often discovered incidentally on a radiographic study.

Postoperative Course

The patient has undergone reduction of the hernia and primary closure of the defect in the diaphragm. Postoperatively, the patient is slow to ambulate. On the third postoperative day, the patient is noted to cough excessively and to have severe upper abdominal pain. Chest x-ray demonstrates a density along the right heart border.

Approach

Based on the postoperative clinical findings, a disruption in the diaphragmatic repair is strongly considered. There may have been excessive tension of the primary repair, especially if the repair was large and patch material was not used. An upper GI study or repeat CT scan of the chest is necessary to confirm the diagnosis. Reoperation and repair of the hernia is indicated.

Presentation

A 72-year-old man presents with the chief complaint of shortness of breath. His symptoms have been progressive over the past year. He is able to climb two flights of stairs before having to stop and rest. His past medical history includes hypertension and hypercholesterolemia. In a review of systems, he denies chest pain, coronary artery disease, fever, cough, hemoptysis, or weight loss. He has an 80-pack-per-year history of smoking but quit 10 years ago.

The physical examination reveals a slender, pleasant gentleman in no respiratory distress. His vital signs are within normal range. The cardiac tones are normal, and his breath sounds are diminished throughout his lung fields. There is no cervical adenopathy. The rest of the examination is unremarkable. Basic laboratory studies revealed neither electrolyte abnormalities nor anemia.

Case Continued

Some of the differential diagnoses for shortness of breath include obstructive airway disease, parenchymal lung disease, and cardiogenic causes. Given the patient's clinical symptoms, the following chest x-rays and computed tomography (CT) scans are obtained.

Chest X-rays

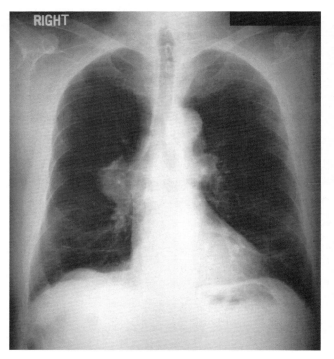

Figure 37-1

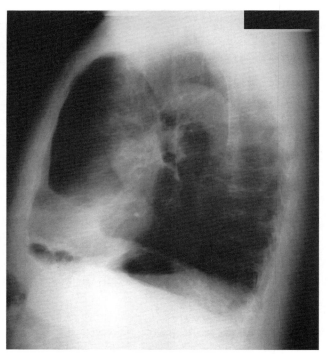

Figure 37-2

Chest X-ray Report

A large mass in the right hilar location is noted. The diaphragms are flattened, and the anteroposterior dimension is enlarged. There are no pleural effusions. The heart size is normal.

CT Scans

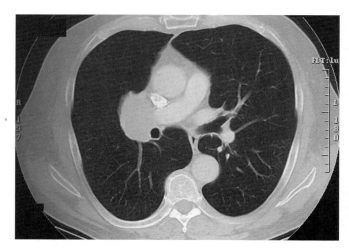

Figure 37-3

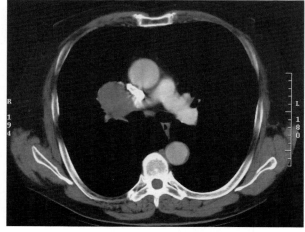

Figure 37-4

CT Scan Report

There is a large, lobulated, 6 cm × 4 cm soft tissue mass in the right hilar region in close proximity to the right upper lobe bronchus. There does not appear to be direct invasion into the superior vena cava or right main pulmonary artery, but the tumor is immediately adjacent to these structures. There are no other abnormal mediastinal or perihilar masses. There are no enlarged lymph nodes. There are no pleural or pericardial effusions.

Discussion

There are many types of lung masses, but a lesion such as this is most likely a bronchogenic carcinoma. A tissue diagnosis should be obtained. Because of the close proximity to the right upper lobe bronchus, bronchoscopy will most likely provide adequate tissue for analysis.

Case Continued

During the bronchoscopy, mucosal congestion is evident in the anterior segment of the right upper lobe. No other abnormalities are noted. This area is brushed and biopsy performed. The pathology is positive for non–small cell lung cancer.

Additional testing is performed with the following results:

Arterial blood gases: pH, 7.44; partial pressure of carbon dioxide (P_{CO_2}), 37; partial pressure of oxygen (P_{O_2}), 64; oxygen saturation, arterial (Sa_{O_2}), 93% (room air)

Pulmonary function test: forced expiratory volume in 1 second (FEV_1); 1.76L (50%), diffusing capacity of lung for carbon monoxide (D_{LCO}), 15 (45%)

Perfusion scans: left lung, 57% perfusion, 51% ventilation

CT scan of the head: no metastatic disease

Bone scan: no metastatic disease

Positron-emission tomography (PET) scan: a large focus of increased fluorodeoxyglucose (FDG) accumulation in the perihilar portion of the right lung

Recommendation

Mediastinoscopy.

Case Continued

Mediastinoscopy is performed and is negative for tumor.

Discussion

Most patients with lung cancer0 present at an advanced stage, and the disease is not curable. Smoking is implicated as the cause in 80% of the cases.

Squamous cell cancer tends to present as a large central mass, sometimes with areas of central necrosis. Adenocarcinomas are usually found in the periphery, whereas small cell carcinomas are usually found centrally and metastasize early.

The staging of lung cancer is based on the TMN classification. T1 lesions are 3.0 cm or less. T2 lesions are greater than 3.0 cm or invade the visceral pleura. A T3 lesion invades the chest wall, mediastinal pleura, or pericardium. T4 lesions involve the cardiac structures, esophagus, vertebral body, trachea, or carina. The presence of a malignant pleural effusion also signifies a T4 lesion.

The nodal involvement is subtyped based on mediastinal involvement. N0 represents no lymph node metastasis. N1 includes peribronchial or ipsilateral hilar lymph node involvement. N2 disease is confined to ipsilateral mediastinal and subcarinal regions. N3 nodes are remote and involve contralateral hilar or mediastinal, scalene, or supraclavicular lymph nodes. The M1 or M0 distinction is determined by the presence or absence of metastatic disease.

The staging is grouped based on the degree of involvement of the above subsets. Stage I is T1-2 N0. Stage IIA is T1 N1. Stage IIB is T2 N1 or T3 N0. Stage IIIA is T3 N1-2 or T1-3 N2. Stage IIIB is T4 or N3. Stage IV is metastatic involvement. In general, stages IIIB and IV are not treated surgically.

Case Continued

After consultation with an oncologist, the patient receives chemoradiotherapy, which consists of paclitaxel (Taxol) and carboplatin and 43 Gy of radiation to the tumor. The tumor responds by shrinking from 6 cm × 4 cm to 3 cm × 2 cm. Neoadjuvant therapy is given because of poor long-term prognosis associated with centrally located T3 N0 lung cancers.

Discussion

This patient has a locally advanced non–small cell lung cancer. The tumor measures 6 cm in greatest dimension and is immediately adjacent to the superior vena cava (T3). There are no enlarged lymph nodes on CT scan and no lymph node uptake on PET scan. Because there is no evidence of metastatic involvement (N0 M0), this patient has a clinical stage IIB (T3 N0 M0) lung tumor. However, the large tumor mass may overlie hilar (N1) lymph nodes, and this may be a clinical stage IIIA (T3 N1 M0).

The treatment regimen for non–small cell lung cancer depends on the stage of the disease at presentation. Surgical therapy for non–small cell lung cancer is directed at complete removal of the tumor and involved lymph nodes. Stage I (T1-2 N0) and stage II (T1 N1) should be treated surgically. No preoperative or postoperative chemotherapy or radiotherapy is typically required.

Neoadjuvant therapy is the application of chemoradiotherapy or chemotherapy preoperatively. This is typically applied to stage IIIA lesions and can be considered for central T3 lesions. Complete surgical resection of locally advanced tumors is critical in determining long-term outcomes. Preoperative therapy may also enhance resectability and may help control micrometastasis earlier, without delay of perioperative recovery.

The most common locations of metastatic spread of non–small cell lung cancer are the liver, adrenal gland, brain, bone, and kidney. The extent of lymph node involvement also dictates survival. If metastatic disease is present, the tumor is a stage IV lesion and is usually not curable. An isolated brain metastasis from the lung is a special circumstance. In such a scenario, if the brain lesion is surgically resectable and the lung primary is early stage, there is a potential for cure (38% 2-year survival rate). The brain lesion is approached first, and if the tumor can be resected successfully, the lung tumor is then resected at a second stage; radiation to the brain is usually administered.

Case Continued

The patient completes his neoadjuvant therapy and subsequently presents with a cough and fever. Sputum and blood cultures are negative. The chest x-ray demonstrates a new infiltrate. Repeat CT scans are obtained.

CT Scans

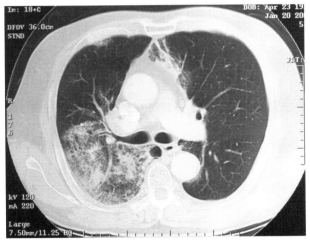
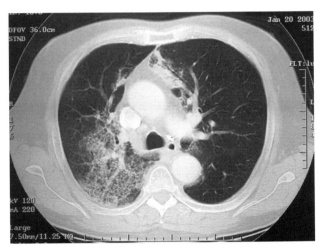

Figure 37-5   **Figure 37-6**

CT Scan Report

Although the tumor is now smaller, there is a large area of ground-glass opacification.

Diagnosis

Radiation pneumonitis.

Discussion

The patient has developed radiation pneumonitis. The effects of radiation on the lung can be divided into early and late phases. The early effect is a pneumonitis and occurs within weeks or months after radiation has been administered. The symptoms vary from shortness of breath to acute respiratory distress syndrome (ARDS). The diagnosis is confirmed by a diffuse opacity mostly involving the irradiated tissue. High-dose steroids may partially reverse the process. The late manifestation of radiation damage is fibrosis, which may produce variable symptoms based on the degree of lung involvement. Linear densities can be seen on x-rays that may be confused for pneumonic infiltrates or recurrent cancer.

Case Continued

The patient is treated with high-dose steroids and gradually recovers over the next 2 months. He then undergoes a right thoracotomy and right upper lobectomy and mediastinal lymph node dissection. Postoperatively, the patient requires prolonged respiratory support but is slowly weaned from the ventilator over 4 days. The pathology demonstrates a poorly differentiated squamous cell carcinoma with positive (N1) lymph nodes. Mediastinal lymph nodes are free of metastatic disease, and a complete resection is achieved.

Presentation

A 53-year-old-man presents to his primary care physician complaining of weight loss, chest pain, and cough. On physical examination, the physician notes decreased breath sounds over the left chest. X-rays are performed, and the patient is referred to your office.

Chest X-rays

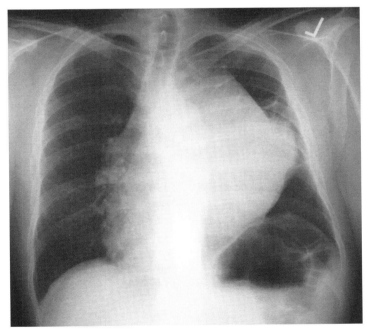

Figure 38-1

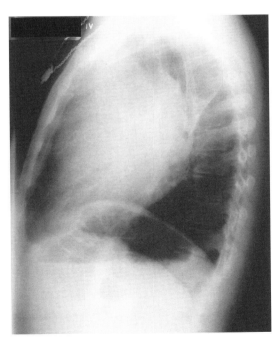

Figure 38-2

Chest X-ray Report

There is a large anterior mediastinal mass projecting to the left side. There is atelectasis of portions of the left lung. The cardiac contour and trachea are displaced to the right side. On the lateral x-ray, the left hemidiaphragm is elevated, which also suggests volume loss, possibly owing to atelectasis in the left lung or diaphragmatic paralysis. ▪

Differential Diagnosis

The major lesions occurring in the anterior mediastinum in the adult include thymoma, lymphoma, thyroid goiter, and germ cell tumors. Less commonly, mediastinal masses may be tumors of vascular or mesenchymal origin or displaced parathyroid tissue.

Discussion

The mediastinum is generally divided into three compartments: the anterior compartment, the visceral compartment, and the paravertebral sulci. The innominate vessels limit the anterior compartment superiorly, with the heart and great vessels limiting it posteriorly. At the thoracic inlet, only the visceral and paravertebral compartments are found. All three compartments extend to the diaphragm. The mediastinal surface of the parietal pleura limits all three compartments laterally.

As mentioned earlier, the major tumors occurring in the anterior mediastinum are thymomas, lymphomas, germ cell tumors, and thyroid goiter. In the visceral compartment, foregut cysts (bronchogenic, esophageal, and gastric) and primary as well as secondary tumors of the lymph nodes constitute most of the masses in this compartment. Also included in visceral compartment masses are pleuropericardial cysts. Most masses arising in the paravertebral sulci are tumors of neurogenic origin (Table 38-1).

In infants and children, the most common masses, in decreasing order of frequency, are neurogenic tumors, enterogenous (foregut) cysts, germ cell tumors, lymphomas, angiomas and lymphangiomas, thymic tumors, and pericardial cysts. In adults, the most common masses, in decreasing order of frequency, are

Table 38-1: Primary Tumors and Cysts of the Mediastinum

Anterior Compartment	Visceral Compartment	Paravertebral Sulci
Thymoma	Enterogenous cyst	Neurilemoma (schwannoma)
Germ cell tumor	Lymphoma	Neurofibroma
Lymphoma	Pleuropericardial cyst	Malignant schwannoma
Lymphangioma	Mediastinal granuloma	Ganglioneuroma
Hemangioma	Lymphoid hamartoma	Ganglioneuroblastoma
Lipoma	Mesothelial cyst	Neuroblastoma
Fibroma	Neuroenteric cyst	Paraganglioma
Fibrosarcoma	Paraganglioma	Pheochromocytoma
Thymic cyst	Parathyroid cyst	Fibrosarcoma
Parathyroid adenoma	Pheochromocytoma	Lymphoma
Aberrant thyroid	Thoracic duct cyst	

From Shields TW. Overview of primary mediastinal tumors and cysts. In: Shields TW, LoCicero J, Ponn RB, eds. *General thoracic surgery*, 5th ed. Philadelphia: Lippincott Williams & Wilkins, 1999:2105, with permission.

thymic tumors, neurogenic tumors, lymphomas, germ cell tumors, foregut cysts, and pericardial cysts.

In children, most of the mediastinal tumors and cysts are symptomatic; in contrast, in adults, only one third of the mediastinal tumors are symptomatic. This is thought to be due to the relatively small size of the thoracic cavity. In children, respiratory symptoms are the most common presentation, even with small masses. In children, fever, lethargy, and pain can be symptoms associated with malignant mediastinal masses. In adults with benign lesions, signs and symptoms from compression of vital structures are uncommon. When malignant disease is present, distortion and fixation may also be present, which result in more prominent and localized symptoms, such as superior vena cava obstruction, chest wall pain, or diaphragmatic paralysis.

In adults, less than 40% of anterior mediastinal masses are malignant. About 25% of all thymomas, all lymphatic tumors, and about 20% of germ cell tumors are malignant. In the visceral compartment, all cysts are benign. Masses of the lymphatic system in the visceral compartment may be benign or malignant. In the paravertebral sulci, less than 3% of neurogenic tumors in adults are malignant.

In children, the incidence of malignancy of a mediastinal mass is greater than in adults. This likelihood decreases with increasing age of the patient. About 45% of the anterior mediastinal lesions are malignant lymphomas, whereas only a small percentage of the germ cell tumors are malignant. In the visceral compartment, most of the lymph node lesions are malignant, whereas most other lesions and cysts are benign. In the paravertebral sulci, more than 60% of the neurogenic tumors are malignant.

Recommendation

Computed tomography (CT) scans of the chest are needed to determine the exact anatomy and character of the lesion and the anatomy of the mediastinum.

CT Scans

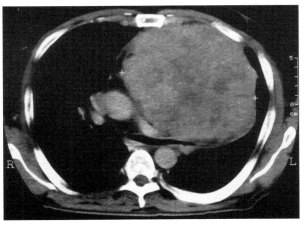

Figure 38-3

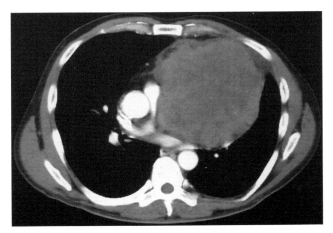

Figure 38-4

CT Scan Report

There is a 15-cm diameter anterior mediastinal mass in the left hemithorax extending from the sternum to the cardiac apex. The mass compresses the main pulmonary artery, left pulmonary artery, and the left main-stem and upper lobe bronchi. There is no evidence of invasion of the mass into any mediastinal structures. The mass is associated with atelectatic changes in the middle and lower portions of the left upper lobe. There is no evidence of lung lesions, masses, or mediastinal adenopathy.

Recommendation

The patient has a large anterior mediastinal mass that is most likely of thymic or germ cell origin. Although a thymic lesion is more likely in this age group, germ cell pathology cannot be excluded. To plan therapeutic intervention, tissue diagnosis should be obtained. Core needle biopsy can be considered; however, needle biopsy may not provide proper adequate tissue quantity for histologic diagnosis and differentiation of various lymphoma types and germinal cell histologic types. Laboratory evaluation of serum α-fetoprotein and β-human chorionic gonadotropin levels should also be obtained.

Case Continued

An anterior mediastinotomy (Chamberlain's procedure) is performed by excising the second costal cartilage and incising the posterior perichondrium; adequate tissue sample is obtained and sent to pathology for examination. Pathology reveals squamous cell carcinoma of thymic origin.

Discussion

Thymic carcinomas are extremely rare. About one third of thymic carcinomas are low-grade malignancy lesions, and two thirds are high-grade malignancy lesions. Only a few patients with low-grade malignant lesions of the thymus die of their disease, whereas more than 85% of those with high-grade tumors die of their disease despite therapeutic intervention.

Squamous cell carcinoma is the most common variant of thymic carcinoma. It is seen more often in men than in women. Most commonly, it affects individuals in their fifth or sixth decade of life. Grossly, the tumor is partially encapsulated and has the appearance of an invasive thymoma. Low-grade, well-differentiated tumors mostly remain localized. The high-grade, poorly differentiated tumors have a propensity to spread to the anterior mediastinal lymph nodes and to extend to the pleura, lungs, and pericardium. The tumor resembles typical squamous cell carcinoma. It may arise *de novo* or in a preexisting thymoma. The well-differentiated tumor may be locally invasive, and necrosis is not often apparent. The poorly differentiated tumor is locally aggressive and may metastasize.

Recommendation

Because there is apparent absence of local invasion of surrounding vital structures on the CT scan, surgical resection is the primary modality of therapy. The tumor is primarily a left-sided mass; thus, a left posterolateral thoracotomy will provide adequate exposure. Flexible fiberoptic bronchoscopy should be performed to evaluate the tracheobronchial tree for tumor extension and invasion. Finally, because the left diaphragm is elevated on the chest x-ray, fluoroscopic evaluation of movement of the left diaphragm will aid in diagnosing phrenic nerve paralysis.

Discussion

The treatment of thymic carcinoma is not well defined. Fewer than 200 cases are reported in the literature, with varied approaches and results. Treatment of squamous cell carcinoma of the thymus is surgical resection. The tumors are highly sensitive to radiation therapy. This modality should probably be used postoperatively, even if complete resection of the tumor mass is obtained. If the lesion is deemed nonresectable or the mass is partially excised, radiation is warranted. There are varying reports of the utility or futility of combination chemotherapy regimens for undifferentiated and advanced lesions. All the chemotherapy regimens are platinum based.

Case Continued

The patient is taken to the operating room. A right radial arterial line and a right central venous catheter are placed. The patient is adequately hyperoxygenated. The anesthesiologist administers propofol as the induction agent. The patient becomes moderately hypotensive. The anesthesiologist rapidly intubates the patient to secure the patient's airway in the face of this hemodynamic instability and institutes positive pressure ventilation. The patient's blood pressure further declines. You notice that the patient's central venous pressure is now elevated above baseline.

Recommendation

Immediate auscultation over the stomach followed by auscultation of the left and right lung at both axillae.

Case Continued

You auscultate equal breath sounds bilaterally.

■ Approach

The patient's body must be secured to the bed and the bed maximally tilted with the left side down. Moderately aggressive volume resuscitation can be used if the patient is thought to be hypovolemic. Intravenous α- and β-adrenergic agents, such as epinephrine and norepinephrine, should be started immediately for hemodynamic support.

Discussion

Compression of the right ventricular outflow tract or main pulmonary artery is the most likely cause of this patient's hemodynamic deterioration. In the supine position, the right ventricular outflow tract is the most superior cardiac structure. The right heart is a low-pressure chamber and is therefore sensitive to external compression. Adverse position, induction of anesthesia, hypovolemia, and reduced contractility are factors that may attenuate compensatory mechanisms.

History and physical examination may elicit positional dyspnea, tachyarrhythmia, and syncope, with elevated jugular and hepatic venous pressures. Right ventricular obstructive symptoms can mimic tracheal or bronchial obstruction. It is therefore imperative not to limit assessment to the tracheobronchial tree.

Patients with an anterior mediastinal mass may develop severe hemodynamic compromise caused by compression of the heart and great vessels after induction of anesthesia and institution of positive pressure ventilation, especially when the patients are in the supine position. Positive pressure ventilation can cause dynamic hyperinflation autopositive end-expiratory pressure because of expiratory gas flow obstruction. With sufficient elevation of intrathoracic pressure, the gradient for venous return is reduced, and right ventricular pressure is reduced, worsening the extent of vascular obstruction.

Hemodynamic support using α- and β-adrenergic agents may be more beneficial than intravascular volume loading in reversing the hemodynamic decompensation.

Case Continued

The patient is stabilized with a 500-mL bolus of normal saline. A posterolateral thoracotomy is performed and the mass excised. The mass involves the left phrenic nerve, which is resected with the mass. Final pathology reveals low-grade squamous carcinoma of the thymus.

Presentation

A 63-year-old woman presents to your office with a 3-month history of dysphagia and a 25-pound weight loss. She has an extensive history of tobacco and alcohol abuse. There is no other pertinent past medical or surgical history. On examination, she has no palpable adenopathy, clear lungs, and no hepatomegaly.

Differential Diagnosis

The most likely diagnosis in a patient with dysphagia, weight loss, and social risk factors such as tobacco and alcohol abuse is esophageal cancer. Other possibilities include mediastinal lymphoma with esophageal obstruction and lung cancer with extensive mediastinal adenopathy.

Recommendation

Upper barium swallow, endoscopy, and chest computed tomography (CT) scan.

▨ Barium Swallow

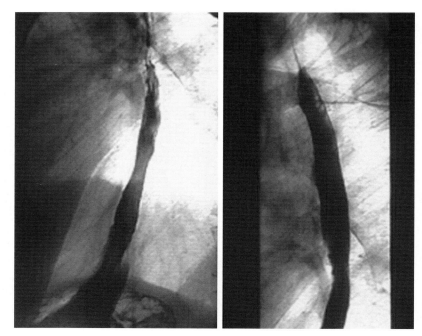

Figure 39-1

Barium Swallow Report

Compression of the esophagus at upper portion. ▨

▨ Endoscopy

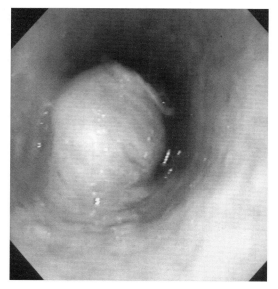

Figure 39-2

A noncircumferential, moderately obstructing mass in upper thoracic esophagus; biopsies performed.

CT Scan

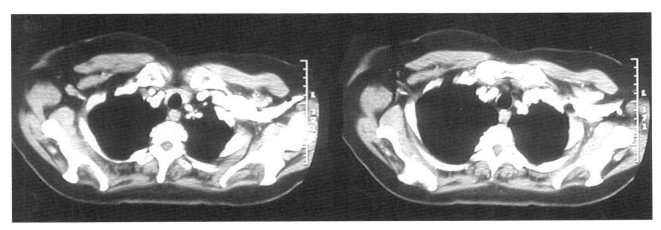

Figure 39-3

CT Scan Report

Mass in the upper thoracic esophagus with narrowing of the esophageal lumen. No evidence of adenopathy or organ metastases.

Pathology Report

Malignant cells, most consistent with squamous cell cancer.

Diagnosis and Recommendation

Squamous cell cancer of the esophagus with moderate esophageal obstruction. Recommendations include endoscopic ultrasound (EUS) and bronchoscopy.

Discussion

Bronchoscopy should be performed in any patient being considered for esophagectomy in whom the primary tumor is adjacent to the trachea or a mainstem bronchus. This is necessary to eliminate the possibility of airway involvement, which would make the cancer unresectable.

EUS is valuable in assessing the depth of penetration of the primary tumor and in defining the status of regional and nonregional lymph nodes. EUS allows evaluation of node size, shape, and internal architecture, each of which helps determine the likelihood of nodal involvement by esophageal cancer.

Bronchoscopy Report

Normal tracheobronchial tree. ■

EUS Report

Tumor invading into but not through the muscularis propria. No abnormal lymph nodes identified. ■

Discussion

There are many options for the management of localized esophageal cancer, including resection, radiation therapy, and multimodality therapy (neoadjuvant chemotherapy and radiation therapy followed by resection). Radiation therapy alone results in relatively poor long-term survival, a high risk for local recurrence, and benign stricture in a large percentage of surviving patients. In patients without nodal involvement and without transmural tumor growth, the addition of neoadjuvant therapy to standard resection has not been shown to have a survival benefit.

Recommendation

Transthoracic esophagectomy, cervical esophagogastrostomy, and feeding jejunostomy.

Case Continued

You perform a transthoracic esophagectomy with gastric pull-up and cervical esophagogastrostomy. The anastomosis is hand sewn with a single-layer 4-0 PDS suture. A jejunostomy feeding tube is placed. The operation is uneventful, and the patient is discharged on tenth postoperative day tolerating a soft solid diet.

Pathology Report

T2 N0 M0 stage IIA squamous cell carcinoma of the esophagus with negative proximal, distal, and lateral margins. ■

Discussion

Postoperative adjuvant therapy has not been shown to provide survival benefit for patients who have had complete resection of their esophageal cancer. Such therapy may be appropriate for patients who have residual local disease or nodal involvement outside of regional lymph nodes. Periodic follow-up surveillance is necessary.

Case Continued

In the first postoperative month, the patient returns for her initial two postoperative visits and reports no problems. Her wounds have healed, she is tolerating a diet, and her physical examination is unremarkable. Six weeks after surgery, the patient complains of progressive dysphagia to solids. An endoscopy is scheduled, but the patient misses her appointment. She eventually undergoes endoscopy 12 weeks after surgery, at which time she has a high-grade stricture in the region of her anastomosis. Biopsies are obtained and demonstrate fibrosis and chronic inflammation. Dilation is attempted but is quite difficult owing to the degree of fibrosis present.

The patient is brought back 1 week later, and additional pneumatic dilation is performed, which adequately opens the esophageal lumen. While in the recovery area, the patient experiences a severe cough. She is admitted to the hospital for observation. Her cough fails to improve overnight. A contrast swallow is performed.

■ Contrast Esophagram

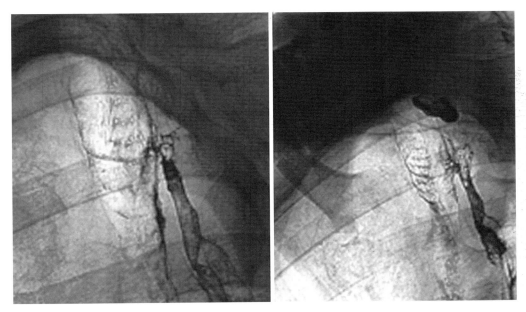

Figure 39-4

Contrast Esophagram Report

Patent fistula between the trachea and the esophagus at the level of the gastric anastomosis. ■

Discussion

The development of an anastomotic-tracheal fistula may be due to erosion into the trachea from a persistent anastomotic leak, trauma from esophageal dilation, or tumor recurrence. Given the proximity in time between the esophagectomy and the development of a fistula in this patient, the most likely etiology is a combination of erosion from the anastomotic leak and trauma from anastomotic dilation. The fact that the biopsies demonstrate no evidence of recurrent tumor supports this diagnosis.

Additional attempts at dilation are likely to enlarge the fistula. The degree of stricturing is sufficiently advanced that continued dilation is not likely to result in palliation of dysphagia. Options for management include stent placement to open the stricture and occlude the fistula or closure of the fistula and patch repair of the esophagus with autologous tissue. A stent is particularly useful when a fistula arises from recurrent tumor, making surgical closure difficult or impossible. When fistulas are a result of benign causes, direct repair is usually most appropriate.

Recommendation

Takedown of esophagotracheal fistula, closure of tracheal defect, and esophagoplasty with pectoralis muscle flap.

Case Continued

The anastomosis is divided from the trachea, and a small defect in the trachea is sutured with interrupted 4-0 Vicryl sutures. The anastomosis is opened longitudinally, and a temporary Silastic stent is inserted. A pectoralis muscle flap develops through a separate incision, and the muscle is tunneled subcutaneously over the clavicle and sutured to the edges of the anastomosis. Postoperatively, the patient's cough resolves. She is discharged 12 days after surgery with jejunostomy tube feedings.

A contrast esophagram is performed 3 weeks after surgery and does not demonstrate any evidence of leak or fistula. Endoscopic evaluation demonstrates normal healing of the anastomosis and a normal trachea. The stent is removed. The patient resumes a regular diet and undergoes routine subsequent follow-up for her cancer with periodic esophageal dilation.

Presentation

You are consulted to evaluate a patient who presents to the oncology service. The patient is a 37-year-old woman with a history of leukemia. She completed her treatment regimen 1 month before her admission. During the past 3 weeks, she has been experiencing low-grade fever and a cough that is productive of mostly clear phlegm. On admission, a chest x-ray is obtained, and the patient is treated with broad-spectrum antibiotics for a presumed pneumonia. Blood and sputum cultures are negative for bacteria and fungi.

■ Chest X-rays

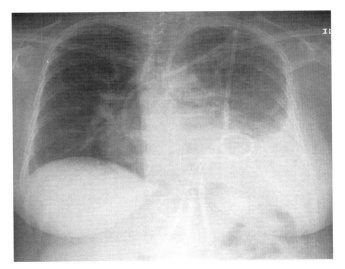

Figure 40-1

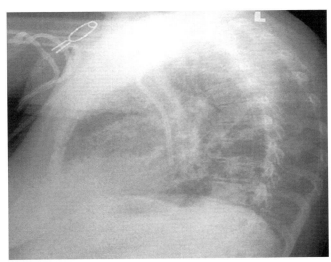

Figure 40-2

Chest X-ray Report

The chest x-rays demonstrate a consolidation of the left lower lobe obscuring the left heart border and left hemidiaphragm. The tip of the central venous catheter is in the right atrium. ■

Discussion

The patient is postchemotherapy and is exhibiting signs, symptoms, and chest x-ray evidence of a pulmonary infection. Blood and sputum studies have not revealed any organisms, and sputum production has been scant despite the chest x-ray findings.

Recommendation

Flexible fiberoptic bronchoscopy.

Case Continued

Flexible fiberoptic bronchoscopy reveals left lower lobe bronchial erythema and minimal acute inflammation of the posterior segmental bronchus. Scanty secretions are present. Bronchial washings reveal many leukocytes and no bacteria. Cultures from the bronchoscopy specimen recover *Aspergillus* species. Further evaluation of the patient reveals a past history of recurrent chest infections. Repeat chest x-rays do not indicate improvement from the initial admission x-ray. The patient continues to have low-grade fever on broad-spectrum antibiotics.

Recommendation

The patient's clinical scenario is consistent with that of a left lower lobe fungal infection with possible cavitation. The extent of radiographic lung disease prompts further diagnostic evaluation. Although there is no evidence of a lung abscess on the chest x-ray, computed tomography (CT) scans of the chest provide a better anatomic definition of the inflammatory process.

CT Scans

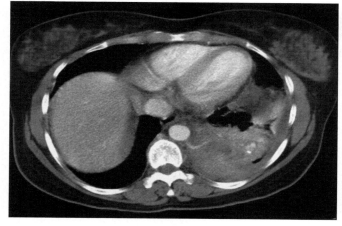
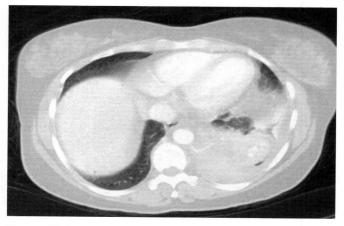

Figure 40-3   **Figure 40-4**

CT Scan Report

CT scans of the chest reveal left lower lobe consolidation with several areas of cavitary lesions. There is a small left pleural effusion. Also evident is an anomalous artery originating from the descending thoracic aorta and entering the left lower lobe. ▪

Diagnosis

Pulmonary intralobar sequestration.

Discussion

Pulmonary sequestration is a congenital anomaly in which normal pulmonary tissue develops without direct connection to the tracheobronchial tree. The vascular arterial supply of the sequestration is from the systemic arterial system, most commonly a branch of the aorta. The venous return from the pulmonary sequestration is through the systemic or pulmonary venous system. Anatomically, pulmonary sequestration is divided into two entities: extralobar sequestration (ELS) and intralobar sequestration (ILS).

ELS forms separately from the rest of the lung and has its own pleural envelope. It makes up 25% to 30% of all sequestrations and is three to four times more common in men. ELS is found in the left hemithorax in 80% to 90% of patients. The mass is usually triangular in shape and is usually positioned at the posterior costophrenic angle. The arterial supply is usually through small-caliber vessels. The systemic venous return of this lesion is through either the portal or the azygous system. CT is usually adequate to identify both arterial supply and venous drainage. Clinically, ELS is most likely to be diagnosed initially on routine prenatal ultrasound early in gestation or as an unexplained density by chest x-ray during childhood. Symptomatic ELS frequently presents in neonates and early childhood with respiratory distress, cyanosis, and feeding problems. About 60% of ELS patients have other associated congenital abnormalities, including diaphragmatic hernia, cardiac defects, diaphragmatic eventration, pericardial cysts, esophageal achalasia, skeletal deformities, renal problems, and esophagobronchial diverticula.

ILS forms within the normal lung parenchyma. It therefore lacks its own pleural envelope. As with ELS, it usually does not have a connection to the tracheobronchial tree. It makes up 70% to 75% of the pulmonary sequestrations and has an almost equal gender distribution. More than 98% of these lesions occur in the lower lobes of the lungs, with 60% occurring on the left side. The systemic arterial blood supply of ILS is usually through a large-caliber systemic arterial branch. Seventy percent of the arteries originate from the thoracic aorta, and 30% are from the abdominal aorta or its branches. These vessels course through the inferior pulmonary ligament to enter the lung. The venous drainage of ILS is through the pulmonary venous system. CT is usually adequate to identify both arterial supply and venous drainage. Only 15% of ILS patients are asymptomatic when the lesion is discovered. A chest x-ray reveals a homogenous opacity in the lung base. More than 50% of patients develop symptoms after 20 years or age, most commonly with cough, sputum production, recurrent infections, and hemoptysis. Communication of this lesion through the pores of Kohn may lead to infection. The inflammatory process affects adjacent normal lung tissue to result in sputum production. Infection may lead to abscess formation. The inflammatory process may also lead to erosion and resultant direct communication of the sequestration with the tracheobronchial tree. Only 12% of ILS patients have associated congenital lesions.

Recommendation

The procedure of choice for this patient is a left lower lobectomy. The operative approach is to dissect the inferior pulmonary ligament and ligate the aberrant artery supplying the sequestration. Given this patient's history of leukemia and chemotherapy, special attention to the patient's nutritional status, immune compromise, and history of steroid use are essential in preparing this patient for surgery.

Discussion

The treatment of intralobar pulmonary sequestration by resection is curative. Segmental resection may be performed; however, inflammatory changes may prevent resection of the sequestration as a segment. In such cases, a lobectomy that includes the sequestered lung should be performed. The arterial supply should be carefully identified and ligated to prevent disruption and hemorrhage.

With respect to extralobar sequestrations, resection should be possible without resecting normal lung tissue. Initial identification and ligation of the arterial supply and venous drainage is necessary.

Case Continued

A left posterolateral thoracotomy is performed. The left lower lobe is adherent, and mobilization of the left lung is difficult. During the initial dissection of the inferior pulmonary ligament, the arterial branch is inadvertently transected close to the diaphragm. The vessel retracts into the abdomen.

Recommendation

Initial direct retrieval of the artery should be attempted; if necessary, the diaphragmatic hiatus should be enlarged to identify and ligate the aberrant artery. In rare instances in which the artery has retracted and cannot be found through the chest, the abdomen should be opened, the aorta exposed, and the aberrant artery ligated. The abdomen is then closed, and the thoracic operation is completed.

Presentation

A 49-year-old man presents to the emergency department with complaints of shortness of breath. He describes persistent and worsening symptoms of shortness of breath and wheezing over several years. He relates a longer than 20-year history of respiratory problems, including a previous pneumothorax requiring tube thoracostomy. He reports a 35-pack-per-year smoking history. On physical examination, you find that he is thin, and although not in respiratory distress, his respiratory rate is elevated (34 breaths/min), with an oxygen saturation of 90%. On auscultation, both lung fields have diminished breath sounds and bilateral wheezing. There is egophony and hyperresonance bilaterally. The emergency department physician obtains chest x-rays and requests an immediate thoracic surgery consult.

Chest X-rays

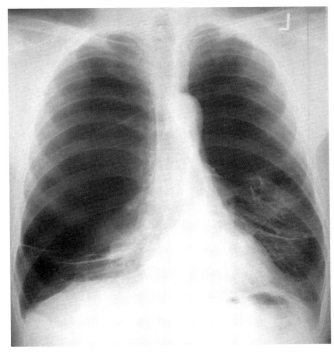

Figure 41-1

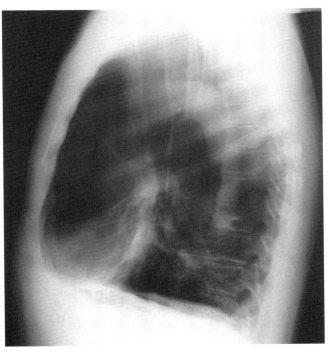

Figure 41-2

Chest X-ray Report

There is a lack of lung markings in both the right and left lung fields. There are bilateral transverse markings suggestive of septation in a giant bulla. The diaphragms are flattened, and the anteroposterior diameter is widened, suggestive of chronic obstructive pulmonary disease. The heart is normal in size. There are no pleural effusions. ▪

Differential Diagnosis

Often, the absence of lung markings is associated with the diagnosis of pneumothorax. It is important not to make this general assumption. A pneumothorax of this size would require a tube thoracostomy, which in this case would be erroneous and would subject the patient to unnecessary complications, such as a significant air leak and loss of tidal volume. Tension pneumothorax may also be present in a patient who lacks lung markings on chest x-ray. When evaluating an x-ray of a patient with a suspected diagnosis of tension pneumothorax, the position of the trachea should be noted. In this case, the positions of the trachea and mediastinum are midline, which suggests against the diagnosis of a tension pneumothorax. Furthermore, bilateral pneumothorax, although possible, is very rare.

Discussion

Pulmonary blebs are due to subpleural alveolar rupture, which results in an intrapleural air space. They are small and are usually located in the apices of the upper lobes; they can also be found at the apices of the lower lobe. Blebs can be acquired as a consequence of chronic obstructive lung disease or can be present at birth and enlarge over time. Typical presentation includes a tall, thin male between the ages of 20 and 40 years who presents with shortness of breath and is found to have a unilateral spontaneous pneumothorax. The first occurrence of a spontaneous pneumothorax can be observed if the pneumothorax is small; in patients with a large pneumothorax, a tube thoracostomy is necessary. The incidence of a second pneumothorax is 20%, and it is 50% for a third pneumothorax. Patients with recurrent pneumothoraces require excision of the bleb to prevent recurrences. In contrast to blebs, bullae are larger than 1 cm and are not sharply demarcated from surrounding lung. Instead, the walls are made up of destroyed lung and a thin membrane composed of visceral pleura and connective tissue. Bullae communicate with bronchi at the base of the bullae. They can form anywhere in the lung but are usually found in the upper lobes. Typically, bullae are divided into two groups: they may be associated with normal lung parenchyma (20%) or with diffuse emphysema (80%). Patients with bullae and normal lung parenchyma have some compression of adjacent lung but near-normal pulmonary function. Bullae with diffuse emphysema may be the result of severe diffuse panacinar emphysema and can be multiple and bilateral. Giant bullae fill at least one half of the hemithorax.

The pathophysiology of giant bullae involves the disparity of compliance between the surrounding lung and the bullae. Adjacent emphysematous lung tissue associated with this disease is less compliant than the bullae. The pressure required to inflate the bullae is therefore far less than the pressure required to inflate the adjacent lung. Therefore, the bullae are preferentially inflated when exposed to negative intrathoracic pressure. As a result, the adjacent lung is retracted away from the bullae. Eventually, the nonfunctioning bullae can occupy much of the hemithorax, leaving little room for functioning lung to inflate. Large intrapulmonary shunts develop, and hypoxia ensues. Surgical excision of giant bullae is based on the theory that by removing the bullae, the remaining functional lung will expand and assist in ventilation.

Recommendation

To evaluate the extent of the bulla and plan for further treatment, a computed tomography (CT) scan of the chest is necessary. Furthermore, CT scanning is helpful in distinguishing a giant bulla from pneumothorax in cases in which septation is not evident on a chest x-ray. CT scan also provides a more accurate assessment of the quality and quantity of remaining viable lung tissue.

A bronchoscopy should be performed to examine the bronchial tree for an obstructive lesion. Pulmonary function tests can be used to establish a preoperative baseline as a means for comparative follow-up. However, pulmonary function tests are not useful in selecting surgical candidates. Good results from bullectomy occur in patients who preserve their diffusing capacity of lung for carbon monoxide (D_{LCO}) and maintain a normal blood gas during exercise.

CT Scans

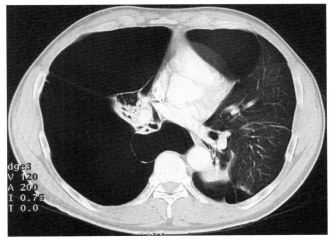 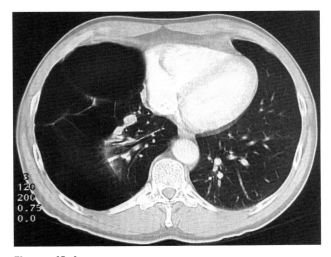

Figure 41-3 **Figure 41-4**

CT Scan Report

Giant bullae are seen bilaterally. Septations are noted within the bullae. In the right chest, viable lung tissue is compressed medially. The left lower lobe is inflated.

Discussion

In patients with bullous disease who are not dyspneic, surgery should be reserved for complications of the disease. Complications that may be associated with bullous disease include pneumothorax, lung abscess that has failed medical therapy, hemoptysis, and persistent pain due to air trapping. In some cases, suspicion of lung cancer is an indication for an operative approach in these patients. In a patient who is dyspneic, resection of a bulla is justified when the bulla occupies one half or more of the hemithorax, there is enlargement of the bulla over a period of time, or there is significant compression of adjacent lung. In patients with bullous disease who are dyspneic, surgical resection of the bulla removes a space-occupying lesion that is compressing viable lung. Removal of the bulla also aids in reducing airway resistance and dead space.

The operative approach to bullous disease is through a posterolateral or a lateral thoracotomy depending on the need for exposure. Sternotomy has also been used in patients with bilateral bullous disease, with satisfactory results. The mortality rate associated with resection of a bulla is 1.5% for patients with normal underlying lung and 11% for patients with diffuse emphysema.

Case Continued

The patient undergoes a right posterolateral thoracotomy through the fifth interspace. The bulla is excised, leaving as much viable lung to allow the lung to expand and fill the space. Careful attention is given to avoid air leaks. Excision of the bulla is performed using multiple applications of a stapler technique in which the stapler is reinforced with Gore-Tex (W. L. Gore & Associates, Flagstaff, AZ) strips to minimize air leaks. After the lung is inflated, two chest tubes are placed to allow expansion of the lung.

Postoperatively, there is a large air leak. The patient remains hemodynamically stable and after 24 hours is successfully weaned from the ventilator. Chest x-ray demonstrates a persistent apical pneumothorax on the operative side.

Discussion

The initial step in the management of persistent air leaks is conservative. Most surgeons would observe a small but persistent air leak for at least 2 weeks before contemplating intervention; large air leaks may require early intervention. Most air leaks seal within a 2-week time frame. Small and moderate air leaks can be managed with a Heimlich valve for earlier hospital discharge.

Use of sealants during an operation can minimize postoperative air leaks and has been reported to eliminate up to 80% of air leaks. Sealants vary in the method of application and ease of use. Tissue adhesives are separated into five categories: (a) fibrin sealants, (b) albumin-based compounds, (c) cyanoacrylates, (d) hydrogels, and (e) collagen-based adhesives.

Fibrin sealants are combinations of thrombin and fibrinogen. Some include calcium chloride and factor XIII or antifibrinolytics, such as aprotinin. They produce a deliverable clot that is a bioabsorbable sealant. Because fibrin sealants incorporate the use of plasma, there is a small risk for viral transmission. Fibrin sealants are used for sealing air leaks and can be used as a treatment for bronchopleural fistulas. Commercial fibrin sealants are Hemaseel APR (Haemacure Corp., Quebec, Canada) and Tisseel VH (Baxter Healthcare Corp., Deerfield, IL).

Albumin-based sealants, also known as glutaraldehyde glues, are based on the combination of albumin and adhesion compounds. Bioglue (Cryolyfe Inc., Kennesaw, GA) uses the combination of bovine albumin and gelatin-resorcinol-glutaraldehyde. Glutaraldehyde glues are strong and biodegradable, with a half-life of about 30 days. Currently, these sealants are approved by the U.S. Food and Drug Administration (FDA) for aortic dissection; however, they are being explored for use in thoracic procedures.

Cyanoacrylates are composed of the compound 2-octylcyanoacrylate. They are commercially available as Dermabond (Ethicon, Inc., Somerville, NJ) and Tru-fill n-BCA (Cordis Neurovascular, Inc., Miami Lakes, FL). These compounds are stronger than fibrin sealant but are also more brittle. They are not bioabsorbable; therefore, the body reacts to them as a foreign body. For this reason, there are associative risks for tissue necrosis, inflammation, and infection. At this time, the use of cyanoacrylates is limited to skin applications.

Hydrogels are made up of polyethylene glycol polymers. They are water soluble, light activated, and bioabsorbable over 3 months. Their application process is more complex. FocalSeal-L (Genzyme Biosurgery, Inc., Cambridge, MA) uses a light source to photopolymerize the substance and activate it after it has been applied. FocalSeal-L has been shown to be useful in reducing the air leaks and bronchopleural fistulas.

Collagen-based adhesives Floseal (Sulzer Spine-Tech, Anaheim, CA) and Proceed (Fusion Medical Technologies, Mountain View, CA) are combinations of bovine collagen and bovine thrombin. These compounds provide a matrix for clot and deliver fibrinogen to help with coagulation. They are designed to control surgical bleeding and are mostly used in vascular surgery and neurosurgery. Their use for air leaks and bronchopleural fistulas has not yet been explored.

Case Conclusion

The patient is observed for 2 weeks without resolution of the air leak. He is taken back to surgery, and disrupted lung tissue from the right lower lobe is identified and stapled with reinforcing strips.

case 42

Presentation

A 17-year-old girl presents with no significant past medical history. She denied a history of fever, chills, night sweats, or weight loss during the 6 months before her office visit. She is a nonsmoker who reports no travel outside of Illinois. She has had the usual respiratory tract infections over the course of her youth. She is referred with the following chest x-rays, which were obtained during admission to the emergency department for abdominal pain, which was subsequently found to be due to appendicitis.

Chest X-rays

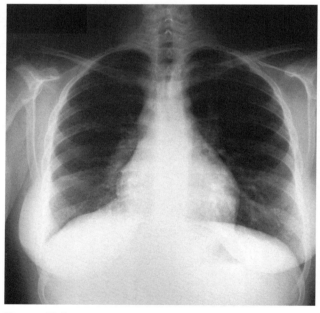

Figure 42-1

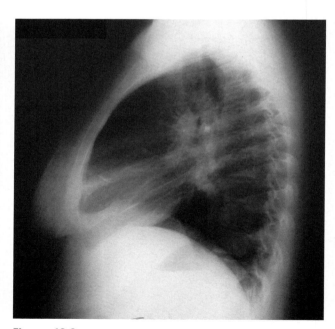

Figure 42-2

Chest X-ray Report

There is a soft tissue mass in the right paratracheal region. The carina is splayed. The lung fields are clear. There are no pleural effusions. ■

Recommendation

Chest computed tomography (CT) scans of the chest to characterize the abnormality found on chest x-ray.

CT Scans

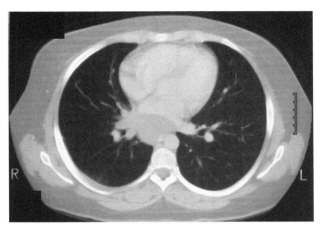

Figure 42-3

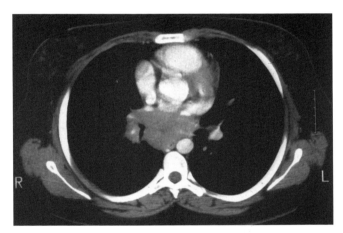

Figure 42-4

CT Scan Report

Enlarged right paratracheal, subcarinal, and right hilar lymphadenopathy are demonstrated. Lung fields are clear.

Differential Diagnosis

The differential diagnosis of a paratracheal (middle) mediastinal mass in a young woman includes infection, malignancy, granulomatous disease, bronchogenic cyst, and esophageal duplication cyst. Infectious causes include bacterial, such as tuberculosis, and fungal, such as histoplasmosis. Malignant causes include lymphoma, lung cancer, and esophageal cancer. Noninfectious granulomatous diseases include sarcoidosis and Wegener's granulomatosis. Histoplasmosis and sarcoidosis frequently present as asymptomatic granulomatous mediastinal lymphadenopathy.

Recommendation

The CT scan finding is most consistent with mediastinal lymphadenopathy; thus, an outpatient mediastinoscopy with biopsy of the enlarged mediastinal lymph nodes is necessary to obtain tissue diagnosis. The specimens should be sent for fungal and tuberculosis culture in addition to histology.

▨ Surgical Approach

Mediastinoscopy is performed by positioning the patient's head at an extended position. A 1-inch transverse incision is made 1 cm above the sternal notch. The strap muscles are divided in the midline, and the pretracheal fascia is incised horizontally, taking care to avoid injury to the inferior thyroid veins. A finger is used to dissect the fascia off of the anterior surface of the trachea. A mediastinoscope is inserted in the pretracheal plane, and using suction-dissection, a right paratracheal mass is partially freed from surrounding tissues. After first aspirating the mass and finding there is no blood return, several biopsies are obtained. During the biopsy, dark blood fills the interior of the mediastinoscope.

Recommendation

A sponge is inserted down the mediastinoscope, and the scope is withdrawn to allow tamponade of the bleeding vessel. If after several minutes of tamponade the bleeding does not stop, sternotomy and repair of the injured vessel is warranted.

Case Continued

The sponge is left in place for several minutes; the mediastinoscope is then reinserted, and the site is noted to have stopped bleeding. No further biopsies are taken. The patient is closed in standard fashion.

Discussion

Bleeding is a well-recognized complication of mediastinoscopy that occurs in 0.1% to 0.2% of the patients. Vocal cord paralysis and pneumothorax occur more frequently than bleeding. Bleeding can result from injury to the azygous vein or apical branches of the right pulmonary artery (in the right lower paratracheal region), or to the bronchial arteries or the main pulmonary artery (in the subcarinal region). Bleeding from the azygous vein usually results from a portion of the wall of the vein being avulsed during performance of a lymph node biopsy when the node is adherent to the vein. The risk can be minimized by attempting to dissect out the entire node from surrounding tissues. Excessive pulling of nodal tissue should be avoided. Venous bleeding usually tamponades with mechanical pressure. Topical hemostatic agents, such as Surgicel or Gelfoam, can be used, but often, a sponge temporarily placed on the bleeding vessel will provide sufficient pressure to tamponade venous bleeding. Bleeding from either bronchial arteries or the pulmonary artery is handled initially by gauze tamponade followed by immediate right thoracotomy. The patient is typed and cross-matched while being prepped and draped.

Histologic Specimens

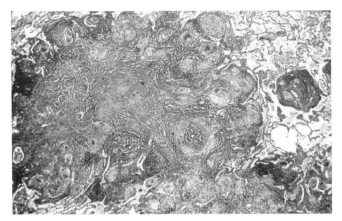

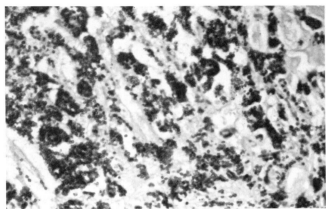

Figure 42-5 See Color Plate 18 following page 114.   **Figure 42-6** See Color Plate 19 following page 114.

Histologic Report

The image on the left is a hematoxylin and eosin staining demonstrating the presence of a granuloma. A Gomori methenamine silver (GMS) staining reveals budding yeast organisms. These findings are consistent with *Histoplasma capsulatum* organisms.

Discussion

Histoplasmosis is caused by the fungus *H. capsulatum*. The fungus is endemic to the river valleys of the United States, such as the Mississippi river, and is supported by the droppings of bats, chickens, and pigeons. Although birds do not harbor the fungus, bats can be infected by the fungus because of their lower body temperature and can excrete the fungus in their droppings. Spores are inhaled into the lungs, where they are phagocytized by alveolar macrophages. In the lungs, the macrophages provide the organisms with both nutrients and mobility. It is difficult to establish the frequency of fungal infections involving the mediastinal lymph nodes because of the large number of subclinical cases, but histoplasmosis is believed to be the most common mediastinal fungal infection.

Most patients who live in endemic areas and are exposed to *H. capsulatum* do not have symptoms. Their only evidence of infection may be positive complement fixation and skin tests. Some patients develop a solitary pulmonary nodule with calcification, which may be evident on radiographic studies. Immunocompromised patients may develop chronic opportunistic lung infections with interstitial pneumonitis and necrosis. Because these patients are anergic from their primary disease process, negative skin tests cannot exclude the diagnosis. Several sputum cultures should be obtained in these patients to culture the fungus.

Treatment of cavitary histoplasmosis includes itraconazole and ketoconazole. Amphotericin B is used in a more severe and disseminated infection. Response rate of medical treatment varies from 65% to 86%. Surgical intervention is reserved for patients with localized disease who failed to respond to several drug treatments.

Fibrotic reaction to *H. capsulatum* may cause significant enlargement of mediastinal and hilar lymphadenopathy. Complications of enlarged lymphadenopathy include superior vena caval syndrome, stenosis of main-stem bronchi, or pulmonary artery and pulmonary vein obstruction. Antifungal treatment of enlarged mediastinal and hilar lymph nodes may be beneficial, especially in cases in which organisms are cultured from biopsy specimens.

Case Continued

Given the finding of asymptomatic, enlarged subcarinal lymph nodes, as a consequence of a fibrogenic response to *H. capsulatum*, the patient is managed nonoperatively with follow-up CT scans of the chest.

Presentation

A 65-year-old woman presents for preoperative evaluation for elective knee replacement. The patient suffers from arthritic degeneration of her right knee and is severely limited in her ability to walk without pain.

Her past medical history includes hypertension and diabetes. She is a long-time smoker of 30 pack-years, but quit 10 years ago. She denies chest pain and shortness of breath, but she is limited in her activity because of her arthritis. She denies weight loss.

On physical examination, the patient is in no acute distress. Her pulse is 80 beats/min, and her blood pressure is 100/60 mm Hg. She has no cervical adenopathy. There are normal breath sounds heard upon auscultation of her chest, and her cardiac examination reveals only a displaced point of maximal impulse (PMI). The right knee is enlarged and somewhat tender and has a limited range of motion.

As part of her preoperative evaluation, routine chemistries and hematologic profiles are drawn and found to be normal. Chest x-rays are performed.

■ Chest X-rays

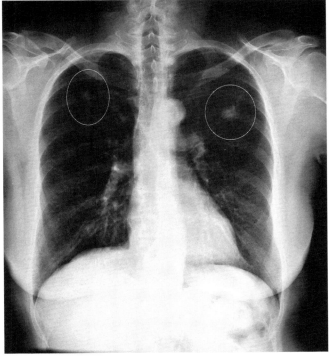

Figure 43-1

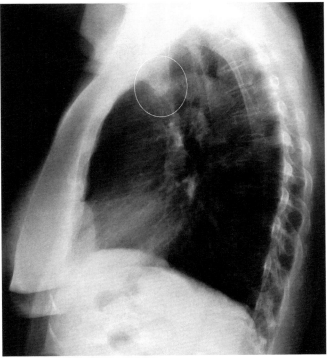

Figure 43-2

Chest X-ray Report

Two nodules are present in both lung fields. One nodule is in the left upper lobe, and one is in the right upper lobe. The heart is not enlarged. There are no pleural effusions. ▨

Discussion

Primary lung cancer, metastatic carcinoma, sarcoma, hamartoma, carcinoid, tuberculosis, and histoplasmosis should be considered in this patient. A computed tomography (CT) scan will provide further anatomic localization as well as evaluate the mediastinum for enlarged lymphadenopathy. A positron-emission tomography (PET) scan can also be obtained to evaluate for metastatic disease.

▨ CT Scans

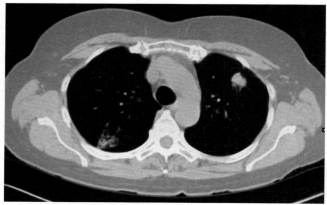

Figure 43-3

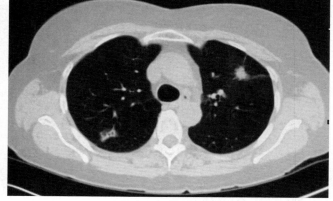

Figure 43-4

CT Scan Report

CT scans demonstrate a 2.0-cm mass in the anterior segment of the left upper lobe and a 2.5-cm mass in the posterior segment of the right upper lobe. No adenopathy is noted in the mediastinum. ▨

PET Scans

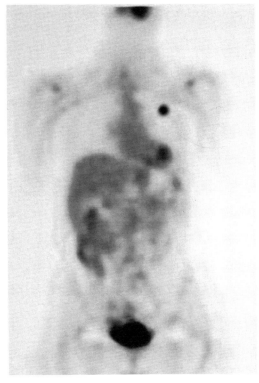

Figure 43-5

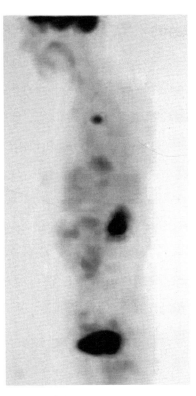

Figure 43-6

PET Scan Report

PET scans reveal intense uptake in the left upper lobe (standardized uptake value [SUV] 5.2). There is faint uptake as well in the right upper lobe (SUV 0.7). There is no evidence of hilar, mediastinal, or distant metastatic disease. Review of a previous magnetic resonance imaging (MRI) study of the knee demonstrates no evidence of malignancy. ▪

Discussion

This patient has two suspicious lung nodules. An asymptomatic lung nodule often represents an early primary lung cancer. It is possible to have two simultaneous tumors. This is thought to occur in 1% of patients with lung cancers. These tumors may be ipsilateral or contralateral.

This phenomenon must be distinguished from metastatic disease, either from the lung as a primary site or from another remote primary site. In this scenario, the PET scan did not demonstrate any areas of increased activity other than the lung, which may represent a primary source or metastatic disease. Satellite tumor nodules may represent interpulmonic metastasis (8% resected ipsilateral lung cancer cases). It is unusual to have contralateral metastasis without mediastinal adenopathy from the primary lung cancer. Because of the heterogeneity of lung tumors, it is sometimes difficult to determine whether two tumors of the same cell types represent metastasis or synchronous tumors. Flow cytometry is helpful in making this distinction.

The 5-year survival rate of patients with synchronous malignant lung tumors, despite early T and N status, is similar to that of patients with stage IIIA disease. This survival is worse than that of patients with either individual tumor. This emphasizes the importance of preoperative metastatic evaluation and planning.

Case Continued

A CT scan of the brain is obtained because the PET scan cannot evaluate brain metastasis; the brain is very metabolically active and always has intense uptake on PET scan examination. Additionally, pulmonary function evaluation is performed. These values were all normal, and the forced expiratory volume in 1 second (FEV_1) is 2.24 (110% if predicted). Bronchoscopy reveals no endobronchial abnormalities.

Recommendation

Left thoracotomy and frozen section with plan for probable left upper lobectomy and mediastinal lymph node dissection. After recovery, resection of the right-sided lesion is performed with a possible segmentectomy.

Discussion

The patient is a suitable candidate for a surgical thoracic procedure. Both lesions are T1, and there is no adenopathy or remote disease. The patient also has excellent pulmonary reserve.

Synchronous lesions may be resected using several different approaches. Unilateral disease is resected by removing both lesions simultaneously. For bilateral disease, especially when bilateral lobectomies are required, careful preoperative planning is necessary. A sternotomy is a well-tolerated incision that may be used for bilateral lesions. However, bilateral lobectomies can be associated with increased morbidity and mortality. Lobectomy through a median sternotomy is tedious and can be unfamiliar for most surgeons. A transverse thoracosternotomy (clamshell incision) gives better bilateral exposure than a sternotomy but is not as well tolerated.

Simultaneous bilateral thoracotomies can be well tolerated if resection is limited. To minimize the magnitude of a complication related to pulmonic surgery, it is prudent to perform both resections in settings separated by several weeks.

Case Continued

The patient is informed that she most likely has bilateral malignancies and that surgical resection offers her the best chance for cure. The patient is taken to the operating room, general anesthesia through a double lumen tube is induced, and the patient is positioned in the right lateral decubitus position. A left thoracotomy is performed, and frozen-section analysis of the left upper lobe mass confirms the diagnosis of non–small cell carcinoma. A left upper lobectomy and mediastinal node dissection are performed. The bronchial margin and all lymph nodes are negative for tumor. The tumor is moderately differentiated squamous cell carcinoma (T1 N0).

The patient's chest tubes are removed on postoperative day 2. She is discharged on postoperative day 4. One week later, she is seen in the clinic and is progressing very well. She is scheduled to have her contralateral lung surgery in 2 weeks.

Discussion

Because the tumor on the left side is larger and may require a more extensive resection, it is recommended that the left side be approached first. The location of the tumor deep in the anterior segment of the left upper lobe makes a conservative segmental resection less likely. The right-sided lesion is anatomically well suited for segmental resection.

Because the patient recovered well after the initial resection, it is reasonable to schedule operation on the right lung 3 weeks later. If any complications develop, the surgery will be postponed.

Case Continued

The patient is taken to the operating room, and a needle biopsy of the left-sided lesion establishes the diagnosis of bronchioloalveolar carcinoma. Biopsy of level 11 and level 4 lymph nodes reveals no evidence of metastatic cancer. Because a left upper lobectomy was previously performed, an appropriate resection would be a posterior segmentectomy of the right upper lobe. The patient is extubated at the completion of the procedure. During transport to the recovery room, oxygen saturation decreases to 84%. With deep breathing and coughing, saturations improve to 92%. Chest x-ray demonstrates no pneumothorax and well-expanded residual right upper, middle, and lower lobes. A large portion of the left lower lobe is atelectatic.

Recommendation

Aspiration bronchoscopy.

Case Continued

Bronchoscopy is performed, and a large mucous plug is aspirated and sent for culture. The patient is able to breathe more comfortably, and saturation is 92% to 94% on 2 L/min of oxygen.

Discussion

Postoperative respiratory complications occur frequently after thoracic surgical procedures. In this case, because of the limited respiratory reserve, very aggressive pulmonary care is necessary. Aggressive pulmonary therapy, early ambulation, inhalational therapy, and incentive spirometry should be instituted early to prevent respiratory problems.

Final Pathology

All lymph nodes are negative for malignancy. The two tumors had different flow cytometry characteristics, indicating synchronous primary lung cancers.

Presentation

A 39-year-old Hispanic woman who immigrated to the United States 18 years ago is referred to you with increasing symptoms of dysphagia, which started with solids 2 years ago and now has progressed to liquids. She has lost 30 pounds in the past 8 months. In addition, she is awakened at night by a worrisome choking sensation and coughing spells. Occasionally, she feels that her food backs up into her throat. The patient denies fever, chills, and night sweats. Past medical history is significant for asthma and a bleeding stomach ulcer 5 years ago, for which she underwent a resection. Her physical examination is only remarkable for severe halitosis. Auscultation of the lungs reveals no wheezing or rhonchi. The heart tones are normal, with no murmurs.

■ Chest X-rays

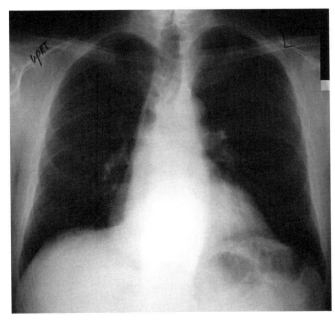

Figure 44-1

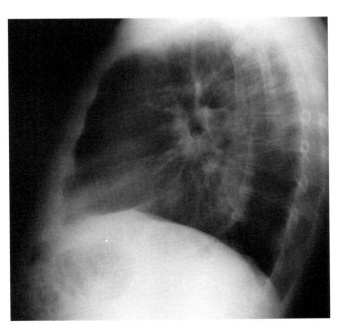

Figure 44-2

Chest X-ray Report

Posterolateral and anterior views of the chest x-ray demonstrate an abnormal shadow posterior and lateral to the right heart border. An air–fluid level in a dilated esophagus is demonstrated on the lateral view. ▪

Recommendation

Upper gastrointestinal (GI) study.

▪ Upper GI Studies

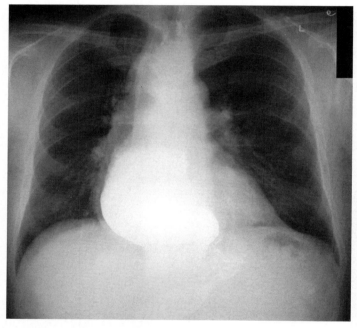

Figure 44-3

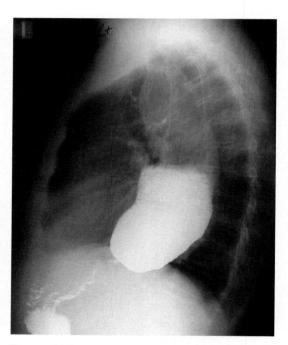

Figure 44-4

Upper GI Report

A late-phase contrast esophagram reveals retained contrast with an air–fluid level in a dilated esophagus. Contrast can be seen trickling into the stomach through an obstructed segment. There is some contrast in the small bowel. ▪

Differential Diagnosis

The symptom complex manifested by this patient may be seen with many pathologic conditions of the esophagus, such as carcinoma, stricture, and dysmotility. Motility disorders may be primary or secondary. Some examples of primary disorders include achalasia, diffuse esophageal spasm, or nutcracker esophagus. Secondary disorders include entities such as diabetes mellitus, Chagas' disease, chronic intestinal pseudoobstruction, scleroderma, and infiltrative diseases.

Chagas' disease is endemic to Central and South America and is caused by a protozoan, *Trypanosoma cruzi*, which infects humans by a bite of an infected insect. The chronic form of the disease affects 10% to 20% of the patients who are infected and affects the colon, heart, and esophagus. The colon is most commonly affected, presenting as megacolon and, in some cases, sigmoid volvulus. The cardiac manifestations include cardiac arrhythmia and cardiomegaly. The esophageal manifestation includes megaesophagus. In addition, the disease may also cause destruction of the myenteric plexus of the duodenum and ureter. The diagnosis of Chagas' disease is confirmed by detection of antibodies by complement fixation or immunofluorescence.

Case Continued

Because the diagnosis of Chagas' disease is considered in this patient, an electrocardiogram and abdominal x-rays are obtained. The electrocardiogram shows a normal sinus rhythm of 82 beats/min. The abdominal x-rays demonstrate a normal bowel gas pattern with no colonic distention.

Recommendation

Upper endoscopy and manometric study.

Case Continued

The upper endoscopy was notable for a dilated esophagus, retained food, and scattered mucosal erythema. No strictures or endoluminal lesions are noted.

Diagnosis

The esophageal manometry identifies an elevated resting pressure and a failure to relax upon swallowing of the lower esophageal sphincter (LES). In addition, there are nonperistaltic contractions of low amplitude involving the body of the esophagus. Diagnosis is achalasia.

Discussion

The different treatment modalities for achalasia include pharmacotherapeutics, botulinum toxin injections, pneumatic dilations, and esophagomyotomy. Botulinum toxin injection results in muscular relaxation at the esophagogastric junction; however, its effect dissipates after 6 to 9 months. Botulinum injection is associated with submucosal scarring, which may complicate future surgical myotomy. Pneumatic dilation could be difficult to perform in this massively dilated esophagus, and esophageal perforation is a concern. Surgical esophagomyotomy offers the best possible results for this patient's long-standing problem.

After the completion of preoperative evaluations, the patient is taken to the operating room and undergoes a left transthoracic Heller's esophagocardiomyotomy with Belsey's fundoplication. The operation and her postoperative course are uneventful until the fourth postoperative day, when the patient develops a temperature of 101.2°F. Her white blood cell count had been steadily rising and is now 16,000 cells/mm^3. On examination, the wound is nonerythematous without drainage. Blood and urine cultures are sent. Chest x-ray shows no pulmonary processes.

Recommendation

Esophagogram to evaluate for a possible esophageal leak.

Case Continued

A contrast esophagram demonstrates extravasation of contrast into the left pleural space with pooling away from the chest tube. The patient is returned to the operating room, where the defect through the mucosa is identified between the diaphragm and the inferior pulmonary vein. The edges of the perforation are débrided and covered with an intercostal muscle flap. The pleural space is copiously irrigated, and a new chest tube is placed in the costovertebral recess adjacent to the repair. Repeat contrast esophagram 10 days later is normal. She is discharged on postoperative day 18.

Discussion

Achalasia is a rare disorder most commonly diagnosed between the third and fourth decades of life. Most cases are of the primary (idiopathic) type, but familial and childhood cases are well documented. It has an estimated incidence of 0.5 cases per 100,000 population, and there is no sex predilection.

The pathophysiologic process is attributable to neuronal abnormalities of various etiologies. The most common postulation is the absence of ganglion cells in the myenteric plexus of the esophagus. Other possibilities include the derangement of postganglionic inhibitory nerve fibers, abnormal extraesophageal vagal innervation, and the loss of vasoactive intestinal peptide (VIP) containing neurons that have potent relaxing effects on the LES.

The patient initially presents with vague symptoms of dysphagia, which then become recurrent and progressive. True regurgitation is rare because of the tight LES, but regurgitation of undigested food from the dilated esophagus is common, especially in the recumbent position, which causes most of the respiratory signs and symptoms.

The two forms of primary achalasia are the more common classic variety and the vigorous type, the main difference being the strength of the amplitude of the tertiary peristaltic waves in the body of the esophagus. Secondary achalasia results from such disease entities as idiopathic intestinal pseudoobstruction, malignancy, postvagotomy achalasia, diabetes mellitus, Chagas' disease, and infiltrative disorders, namely sarcoidosis, amyloidosis, and glycogen storage diseases.

Diagnostic modalities include a chest x-ray, contrast esophagram, upper endoscopy, and manometry. Radionuclide studies may provide an alternative to contrast imaging during follow-up of patients after dilation. The *sine qua non* of diagnosis is the failure of the LES to relax during swallowing.

The four treatment options are palliative at best and seek to relieve the functional obstruction due to an increased LES tone. Treatment with drugs such as the β-agonists, nifedipine, or isosorbide dinitrate is not very effective and has been largely abandoned. These medications are reserved for patients who are too ill to tolerate other treatment modalities. Botulinum toxin injection into the LES provides symptomatic relief for up to 6 months in one half to two thirds of patients, but repeat injections are necessary. Pneumatic dilation under fluoroscopic control disrupts the LES smooth muscle fibers, thereby preventing the sphincter from closing down. Symptomatic relief can be expected in two thirds of patients after a single dilation. Repeat dilations are often necessary. The rate of perforation is estimated at 1.4% to 5%, with a mortality rate of about 1%. Most clinicians initially offer balloon dilation to their patients and refer those who have failed balloon therapy for surgical evaluation.

Surgery employs an open or thoracoscopic approach through the chest or abdomen. Heller described a posterior and an anterior myotomy in 1914. The modified technique employed now is a single anterior myotomy that begins well above the LES and continues 1 cm below it, onto the cardia of the stomach. To be effective, the myotomy must include the circumferential dissection of the mucosa off the inner circular muscle for about 50% of the circumference of the esophagus. The routine addition of an antireflux procedure is controversial. If the myotomy is too short, the risk for persistent dysphagia is high, whereas severe reflux is inevitable when the incision is extended too far below the LES. The decisions and the success of the operation depend largely on the preference and experience of the surgeon. Transhiatal esophagectomy provides an excellent alternative to those patients who fail myotomy. Surgery is the most invasive, yet the most effective, of all the management options because many patients experience permanent relief.

Achalasia, especially if long-standing, is associated with a 5% to 7% risk for esophageal carcinoma that is not favorably altered by any form of treatment. Barrett's epithelial changes may result from postoperative reflux, also increasing the patient's risk for eventually developing esophageal carcinoma. Long-term surveillance of these patients is highly recommended.

case 45

Presentation

A 32-year-old woman who recently immigrated to the United States from Europe received a chest x-ray for the immigration process. She is a nonsmoker and worked as a kindergarten teacher in her homeland. She has no pain and denies cough. There is no family history of cancer. Vital signs are normal. Physical examination is unremarkable.

▪ Chest X-rays

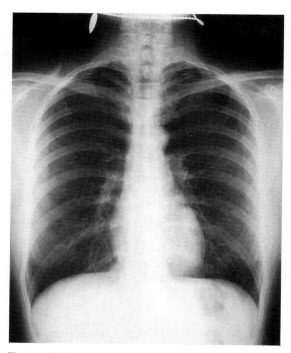

Figure 45-1

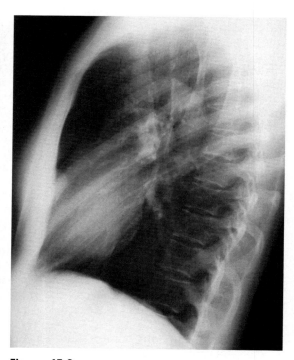

Figure 45-2

Chest X-ray Report

The x-rays show a 2-cm, well-circumscribed nodule in the left lung field. The rest of the lung fields are clear with no other masses or atelectasis. There is no pleural effusion, and the heart size is normal. ▪

Differential Diagnosis

The differential diagnosis includes a number of benign, inflammatory, and malignant conditions. Hamartoma is the most common benign lung tumor, composing 5% of resected nodules. Other benign conditions of the lung include clear cell tumor, chondroma, fibroma, fibromyxoma, sclerosing hemangioma, and granular cell myoblastoma. Inflammatory nodules are more common than benign neoplastic tumors. Most are granulomas that result from prior infection of tuberculosis or fungi, such as *Histoplasma*, *Coccidioides*, or *Blastomycosis* species. Other causes of granulomas that can be multiple or solitary are sarcoidosis, Wegener's granulomatosis, or eosinophilic granuloma.

Recommendation

If available, previous chest x-rays should be obtained for comparison; in addition, computed tomography (CT) scans are indicated to localize the nodule and plan a diagnostic and therapeutic approach.

◼ CT Scans

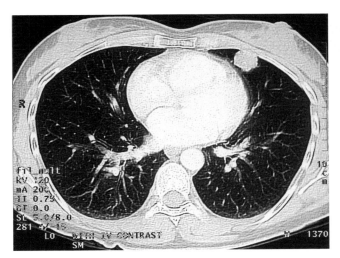

Figure 45-3

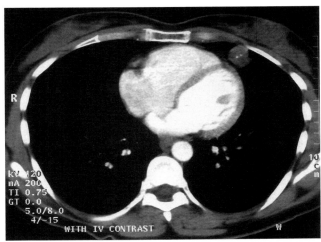

Figure 45-4

CT Scan Report

A 2-cm, well-circumscribed mass with smooth borders is seen. There is discrete central calcification. There are areas of fatty consistency. The rest of the lung fields are clear. There are no enlarged mediastinal lymph nodes. ◼

Discussion

Because the clinical suspicion of malignancy is low, but the patient does not have any previous x-rays, the options are to follow the lesion with repeat CT scan in 4 months, establish a diagnosis by a less invasive approach such as needle biopsy, or proceed with surgical resection. Calcifications demonstrated on CT scan may be present in up to 30% of hamartomas, and fine-needle aspiration may yield a diagnosis in up to 85% of these lesions. However, complications of pneumothorax during CT-guided needle biopsy can occur. Sputum cytology and bronchoscopy have low yield owing to the peripheral location of this mass.

Case Continued

You discuss therapeutic options with the patient. She just moved to this country from Europe and recently married. She plans to start a family and would like to know the diagnosis. You recommend that she undergo surgical resection.

Discussion

The options for surgical excision include video-assisted thoracic surgery (VATS) or open thoracotomy. Given the peripheral location of the tumor and the low suspicion that the tumor is malignant, VATS is a feasible option in this case. VATS will allow adequate nodule resection and tissue diagnosis using small incisions and no rib spreading. The benefits of VATS include decreased postoperative pain, decreased hospital length of stay, and earlier return to normal activities. Intraoperatively, the tumor is sent for frozen-section analysis, and if it is proved malignant, completion lobectomy can then be performed through a lateral thoracotomy or by a VATS technique.

Case Continued

After double-lumen intubation, the patient is positioned in the right lateral decubitus position, and three ports are inserted into the left chest. During the VATS, many thin pleural adhesions are seen and are dissected sharply. The tumor is peripherally located, and although not directly visible, the tumor is marked by some puckering of the visceral pleura. A wedge resection is performed with an endoscopic stapler. The specimen is removed in a plastic bag to avoid contamination. The preliminary frozen-section finding is condromyxoid hamartoma. The left lung is insufflated, and irrigation is used to ascertain that there is no air leak. A single chest tube is placed, and bupivacaine (Marcaine) is injected close to the intercostal nerve to decrease incisional pain after surgery.

The patient is extubated and transferred to a stretcher, at which time the patient begins to have a grand mal seizure lasting 90 seconds. The anesthesiologist administers 5 mg of diazepam intravenously, and the patient is in a postictal state. The patient's airway and ventilation are adequate, and she does not require intubation. Her blood pressure is 120/60 mm Hg, pulse is 106 beats/min and regular, and oxygen saturation is 98% on 2-L nasal canula. She fully awakens 2 hours later, and repeat examination shows no neurologic deficits. Neurology consultation recommends administration of phenytoin (Dilantin) and an electroencephalogram (EEG).

Discussion

The patient most likely had intravascular injection of the bupivacaine at the conclusion of the procedure. The maximum dose of bupivacaine is 3 mg/kg, compared with lidocaine (Xylocaine), for which the maximum dose is 7 mg/kg. Administration of epinephrine (1:100,000) with these drugs provides vasoconstriction, thus delaying absorption of the drug and prolonging the anesthetic effect. Use of epinephrine with lidocaine increase the maximum dose from 4 mg/kg to 7 mg/kg. If accidental intravenous or intraarterial injection occurs, neurologic or cardiovascular effects may occur. In addition to seizures, headache, tinnitus, and confusion may also occur. Cardiovascular complications are the most serious and include severe hypotension from vasodilation, and ventricular fibrillation.

Case Continued

The patient remains in the intensive care unit and is transferred to the floor the next day. She has an uneventful recovery and is discharged on the third postoperative day.

case 46

Presentation

A 48-year-old man who has been living in homeless shelters for the past 3 years presents to the emergency department with a 1-week history of cough and hemoptysis. He was previously diagnosed with tuberculosis (TB) but has been noncompliant with multidrug therapy. Chest x-rays are performed on admission.

Chest X-rays

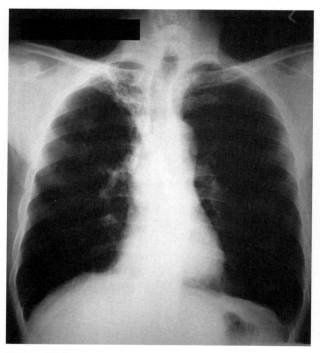

Figure 46-1

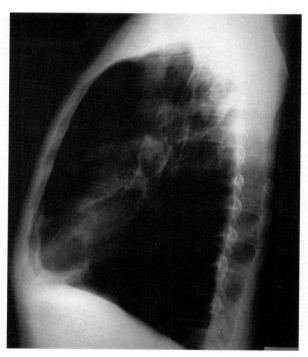

Figure 46-2

Chest X-ray Report

The chest x-rays demonstrate airspace disease in a collapsed right upper lobe with cephalad displacement of the major and minor fissures. There are no pleural effusions. The heart size is normal.

Discussion

These findings are consistent with a chronic infectious process involving the right upper lobe and resulting in the destruction of lung parenchyma. This finding on the chest x-ray is most likely the result of untreated or inadequately treated TB in this middle-aged man who has lived an impoverished lifestyle. Hemoptysis might be due to TB infection, a coexisting bacterial infection, or bronchiectasis in the destroyed lung. A superinfection with fungus, such as *Aspergillus* species, might also account for the hemoptysis. An underlying malignancy should also be considered.

In the United States, the incidence of TB declined at a rate of 6% per year between 1953 and 1984, but since 1985, there has been an increase in the number of cases. This rise in incidence of TB has been attributed to the following factors: (a) the increased incidence of human immunodeficiency virus (HIV) infection, (b) immigration of people from areas of high prevalence of TB to the United States, and (c) social conditions such as homelessness and increased crowding in shelters, nursing homes, and prisons.

In the absence of massive hemoptysis (more than 600 mL within a 24-hour period), chest computed tomography (CT) scans with contrast infusion should be obtained for further evaluation.

CT Scans

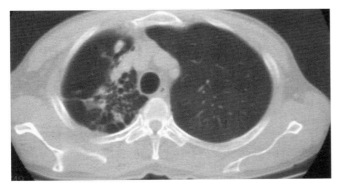

Figure 46-3

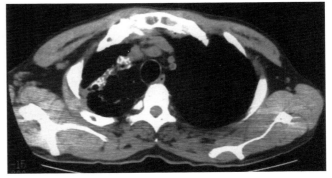

Figure 46-4

CT Scan Report

The chest CT confirms a largely destroyed right upper lobe with evidence of bronchiectasis. There are no enlarged mediastinal lymph nodes, and there is no evidence of pneumothorax or pleural effusions.

Discussion

Although medical therapy offers a complete response with a 5% lifetime risk for relapse, noncompliance with therapy and immunocompromised states are the most common causes of treatment failures. Medical therapy involves 6 months of treatment with isoniazid (INH) and rifampin. In addition, pyrazinamide is administered for the first 2 months of therapy (until the sputum cultures are negative). Occasionally, ethambutol or streptomycin is used as well, in which case the duration of therapy can be shortened to 4.5 to 5 months. Compliance with treatment is the major challenge, especially in patients who are homeless or live in shelters and in patients who are unable or unwilling to participate in a directly observed therapy (DOT) program.

Multiagent treatment is advocated because the incidence of resistance increases with the size of the inoculum as the tubercle bacillus undergoes random spontaneous mutation, making it resistant to single agents fairly readily. In addition, the use of multiagent therapy has been found to accelerate the response and thereby shorten the duration of treatment.

In patients with HIV who have had TB, the relapse rate is about 10% per year. HIV infection is also associated with an increased risk for developing new infection with TB. Most investigators believe that the duration of therapy for primary infection with TB in the HIV-positive group of patients should be 9 months, as opposed to 6 months in HIV-negative patients. A clinical trial is currently underway to assess the optimal duration of therapy in HIV-positive patients with TB.

Before the introduction of effective drug therapy for TB, collapse therapy was used to control the disease. Alexander first proposed collapse therapy in 1925. Thoracoplasty was the form of therapy he described. With the advent of effective drug therapy, the indication for surgical management of TB has waned, and thoracoplasty is rarely used any more. Current indications for surgery include (a) massive hemoptysis (more than 600 mL in 24 hours), (b) bronchopleural fistula, (c) bronchial stenosis, (d) trapped lung, (e) destroyed lung with persistently positive sputum (usually due to resistant organisms), and (f) resection for suspicion of malignancy. When a surgical approach is indicated, surgical resection of the involved lobe or lung is most often required.

Massive hemoptysis can result from bleeding from either a bronchial artery or less often a branch of the pulmonary artery. Emergency surgery is recommended after adequate resuscitation. Bronchoscopy is performed first to identify the source of bleeding. Protection of the uninvolved lung with either a bronchial blocker or double-lumen endotracheal tube is important to minimize aspiration pneumonia. Drug therapy is instituted empirically until intraoperative culture results are available.

In cases in which a bronchopleural fistula (BPF) is found, resection of the involved portion of the lung with muscle flap reinforcement of the bronchial stump is strongly recommended. Either the serratus anterior or latissimus dorsi muscles can be used for this purpose. Occasionally, collaboration with a plastic surgeon is helpful. Whenever possible, surgery should be postponed until multidrug therapy has been administered for 3 months.

Bronchial stenosis is uncommon but, if symptomatic, can be treated with stenting when proximal airways are involved and resection when more distal airways are involved. Whenever possible, multidrug therapy should be started 3 months before resection.

Trapped lung is also an uncommon complication of TB and tuberculous effusions. Tuberculous effusions should be aspirated as completely as possible and multidrug therapy started. Chest tube drainage should be avoided to minimize the risk for secondary bacterial infection and subsequent development of a bronchopleural fistula or trapped lung. When a trapped lung is diagnosed, decortication alone, or more often resection and obliteration of the potential pleural space with a pleural tent or muscle flap transposition, is recommended.

The most common current indication for surgery is the development of resistant microorganisms associated with destroyed lung. When possible, multidrug therapy is recommended before surgery to decrease the number of viable organisms. Despite 3 months of multidrug therapy, about one half of the patients operated on will have a positive sputum culture. Optimizing nutritional status during the preoperative phase has decreased the risk for complications in the postoperative period.

Case Continued

Because the patient has been noncompliant with medical therapy and because of his social situation, he is at a higher than normal risk for recurrent disease, and surgical management of his right upper lobe disease is recommended.

Discussion

Preoperatively, a chest CT scan, pulmonary function testing, and in some cases, a quantitative ventilation-perfusion scan are completed. A double-lumen endotracheal tube and general anesthesia are used. Epidural catheters are placed for postoperative analgesia, and multidrug therapy is continued for 1 to 2 years after surgery (depending on sputum culture results). Extrapleural dissection may be required if extensive inflammation is encountered. Muscle flap reinforcement of the bronchial stump or pneumonectomy stump should be strongly considered in order to minimize the likelihood of a postoperative BPF or a residual pleural space. A muscle flap should be performed if the sputum is positive, there is a preexisting BPF, or if polymicrobial contamination complicates the case.

Case Continued

A right posterolateral thoracotomy is performed through the fourth interspace. A dense inflammatory reaction and destruction of the right upper lobe is evident. The right upper lobe is resected, and the specimen is sent for culture as well as permanent histologic sections. Multidrug therapy is instituted based on sputum culture and sensitivity.

Histologic Evaluation

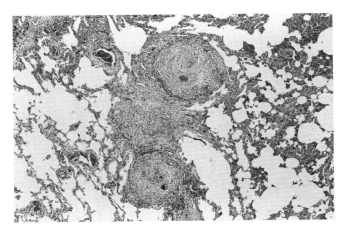

Figure 46-5   See Color Plate 20 following page 114.

Hematoxylin and eosin stain at low power field, demonstrating rounded granulomas within the lung parenchyma.

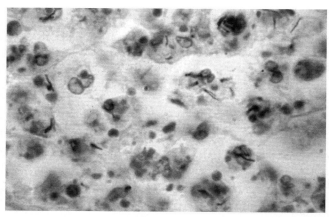

Figure 46-6   See Color Plate 21 following page 114. An acid-fast (Ziehl-Neelsen) stain demonstrating thin, red, rod-shaped mycobacteria organisms.

Presentation

A 78-year-old woman is referred to your office by a primary medical physician with complaints of cough and right shoulder discomfort for the past 8 weeks. Additionally, she relates a history of joint pain and swelling, which has progressively worsened during the past year. The pain is a dull ache and is found in all of her joints. It is worse in her fingers and toes, and she has noticed her nail beds becoming progressively deformed during the same period of time. Her past medical history is significant for two syncopal episodes during the past year, which were found to be hypoglycemic episodes. She denies any history of smoking. There is no history of work-related or environmental exposures. On examination, the lungs are clear, the heart sounds are normal, and there are no murmurs. On examination of the extremities, there is evidence of clubbing of the fingers and toes. She presents with the following chest x-rays.

Chest X-rays

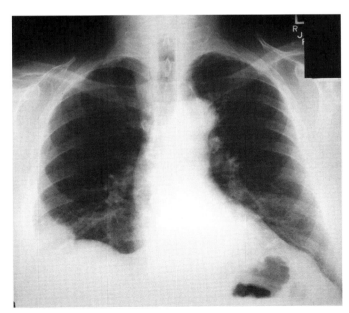

Figure 47-1

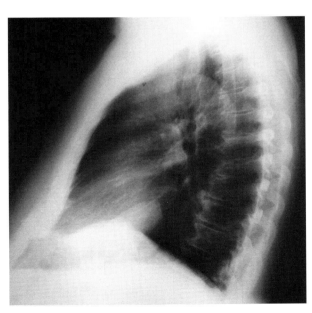

Figure 47-2

Chest X-ray Report

A rounded mass is located in the lateral aspect of the right chest and abuts the right hemidiaphragm. There are no masses in the left lung. The heart size is normal. There are no pleural effusions. ▧

Recommendation

Computed tomography (CT) scans of the chest.

▧ CT Scans

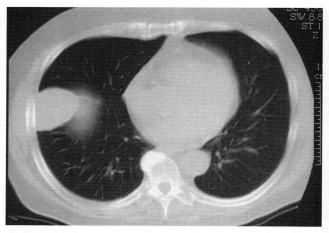

Figure 47-3

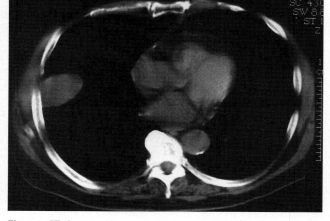

Figure 47-4

CT Scan Report

A smooth, oblong mass is identified in the lateral portion of the right lower lung field. The mass is homogenous and measures 5.4 cm × 4.2 cm in diameter. No other pleural or pulmonary masses are seen. The remaining lung fields are without infiltrate or effusions. The heart and aorta have appropriate opacification without aneurysmal disease. There is no evidence of mediastinal lymphadenopathy. ▧

Differential Diagnosis

The differential diagnosis of this mass includes lung cancer, metastatic tumor, and tumor of pleural origin. The smooth, rounded appearance of the lesion presents a higher likelihood of a benign, slow-growing neoplasm. Metastatic disease may be associated with prior history of a primary neoplasm. The radiologic appearance of a lung cancer is varied and remains a diagnostic possibility. Pleural fibromas are smooth-walled, homogenous masses that can originate from the visceral or, less likely, the parietal pleura. Half of these tumors are pedunculated, enabling them to assume a dependent position. Decubitus x-rays in various positions can identify the tumor's positional changes.

Consideration for histologic diagnosis is made to plan appropriate therapy and further diagnostic evaluation. Because there is no evidence of mediastinal adenopathy, the diagnostic yield of mediastinoscopy is low. Furthermore, bronchoscopy will not yield a diagnosis because the mass is away from the bronchial tree. Other options for obtaining tissue diagnosis include excisional biopsy, or less invasive methods such as fine-needle aspiration or core biopsy with CT guidance. Fine-needle aspiration or core needle biopsy can be performed to obtain histologic confirmation. Additionally, electron microscopy and immunostaining can be performed on a core specimen, which may provide a more specific histologic diagnosis.

Core Needle Biopsy

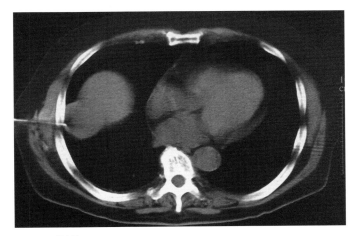

Figure 47-5

Core Needle Biopsy Histologic Report

Sections reveal cylinders of fibrous tissue containing relatively uniform spindle cells with oval nuclei and bland nuclear chromatin. No necrosis is identified. No mitotic activity is identified. Benign mesothelial cells and scant fibrocollagenous tissue are identified. Immunochemical stains are positive for CD34.

Diagnosis

Localized fibrous tumor. No features of malignancy.

Discussion

Fibrous tumors of the pleura are known by a variety of misnomers, including local and fibrous tumors, benign mesothelioma, subpleural or pleural fibroma, and fibromyxoma. These terms suggest the benign nature and mesothelial origin of this tumor. However, histologic and biologic examination of these neoplasms have shown that they have malignant forms and most likely originate in the sub-mesothelial connective tissue of the pleura rather than in the pleura itself. For these reasons, *localized fibrous tumor* is a more proper term. In contrast, diffuse fibrous tumors present as malignant mesothelioma and are related to asbestos exposure. Localized fibrous tumors are not associated with asbestos exposure and are less common. Although invasive forms of localized fibrous tumors exist, most are benign. Benign and invasive forms are determined histologically by the presence of nuclear pleomorphic mitotic activity and high cellularity. Necrosis and hemorrhage are more commonly found in the malignant form.

Localized fibrous tumors of the pleura usually arise from the visceral pleura and are found in various sizes but are commonly larger than 5 cm. These tumors project into the pleural space and compress adjacent lung parenchyma to varying degrees; some may even opacify the entire hemithorax. These neoplasms are rarely intrapulmonary and rarely present as multiple lesions. Most are oblong or spherical in shape and well circumscribed. They are usually attached to the pleura by a vascular pedicle and therefore can fluctuate in the hemithorax with dependency.

Most of these tumors behave in a benign fashion, rarely invading adjacent lung tissue. They are slow growing and in many cases have been followed for several years without resection. Complete surgical excision usually results in a cure; however, recurrences have been reported with inadequate excision. Malignant tumors that are incompletely resected and tumors that recur locally have an unfavorable long-term prognosis. Suggestion of more aggressive tumor behavior includes tumors associated with pleural effusions, tumors arising from the parietal pleura, and tumors with chest wall, mediastinal, and diaphragmatic invasion. Metastasis to extrathoracic structures is rare. Localized tumors of the pleura, which histologically possess atypical cytologic features and a high mitotic rate, are considered malignant; however, some of these tumors can be associated with a favorable prognosis, especially when completely resected.

Patients with pleural fibromas are usually asymptomatic, with the tumor usually found incidentally on chest x-ray. When symptomatic, symptoms of pleural fibromas are related to their large size and compressive effects, such as dyspnea, cough, and chest pain. Moreover, these tumors may manifest paraneoplastic syndromes, such as hypertrophic pulmonary osteoarthropathy and hypoglycemia. Hypoglycemia is caused by secretion of insulin-like peptide and decrease in secretion of glucagons. In this scenario, the patient exhibited symptoms of both. Hypertrophic pulmonary osteoarthropathy is more frequently associated with localized tumors of the pleura than with lung cancer. Excision of the tumor relieves the symptoms of hypertrophic pulmonary osteoarthropathy and hypoglycemia.

Recommendation

Right lateral thoracotomy and excision of the tumor.

Case Continued

Right lateral thoracotomy is performed through the sixth intercostal space. The tumor is found in the major fissure with connections to the visceral pleura of the right lower lobe and the undersurface of the right middle lobe. A GIA stapling device is used to excise the tumor with an adequate margin of lung from the right middle and lower lobes. Anterior and posterior chest tubes are secured in place, and the chest is closed.

Specimen Photograph

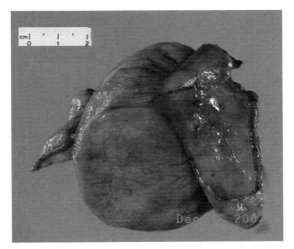

Figure 47-6   See Color Plate 22 following page 114.

Final Pathology Report

Benign localized fibrous tumor of the pleura.

Case Continued

The patient is extubated at the conclusion of the procedure and is transferred to the recovery room. No air leak is present. On the second postoperative day, the chest tubes are removed. The patient is discharged home on the third postoperative day.

Presentation

A 72-year-old man presents with difficulty swallowing and regurgitation of previously swallowed solid foods.

His past medical history is significant for hypertension, coronary artery disease, and stroke. His past surgical history includes a left carotid endarterectomy 3 years ago. Review of systems is significant for weight loss of 15 pounds during the past year. A year ago, the patient suffered a stroke that resulted in right hemiparesis, which has improved with rehabilitation. The patient has had persistent dysphagia and reports feeling that the food is getting stuck in his throat. In addition, he frequently regurgitates undigested food, has foul-smelling breath, and was recently admitted to the hospital for pneumonia.

On physical examination, the patient appears emaciated and debilitated. He is afebrile and hemodynamically stable. There is no cervical adenopathy, and the thyroid gland is not enlarged. A left cervical scar is noted from previous carotid surgery. The lungs are clear, and his cardiac tones are normal. He has moderate right hemiparesis from his stroke. The rest of the examination is unremarkable.

■ Chest X-rays

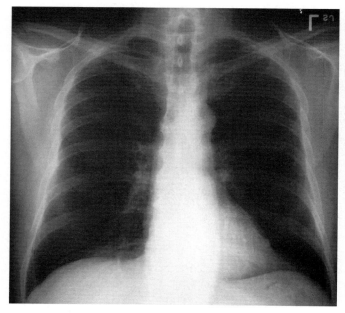

Figure 48-1

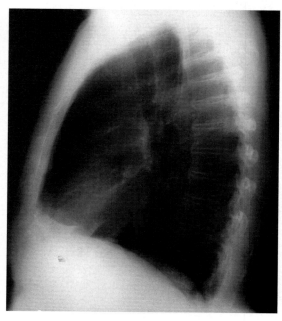

Figure 48-2

Chest X-ray Report

Chest x-rays demonstrate clear lung fields. No masses are evident. The trachea is slightly deviated to the right. ▨

Discussion

Dysphagia and weight loss are common manifestations of esophageal disease.

Achalasia, Barrett's esophagus, diffuse esophageal spasm, diverticula, and esophageal cancers all have to be considered in the differential diagnosis. The characteristics of the refluxed material may be helpful. Spontaneous reflux of undigested food and noisy swallowing are commonly associated with Zenker's diverticulum. The level at which the food bolus appears to lodge may indicate the level of obstruction. An esophagogram is an excellent initial diagnostic modality of choice in patients who present with dysphagia. Computed tomography (CT) scan may also be performed if malignancy is suspected.

▨ Esophagogram

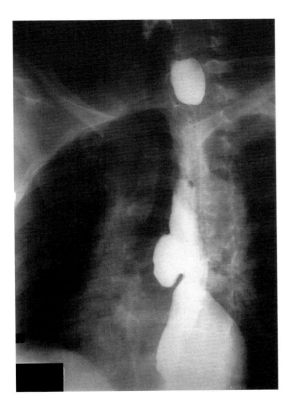

Figure 48-3

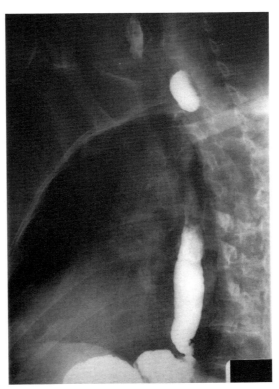

Figure 48-4

Esophagogram Report

The esophagograms seen demonstrate a diverticulum in the proximal esophagus, which remains filled with contrast after most of the contrast has cleared from the esophagus. This finding is characteristic for a Zenker's diverticulum. ▨

Discussion

Diverticula of the esophagus are most commonly acquired and found in adults. Congenital diverticula are rare. These pouches are lined with epithelium and may result from either pulsion or traction forces.

Zenker's diverticulum, or pharyngoesophageal diverticulum, is an acquired disorder that results when the mucosal and submucosal layers herniate through the anatomically weak junction posteriorly between the pharynx and esophagus (Killian's triangle). This may result because of obstructive contractions of the cricopharyngeus muscle. The coordination of all the muscles in deglutition is complex, and the timing of the relaxation of the cricopharyngeus is critical in the normal process of swallowing.

Zenker's diverticulum is a false diverticulum because it does not contain all the anatomic layers of the esophageal wall. The diverticulum extends posteriorly over the cricopharyngeus in the space between the esophagus and the vertebral body and generally enlarges with time; occasionally, it may extend into the mediastinum. Most patients with Zenker's diverticulum are symptomatic. There is a finite amount of space that this sac may occupy before causing extrinsic compression of the esophagus producing symptoms such as dysphagia, regurgitation, and aspiration.

Zenker's diverticula are frequently associated with other esophageal problems such as hiatal hernia, other diverticula, achalasia, or diffuse esophageal spasm.

Epiphrenic, or supradiaphragmatic diverticula are also false diverticula. These occur in the lower esophagus, and many patients are asymptomatic, although some will have dysphagia and regurgitation. Pain may be the clinical feature of epiphrenic diverticula, which may be associated with diffuse esophageal spasm.

Traction diverticula of the mid-esophagus usually result from mediastinal granulomatous diseases, most commonly histoplasmosis and tuberculosis. Because these diverticula contain all the layers of the esophageal wall, including the muscular layer, they are true diverticula. Characteristically, they are much smaller than pulsion diverticula. They have a broad base, and the tapered tip points toward the adhering mediastinal lymph nodes. They are usually asymptomatic. Treatment is usually required if a fistula develops between the esophagus and the tracheobronchial tree. Surgery is directed at division of the fistula and placement of nondiseased tissue between these structures.

Case Continued

The patient is admitted to the hospital for repair of his Zenker's diverticulum, and preoperative laboratory tests and medical clearance are obtained. Because of previous left carotid surgery, the diverticulum is approached through a right cervical approach. The esophagus and diverticulum are difficult to visualize because of their left-sided orientation. With proper retraction and exposure, a cricopharyngeal myotomy and diverticulectomy are performed. A drain is placed, and the patient is transported to the recovery room.

Discussion

No effective medical therapy is available for Zenker's diverticulum. Maneuvers such as sitting upright to assist in postural drainage of the esophagus, or finely chewing the food bolus, may reduce chances of aspiration.

Surgical therapy is indicated in the treatment of Zenker's diverticulum when symptoms are present. Cricopharyngeal myotomy is an important part in the surgical treatment of Zenker's diverticulum. Removal of the diverticulum (diverticulectomy) or suturing the diverticulum (diverticulopexy) to the prevertebral fascia to enable drainage with gravity is performed in addition to a cricopharyngeal myotomy.

Patients with Zenker's diverticulum can have multiple comorbid conditions, and careful preoperative evaluation is required. Surgery should be delayed until treatment of dehydration and evaluation for pneumonia is complete. Although the procedure may be performed with local anesthesia, general anesthesia is preferred to reduce the chances of aspiration with manipulation of the diverticulum.

The patient is positioned supine, and a shoulder roll is placed under the scapulae and the head is turned to the right. A left cervical incision is preferred because the cervical esophagus is to the left side of the neck. The exposure can also be obtained through a collar-type incision; arthritic conditions may limit mobility of the neck.

An incision is made along the anterior border of the sternocleidomastoid muscle and extended through the skin and subcutaneous tissues. The platysma muscle is divided. The incision is centered on the cricoid cartilage (lower than that of a carotid endarterectomy) and extends from the hyoid bone to the jugular notch. The carotid sheath and sternocleidomastoid muscle are retracted laterally. Care must be taken when manipulating the carotid artery and vagus nerve.

The retropharyngeal space is mobilized by creating a plane between the prevertebral fascia and the pharynx. The recurrent laryngeal nerve is found between the esophagus and trachea, and care is required to avoid direct compressive trauma with medial retraction. The inferior thyroid artery, middle thyroid vein, and omohyoid muscle may be divided to facilitate exposure. The cricopharyngeus muscle inserts onto the cricoid cartilage, and the diverticulum arises just proximal to this landmark on the posterior pharynx. The diverticulum can be mobilized by both blunt and sharp dissection.

A cricopharyngeal myotomy is then performed longitudinally through the cricopharyngeus and extended 4 to 5 cm onto the cervical esophagus. A right-angle clamp is used to divide the muscle fibers accurately. The mucosa is separated from the muscle so that half of the circumference of the esophagus is mobilized and the mucosa bulges.

A diverticulectomy is usually performed if the sac is larger than 4 cm. This is done after mobilization of the diverticulum. An automatic stapling device or suture closure may be used. Care must be taken not to retract the pouch aggressively when stapling because this may narrow the esophagus; pouch excision is performed while a 50-French bougie is introduced into the esophagus to prevent lumen narrowing, and a drain is left at the completion of the procedure.

Surgical Approach

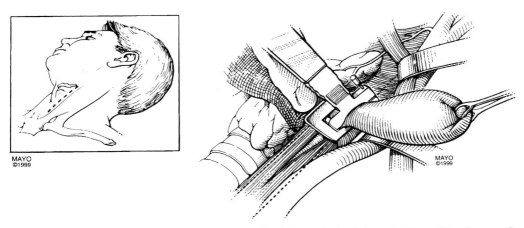

Figure 48-5 Stapled diverticulectomy approached through the left neck. (From Deschamps C, Trastek VF. Esophageal diverticula. In: Shields TW, LoCicero J, Ponn RB, eds. *General thoracic surgery*, 5th ed. Philadelphia: Lippincott Williams & Wilkins, 1999:1843, with permission.)

With diverticulopexy, the sac is sutured with nonabsorbable material to the prevertebral fascia, suspending the diverticulum in the cephalad position (see figure). Diverticulopexy is preferred by some surgeons because the sac is not opened. With this approach, the chance for a leak and contamination of the wound is minimal, and patients may resume their diet on the first postoperative day.

Alternative therapy is peroral pharyngoesophagotomy. This procedure is performed transorally; a GIA stapler is used to divide the tissue between the diverticulum and the esophagus.

Case Continued

On arrival to the recovery room, the patient is experiencing difficulty breathing. Respirations are labored, and he requires reintubation. When passing the endotracheal tube, you notice both vocal cords are in the paramedian position.

Discussion

Recurrent laryngeal nerve injury is the most common postoperative complication following surgery for Zenker's diverticulum, followed by an esophagocutaneous fistula. Patients with single recurrent laryngeal nerve injury usually present with hoarseness with varying degrees of aspiration. Vocal cord injection with Teflon or Gelfoam can be used to mobilize the cord medially. Bilateral cord injury requires control of the airway with endotracheal tube or tracheostomy to prevent inspiratory stridor and aspiration. Nerve function may recover spontaneously in stretch injuries. Permanent tracheostomy or complex laryngeal reconstruction may be required if spontaneous recovery does not occur. Overaggressive retraction from a right-sided approach may have increased the risk for injury of the recurrent nerve in this case.

Presentation

A 14-year-old girl is admitted to the hospital with complaints of a productive cough, fever of 102.3°F, and shortness of breath. The patient has a history of multiple episodes of pneumonia and skin infections due to a diagnosis of Job's syndrome.

Discussion

Job's syndrome, or hyperimmunoglobulin E syndrome, is a disease of abnormal neutrophil and monocyte chemotaxis function manifesting with recurrent infections. Patients experience multiple skin abscesses and recurrent pneumonias. Most infections are caused by *Staphylococcus aureus* and *Candida* species. Pulmonary manifestations can be associated with bronchopleural fistulas and cyst formation. Patients may also have coarse facies, restrictive lung disease, eczematous dermatitis, and scoliosis. The syndrome is inherited by autosomal dominance with variable penetrance.

Case Continued

The patient is admitted to the hospital and started on intravenous antibiotics and oxygen. A chest x-ray is obtained.

◼ Chest X-ray

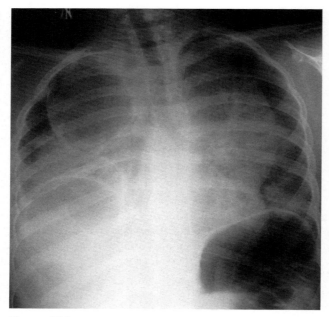

Figure 49-1

Chest X-ray Report

The chest x-ray demonstrates a large cystic mass occupying the upper mediastinum and both pleural spaces. The right costophrenic angle is obscured. A large gastric bubble is demonstrated in the left upper quadrant. ◼

Discussion

Pneumatoceles are thin-walled cavities most often caused by *S. aureus*. Pneumatoceles develop as sequelae of bacterial pneumonias in children. Although less than 3% of bacterial pneumonias in children result in formation of a pneumatocele, more than 80% of *S. aureus* pneumonias result in pneumatocele in the same population. Other organisms associated with pneumatocele formation include *Streptococcus pneumoniae, Haemophilus influenzae, Klebsiella pneumoniae, Serratia marcescens, Escherichia coli*, group A streptococci, *Mycobacterium tuberculosis*, and *Pseudomonas aeruginosa*. Pneumatoceles rapidly develop in areas of previous consolidation. Because of the rapid growth and thin walls, these cavities can rupture into the pleural space, causing a tension pyopneumothorax. In such cases, insertion of a tube thoracostomy can be life saving. Most children present with symptoms typical of pneumonia, such as fever, cough, and dyspnea. The differential diagnosis for children presenting with these symptoms includes bacterial pneumonia, pneumatocele, pulmonary sequestration, cystic adenomatoid malformation, and bronchogenic cyst.

Recommendation

Blood cultures, sputum cultures, and broad-spectrum antibiotics.

Case Continued

By the second hospital day, the patient is still febrile, with a temperature of up to 101.7°F. The white blood cell count is 22,000/mm³, and blood culture grows *S. aureus*.

Recommendations

Computed tomography (CT) scans of the chest to evaluate for abscess.

CT Scans

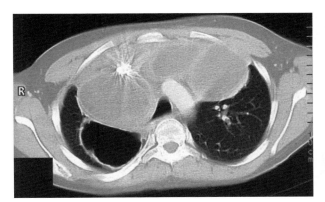 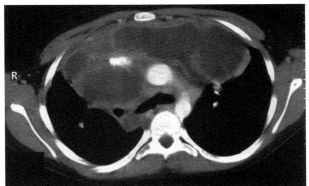

Figure 49-2   **Figure 49-3**

CT Scan Report

CT scans of the chest confirm the presence of a multiloculated cystic mass occupying the anterior mediastinum, extending into both hemithoraces, with compression atelectasis of the right lung. On additional images, the right lung demonstrates the presence of two pneumatoceles, one in the right upper lobe and another in the right lower lobe.

Case Continued

After the CT scan, the patient is more dyspneic, with an oxygen saturation of 82%. She is intubated and transferred to the pediatric intensive care unit for further treatment. Interventional radiology is consulted for possible percutaneous catheter drainage; however, based on the CT scan finding of loculated cysts, percutaneous drainage is not attempted.

Recommendation

The cystic mass is most likely an infected cyst that is occupying a large volume of the chest resulting in hypoxia and dyspnea. Resection of the cystic mass is necessary if the patient is not a candidate for percutaneous drainage. Because the cysts extend into both hemithoraces from the mediastinum, and access to both pleural spaces is necessary, the planned surgical approach is through a bilateral anterior thoracosternotomy (clamshell incision) rather than a standard median sternotomy.

Operative Findings

A bilateral anterior thoracosternotomy is performed. A massive cystic lesion is present that not only involves the anterior mediastinum but also completely wraps around the superior vena cava, trachea, and arch vessels. The cyst fills most of the right chest and the upper aspect of the left chest. The portions of the cyst in the right lower chest are filled with purulent material, but no obvious communication is present with the lung. The cyst is resected in its entirety, with care taken to preserve both phrenic nerves. The pneumatoceles are not resected in order to preserve lung tissue. The expectation is that the pneumatoceles will resolve with long-term conservative management.

Postoperative Chest X-ray

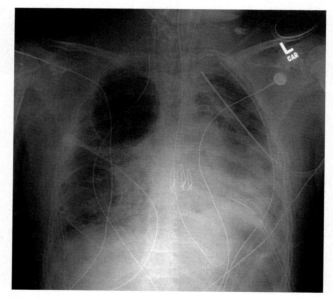

Figure 49-4

Chest X-ray Report

The postoperative films demonstrate a right-sided pneumatocele as well as a right-sided consolidation. Bilateral tube thoracostomy is present. An endotracheal tube is above the carina. Three sternal wires are visible.

Discussion

Pneumatoceles are believed not to represent a true lung abscess. In most circumstances, with control of infection, most pneumatoceles will eventually close, although the time frame can be variable. Surgical resection is not indicated if the cavity has not ruptured into the pleural space and there is no empyema present. In this case, additional concerns are raised regarding potential space issues and postoperative empyema if both of the pneumatoceles are resected. Conserving lung parenchyma is important in patients with a congenital abnormality and a predisposition for future lung infections.

Pathology Report

The final pathology demonstrates a large cystic mass with extensive necrosis, chronic inflammation, and foreign-body giant cell reaction with marked proliferation of foamy histiocytes. ▪

Case Continued

The patient is maintained on the ventilator until her pain management is controlled. Antibiotics are continued, and she is nutritionally supported. The patient's oxygen requirements slowly decrease, and she is successfully extubated on the tenth postoperative day. The patient continues to improve and is discharged home. She is maintained on chronic antibiotic therapy. She continues to complain of mild dyspnea on exertion. Her follow-up chest x-rays continue to demonstrate right-sided pneumatoceles. Surgical resection may be considered in the future.

▨ Chest X-rays

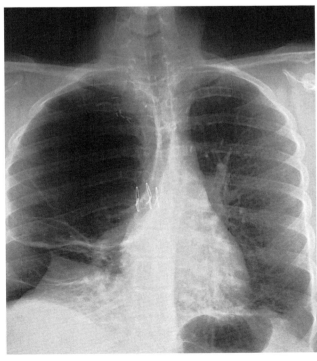

Figure 49-5

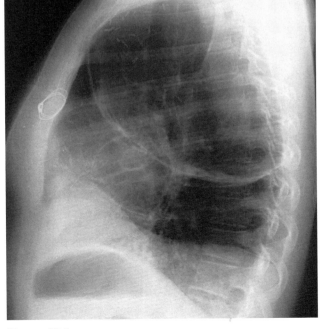

Figure 49-6

case ■ 50

Presentation

A 52-year-old woman with no significant past medical history presents to your office after she was seen by her primary medical doctor with symptoms of ptosis and diplopia. She is a nonsmoker. On examination, there are decreased breath sounds over the left lung field. The patient presents with the following chest x-rays.

■ Chest X-rays

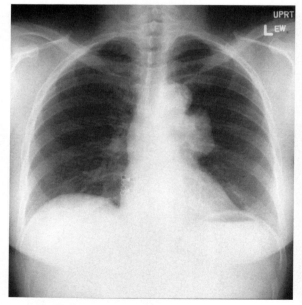

Figure 50-1

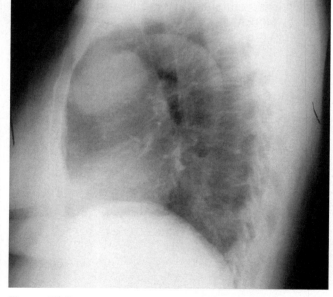

Figure 50-2

Chest X-ray Report

Lung fields are clear; the heart is of normal size. Both diaphragms are visualized. A round anterior mediastinal mass is present. ■

Differential Diagnosis

The differential diagnosis for anterior mediastinal masses in the adult includes thymoma, lymphoma, thyroid, and germ cell tumor. In children, the differential diagnosis for mediastinal masses includes germ cell tumors and lymphoma. In this patient with symptoms of ptosis, diplopia, and an anterior mediastinal mass, one must consider myasthenia gravis to be the primary diagnosis.

Discussion

Fifteen percent of patients with myasthenia gravis have a thymoma. In contrast, 30% to 50% of patients with thymoma have myasthenia gravis. The incidence of thymoma is equal in male and female patients. This is in contrast to myasthenia gravis, in which the female-to-male ratio is 2:1. Symptoms may include ptosis, ophthalmoplegia, dysarthria, and dysphagia. Severity of weakness increases during the day, especially after use of affected muscle groups. The syndrome is characterized by autoantibodies to acetylcholine (ACH) receptors. In addition, the ACH receptor concentration at the neuromuscular end plate is reduced.

The initial diagnostic test is the Tensilon test (edrophonium chloride), which is a short-acting anticholinesterase. Response to the Tensilon test is within 45 to 60 seconds; patients may also experience salivation, sweating, and nausea. Blood tests for antibodies against ACH receptors are elevated in most patients. Normal levels of ACH receptor antibody do not exclude the diagnosis of myasthenia gravis. Other tests may include repetitive nerve stimulation and single-fiber electromyography.

Medical treatment of myasthenia gravis may include the following: pyridostigmine (Mestinon), neostigmine bromide (Prostigmin), steroids, azathioprine (Imuran), cyclosporine, plasma exchange, and intravenous immune globulin. Thymectomy results in remission in up to 50% of patients. Patients with improved outcome after thymectomy are young, female, do not require steroids, and have had a short preoperative medical course. Intraoperative findings include lymphoid hyperplasia in 70%, thymic atrophy in 15%, and neoplastic thymoma in 15%.

Recommendation

Tensilon test as well as computed tomography (CT) scans of the chest.

Case Continued

The patient has a positive Tensilon test, and the following CT scans.

CT Scans

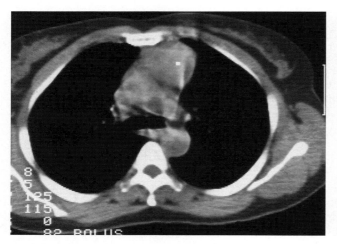

Figure 50-3

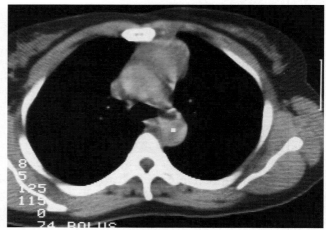

Figure 50-4

CT Scan Report

A 3-cm × 4-cm homogenous mass in the anterior mediastinum, which does not involve the lung or heart structures. ■

Diagnosis and Recommendation

Myasthenia gravis with thymoma. The patient is offered a thymectomy, which will be performed through a median sternotomy. The patient is informed that relief of symptoms is expected in 75% of patients.

It is explained to the patient that symptoms may not improve for an extended period of time and that she will need to continue her current medications postoperatively to control her symptoms. Complications include bleeding, infection, phrenic nerve palsy, and death.

Surgical Approach

It is critical to perform a complete thymectomy to remove the tumor and all thymic tissue in order to provide for the best possible outcome. A median sternotomy is performed, the pleura on both sides are opened, and the phrenic nerves are carefully identified. The thymus is sharply dissected off the pericardium in its entirety. Any area that is involved must be resected. A single 28-French chest tube is placed at the conclusion of the operation, which is usually removed on the first or second postoperative day.

Case Continued

A sternotomy is performed, and the thymus is found to be grossly enlarged. Areas of invasion are apparent at the left phrenic nerve as well as the pericardium on the left side. The patient undergoes a total thymectomy with resection of a portion of the pericardium and the left phrenic nerve.

Discussion

Thymomas are staged based on invasion of surrounding tissue. In stage I, the mass has an intact capsule; most thymomas are in this category. Stage II thymomas have local invasion of the pleura, phrenic nerve, or pericardium. Stage III thymomas have gross invasion, such as to the lung or aorta. Stage IV thymomas have disseminated disease, with stage IVA being intrathoracic and stage IVB being extrathoracic. This patient's thymoma has invasion of the phrenic nerve and pericardium and is categorized as stage II. Radiation is offered to patients with thymomas of stage II or higher. Chemotherapy may be used in stage IV thymomas under clinical protocol.

Case Continued

At the conclusion of the procedure, the patient is extubated and transferred to the recovery room. Two hours after surgery, the patient is noted to be in marked respiratory distress requiring intubation and mechanical ventilation.

Approach

In this patient with myasthenia gravis, two main issues may be contributing to her respiratory distress. Initially, narcotics should be excluded as the cause for respiratory failure. The patient may have received an excessive dose of narcotics in the recovery room for pain management. More importantly, a patient with myasthenia gravis may be experiencing a myasthenic crisis. A neurologic consultation should be obtained urgently, and consideration should be given to treatment with plasma exchange. Finally, because the left phrenic nerve was sacrificed, the patient may be experiencing respiratory distress due to paralysis of the diaphragm. The patient should be transferred to the intensive care unit. A chest x-ray and blood gas should be obtained.

Case Continued

The chest x-ray shows no evidence of pneumothorax; the chest tube is in the proper position. The endotracheal tube is 2 cm above the level of the carina. The patient receives plasma exchange and slowly recovers over the next 3 days. She is then extubated and discharged on her preoperative medications. The patient's neurologist continues a slow taper of her preoperative medications in the ensuing months. She is scheduled to receive radiation therapy by the radiation oncologist.

case 51

Presentation

A young man, 18 years old, is referred to your office by his family physician with a report of an abnormal chest x-ray finding. His chief complaint is progressively worsening weakness of the right hand and numbness of the right triceps muscle area. The patient reports that his right arm is heavy and that the shoulder is painful with exercise. He has fever and night sweats on occasion but no cough, chills, hemoptysis, or weight loss. He has been a one-pack-per-day smoker for the past 5 years. On examination, his vitals are stable except for a temperature of 100.5°F. There is fullness at the right base of the neck but no discrete mass. The breath sounds are decreased at the apex of the right lung field. The right scapular area is raised, and the right arm shows reproducible pain on abduction.

Chest X-rays

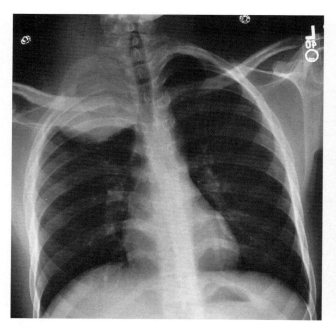

Figure 51-1

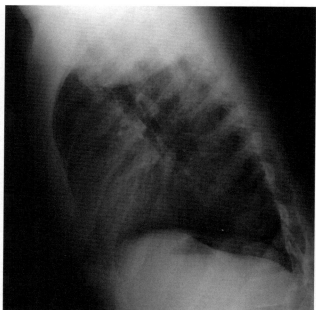

Figure 51-2

A well-circumscribed mass is present in the right upper chest. A soft tissue density is seen at the right side of the neck. There are no other masses, mediastinal abnormalities, or pleural effusions. ▨

Recommendation

Computed tomography (CT) scans.

▨ CT Scans

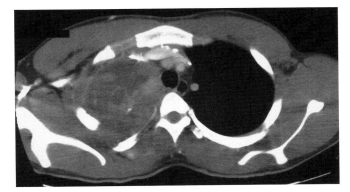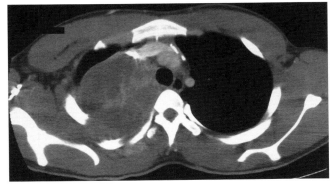

Figure 51-3   **Figure 51-4**

CT Scan Report

The CT scans of the chest demonstrate a large, infiltrative, heterogeneous mass with multiple areas of necrosis arising from the right upper lung. It extends into the adjacent soft tissue of the right upper back between the ribs and the scapula. There is bony destruction of the right transverse processes of T1 and T2, the accompanying ribs, and possibly the scapula. The superior vena cava is distorted, but the arch vessels, although shifted to the left, are otherwise uninvolved. The tumor abuts but does not appear to invade the trachea. ▨

Differential Diagnosis

The patient has a soft tissue shadow at the right neck, tumor occupying the apex of the right lung including the posterior mediastinum, and tumor at the posterior chest wall. Because of the destruction of adjacent bony structures, the tumor is most likely malignant. The differential diagnosis includes neurogenic tumors, chest wall tumors, primary lung carcinoma, osteomyelitis, and metastatic disease. The most common malignant neurogenic tumors include ganglioneuroblastoma, neuroblastoma, malignant schwannoma, malignant pheochromocytoma, and malignant paraganglioma. The list of malignant chest wall tumors includes myeloma, malignant fibrohistiocytoma, chondrosarcoma, rhabdomyosarcoma, Ewing's sarcoma, plasmacytoma, liposarcoma, neurofibrosarcoma, osteogenic sarcoma, hemangiosarcoma, leiomyosarcoma, and lymphoma.

Recommendation

After the history, physical examination, and review of the chest x-rays, it is recommended to the patient that histologic diagnosis is necessary for further treatment planning. Based on the location and the extent of the tumor, specimen may be obtained by incisional biopsy, Tru-Cut needle biopsy, transbronchial biopsy, or fine-needle aspiration.

Discussion

Adequate tissue sampling is mandatory. Small (3 to 4 cm) primary tumors are diagnosed and treated by resection with a 2- to 4-cm margin. If the tumor is found to be malignant on final pathologic examination, a wide radical excision is required, and the patient is returned to the operating room where the biopsy site is completely excised and included in a 2- to 4-cm margin. Primary chest wall or soft tissue masses larger than 4 cm are diagnosed by an incisional biopsy. The skin incision is positioned in a location that will be included in future resection, if more extensive resection is necessary.

Case Continued

The patient is taken to the operating room for bronchoscopy, followed by an incisional or Tru-Cut needle biopsy of the mass. At induction of general anesthesia, the patient becomes profoundly bronchospastic and unresponsive to pharmacologic intervention. Poor visualization of the airway does not enable the anesthesiologist to intubate the patient successfully. Fiberoptic intubation is attempted but abandoned because of oxygen desaturation. A cricothyroidotomy is emergently performed and a 6-French endotracheal tube inserted. After a few seconds, the patient's oxygenation improves. After a normal bronchoscopic examination, the patient is placed in a left lateral decubitus position, and Tru-Cut needle biopsies of the mass are performed at the transverse mid-scapular line just lateral to the vertebral column. The patient is transferred to the recovery room, where he is extubated on the first postoperative day. However, as a precautionary measure, the cricothyroidotomy tube is not removed until the second postoperative day.

Pathology Report

Ewing's sarcoma. ▪

Discussion

Chest wall tumors present as asymptomatic, slowly enlarging masses, but in nearly all malignant tumors, pain eventually occurs. On rare occasions, accompanying signs and symptoms include fever, leukocytosis, and eosinophilia.

Magnetic resonance imaging (MRI) studies and CT scans are complementary in the evaluation of chest wall tumors, but often, it is not necessary to obtain both exams. MRI is preferred because it can distinguish the tumor from nerves and blood vessels. In addition, MRI enables visualization of the tumor in coronal or sagittal planes, which may be useful in preoperative planning. CT scans are better for assessing pulmonary nodules.

Ewing's sarcoma of the rib cage makes up 10% to 15% of all primary malignant neoplasms of the bony thorax. When it presents in this location, it generally has a worse prognosis than a primary in a long bone of an extremity because metastases to the lungs occur in about half of cases. Only one third of all cases of Ewing's sarcoma occur in patients older than 20 years of age. It is most common in adolescence and has a peak incidence in the second decade of life. It is an uncommon tumor in young infants. The male-to-female ratio is 2:1. Signs and symptoms are common and include a painful enlarging mass, fever, malaise, anemia, leukocytosis, and an elevated erythrocyte sedimentation rate (ESR). Radiating spicules on the surface of the bone and "onion peel" appearance of the surface of bone are common but nonpathognomonic features of Ewing's sarcoma.

This tumor is a great masquerader because radiographically it may be confused with osteogenic sarcoma, its clinical presentation may be similar to osteomyelitis, and histologically it may be indistinguishable from lymphoma, embryonal rhabdomyosarcoma, or small cell carcinoma.

Treatment of Ewing's sarcomas includes a trimodality therapy with chemotherapy, surgery, and radiation. Some of the very active chemotherapeutic agents are ifosfamide, mesna, etoposide, doxorubicin, cyclophosphamide, vincristine, and dactinomycin. Both surgery and radiotherapy may control local disease, but without consequent cytostatic chemotherapy, all patients will eventually succumb to distant metastases. Early spread to the bone marrow, other bones, and lungs occurs in 30% to 75% of patients. Overall 5-year survival rate is 40% to 50%.

Case Continued

The patient receives 14 cycles of chemotherapy. Repeat CT scan demonstrates shrinkage of the tumor by 60%. The patient is taken to the operating room, where a right posterolateral thoracotomy and resection of the mass with segments of the second, third, and fourth ribs are performed. No reconstruction is necessary because the scapula is not resected. After surgery, the patient recovers well and is discharged on the fourth postoperative day. After a 2-week recovery, the patient is scheduled to receive 6 weeks of radiation therapy.

case 52

Presentation

A 77-year-old man with a past medical history significant for hypertension presents to his primary care physician with complaints of left-sided chest pain. The patient denies cough, hemoptysis, fever, chills, night sweats, anorexia, and weight loss. He is a nonsmoker. He reports a previous episode of left-sided chest pain, about 10 years ago, at which time he was diagnosed with a chest x-ray abnormality that has been followed with serial computed tomography (CT) scans and no recommended intervention.

▨ Chest X-rays

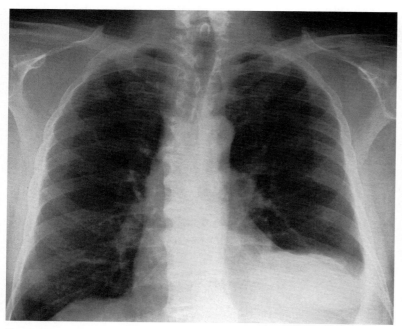

Figure 52-1

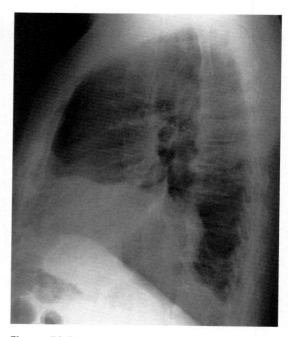

Figure 52-2

Chest X-ray Report

Chest x-rays demonstrate a large density obliterating the left heart border. There are no masses in the lung field. The left costophrenic angle is blunted. Review of previous chest x-rays from 4 years ago demonstrated a smaller density in the left hemithorax. ▤

▤ CT Scans

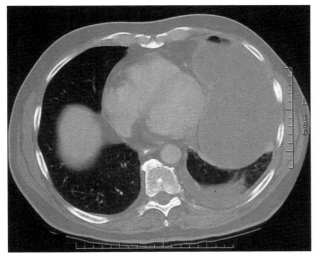 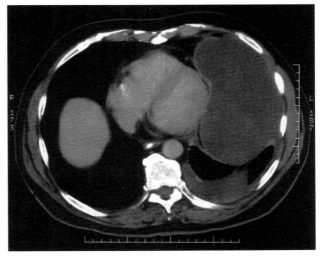

Figure 52-3   **Figure 52-4**

CT Scan Report

There is a loculated fluid collection in the left lower thorax measuring 15 cm × 8 cm. There is a small to moderate amount of free-flowing left-sided pleural fluid. On the CT scan performed 10 years earlier, the cyst measured 5 cm and was associated with minimal atelectasis of the left lower lobe. Serial CT scans are evaluated that demonstrate a gradual increase in size. The last scan, performed 4 years before the current study, measured the cyst at 16.5 cm, which was associated with minimal atelectasis. ▤

Discussion

The mediastinum is divided into superior, anterior, middle (visceral), and posterior compartments. Cystic lesions of the mediastinum can arise from any compartment of the mediastinum but typically are related to structures within the middle mediastinum. The middle (visceral) mediastinum is the area of mediastinum between the anterior and posterior pericardium. The contents of the visceral mediastinum include the heart, pericardium, phrenic nerves, trachea, and lymph nodes. Pericardial cysts appear as well-demarcated densities, less commonly with air–fluid levels when they have a communication with the respiratory or gastrointestinal tracts. Cystic lesions of the mediastinum are more commonly symptomatic in infants and young children because of obstruction of the tracheobronchial tree or esophagus. Most mediastinal cysts in adults are incidental findings not requiring intervention.

Case Continued

The patient is referred to a pulmonologist because of the chest pain and development of a new free-flowing effusion. A thoracentesis is performed and reveals a transudative effusion. The cytologic evaluation of the fluid demonstrates reactive mesothelial cells in a background of chronic inflammation and many eosinophils.

Recommendation

Because the pleural fluid shows no evidence of malignancy and the patient's pain subsides, no intervention is necessary at this time.

Case Continued

In the intervening 2 months, the patient had developed a new atrial tachyarrhythmia and had undergone electrophysiologic evaluation. He received an antiarrhythmic medication. Upon further questioning, the patient admits to persistence of the left-sided chest pain, which increases with respiration. The repeat CT scan is unchanged from the prior study. After further discussion with the patient, surgical management of the cyst is planned.

Approach

Size of the pericardial cyst is the limiting factor in considering a minimally invasive approach. Cystic lesions that have achieved a large size limit visibility in the chest and may require decompression before thoracoscopic resection. The planned approach is to attempt a thoracoscopic decompression and resection; given the size limitation, the possibility of a thoracotomy is discussed with the patient preoperatively.

Case Continued

Intraoperatively, the patient is intubated using a double-lumen endotracheal tube, and the patient is positioned in the right lateral decubitus position. Three ports are used: a lower port in the seventh interspace for the camera and two working ports in the fourth interspace, one in the anterior axillary line and the other in the posterior axillary line. On inspection, a moderate amount of straw-colored pleural fluid is present in the left chest. The cyst itself is thick walled and appears to arise from the cardiophrenic angle. The cyst is grasped with two clamps, and a small opening is created. Thin, dark-brown fluid is drained from the cyst, which decompresses the cyst completely. The cyst is densely adherent to the pericardium and diaphragm but not adherent to the lung. The pericardium is entered in order to resect the cyst completely, with care taken to avoid the phrenic nerve. No intrapericardial abnormalities are identified. Cultures of all fluid specimens are negative. Pathologic analysis reveals a mesothelial cyst with evidence of chronic inflammation and hemorrhage.

Discussion

Mesothelial cysts have an incidence of roughly 1 in 100,000 people. Pericardial or pleuropericardial cysts are located in the right cardiophrenic angle in 50% to 70% of cases, on the left in 20% to 30%, and in other parapericardial locations in the remainder. Anatomically, the anterior cardiophrenic angle is bounded by the pericardium medially, the chest wall anteriorly, the pleura laterally, the phrenic nerve posteriorly, and the diaphragm inferiorly.

The differential diagnosis of abnormalities in this location includes foramen of Morgagni hernia, ventricular aneurysms, mediastinal tumors, and diaphragmatic tumors or eventrations. It has been estimated that only 20% of these cysts are symptomatic, with the most common symptoms being dyspnea and chest pain. It has been observed that symptoms rarely resolve completely unless the cyst is very large.

With the improved resolution of CT scanning, incidentally identified asymptomatic cysts do not require any further intervention. Should the diagnosis remain in question, percutaneous aspiration is performed to confirm the diagnosis. Surgical resection can be performed when the diagnosis is uncertain or when the patient is experiencing symptoms from a large pericardial cyst.

case 53

Presentation

A 73-year-old man is referred to your office because of an incidental finding on a chest x-ray. The patient denies cough, fever, chills, weight loss, and appetite changes. He has a 50-pack-per-year smoking history and a past medical history of diabetes mellitus. On physical examination, there are diminished breath sounds at the bases of the lungs bilaterally. The following chest x-rays and computed tomography (CT) scan are obtained.

Chest X-rays

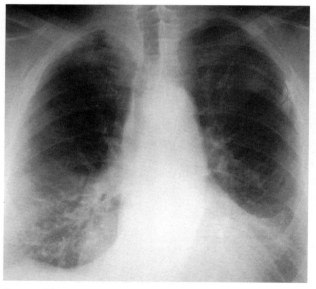

Figure 53-1

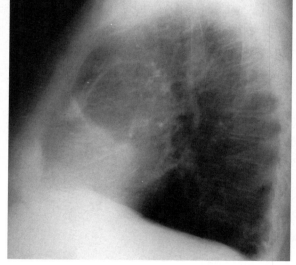

Figure 53-2

Chest X-ray Report

The chest x-rays demonstrate a left upper lobe mass measuring 2.5 cm. There is bilateral apical and pleural thickening along the lateral aspect of the hemithoraces.

CT Scan

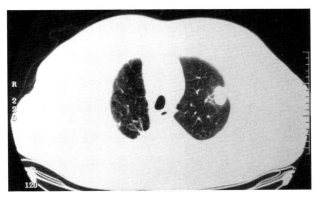

Figure 53-3

CT Scan Report

The CT scan demonstrates a 2.7-cm × 3.2-cm mass in the peripheral portion of the left upper lobe. There are no other masses or infiltrates in the rest of the lung fields, and there are no pleural effusions. On additional images, there is no evidence of mediastinal adenopathy.

Discussion

The lung mass in a 73-year-old smoker is highly suspicious for malignancy. Sputum cytology, diagnostic fiberoptic bronchoscopy, fine-needle aspiration (FNA) of the mass under CT guidance, core needle biopsy under CT guidance, and excisional biopsy are modalities that enable the clinician to obtain tissue for diagnosis. Sputum cytology has a sensitivity of 20% to 70%; however, if the mass is peripheral, the yield for sputum cytology is small. The yield is higher when the tumor involves a main bronchus and when the patient presents with a productive cough or hemoptysis. Squamous cell cancer is more often diagnosed on sputum cytology than adenocarcinoma or small cell cancer. When sputum cytology identifies malignant cells, the specific cell type can be identified in 85% of the patients. Bronchoscopy has a high diagnostic yield if the tumor can be visualized in the endobronchial tree. Biopsy and brushings of a peripheral lesion yield a positive result in 25% of cases. Transthoracic FNA and core biopsy are applicable for peripheral lesions with a diagnostic accuracy of 80% to 95%. All of these diagnostic modalities are acceptable but do have a false-negative rate. For this reason, many surgeons would elect to perform an excisional biopsy either by video-assisted thoracoscopic surgery (VATS) or thoracotomy in order to obtain a proper tissue specimen for diagnosis. Achieving a diagnosis of cancer by less invasive means before thoracotomy allows for clinical staging and proper treatment planning such as preoperative chemoradiation in patients with positive (N2) lymph nodes on mediastinoscopy. Patients with negative needle biopsy may require surgical biopsy to verify that the mass is benign, if the clinical suspicion for cancer is high.

Recommendation

CT-guided FNA to prove the presence of cancer in this older patient.

◾ CT-guided Fine-Needle Aspiration

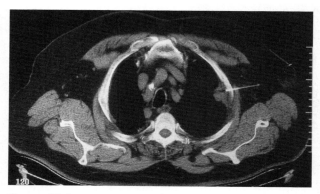

Figure 53-4

Pathology Report

The specimen contains many histiocytes, few lymphocytes, and fibroconnective tissue that are consistent with benign fibrous histiocytic lesion. No malignant cells are identified.

Case Continued

The patient is told that although the needle biopsy was negative for tumor, an open lung biopsy should be performed. The patient refuses to undergo a surgical procedure and returns in 6 months with a dry cough. The following CT scans and PET scans are obtained.

◾ CT Scans

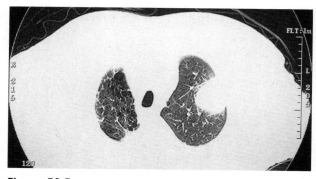

Figure 53-5

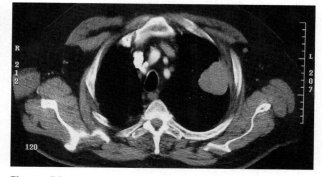

Figure 53-6

CT Scan Report

The mass lesion in the periphery of the left upper lobe has increased in size and is now measuring 5.1 cm × 4.2 cm. There is parenchymal scarring in the right upper lobe. There are no pleural effusions; however, there is pleural thickening within the anterior aspect of the right upper hemithorax.

PET Scan

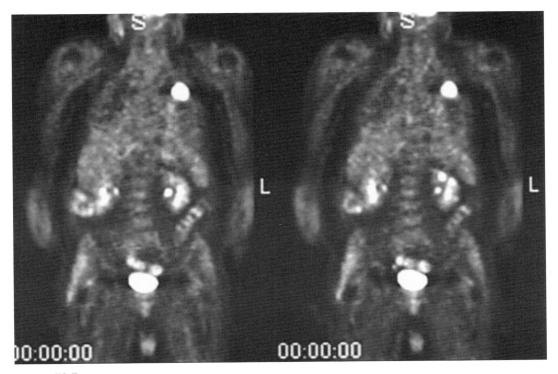

Figure 53-7

PET Scan Report

There is intense uptake of radioactivity in the left upper lobe measuring 8.7 standardized uptake value (SUV), which corresponds to the mass demonstrated on the CT scans of the chest. This finding is highly suggestive of malignancy. There is no evidence of uptake in the mediastinum, right hemithorax, or adrenal glands.

Discussion

When the diagnosis of malignancy is highly suspected and operative resection is contemplated, three questions should be asked:

1. Does clinical staging indicate that a complete resection can be accomplished?
2. How extensive an operation is required to obtain a complete resection?
3. Can the patient withstand the operation?

Pulmonary resection causes many physical and hemodynamic changes. After resection, the size of the pulmonary vascular bed is reduced, which causes increased pulmonary vascular resistance and stress on the right heart. Patients who have marginal cardiac status may decompensate. Additionally, splinting from pain, inability to clear secretions, and increased work of breathing can all contribute to respiratory failure and may potentiate cardiac problems. Lobectomy in a patient older than 70 years of age carries a mortality rate of 5% to 7%. If a patient sustains a postoperative myocardial infarction, the risk for death increases to almost 50%; therefore, preoperative evaluation of a patient's physical status is imperative.

Forced vital capacity (FVC) reflects compliance of the lungs. Forced expiratory volume in 1 second (FEV_1) reflects obstructive disease. These values together are used to diagnose restrictive lung disease. Diffusing capacity of lung for carbon monoxide (DcLO) is performed by holding a breath of dilute carbon monoxide for 10 seconds and then exhaling. This evaluates the integrity of the alveolar capillary membrane and the pulmonary capillary blood volume and reveals decreased surface area for gas exchange. Studies have shown that DcLO is the best predictor of pulmonary complications. Elevated partial pressure of carbon dioxide in the blood (Pco_2) is associated with chronic respiratory insufficiency. Finally, maximal voluntary ventilation is performed by calculating the volume of air ventilated in a period of 12 seconds. This reflects airflow, pulmonary mechanics, respiratory muscle strength, and endurance.

After pulmonary function tests (PFTs) are performed, postoperative function can be extrapolated based on the proposed pulmonary resection. Normally, lung ventilation is 55% on the right and 45% on the left. Each lobe on the left accounts for about 22.5% of lung function, and each lobe on the right roughly accounts for 18.3%. Predicted postoperative PFTs can be determined by reducing the numbers by the percentage of resected lung. This is critical because 800 mL and 35% of predicted postoperative FEV_1 are used as the lower limits of resectability.

A more accurate means of determining predicted postoperative lung function is a quantitative ventilation-perfusion scan. Exercise testing and maximum oxygen consumption (VO_{2max}) are excellent predictors of postoperative morbidity and mortality. In fact, one study showed that a true VO_{2max} of more than 15 mL/kg/min is predictive of increased mortality and complications such as cardiac arrhythmias, pneumonia, and atelectasis. A careful history can identify patients with reduced oxygen consumption. Patients who report the ability to climb three flights of stairs successfully have a shorter length of stay and a reduced number of postoperative complications.

PFTs should be used to screen patients for surgery, but not to exclude them from surgery. Because PFTs are highly variable and dependent on patient cooperation, additional studies should be performed in those patients who perform poorly on PFTs to determine resectability. Patient motivation is also important in assessing operability.

Case Continued

PFTs reveal an FEV_1 of 2.67 L (79% of predicted) and a DLCO of 29.92 (63% of predicted). The patient undergoes a posterolateral thoracotomy through the fifth intercostal space. On examination, the tumor is adherent to the parietal pleura. A needle biopsy is performed, and pathologic analysis reveals adenocarcinoma. The left upper lobe, parietal pleura, and mediastinal lymph nodes are resected. Final pathology reveals poorly differentiated adenocarcinoma. Bronchial and vascular margins are free of any microscopic cancer. All lymph nodes (levels 5, 6, 7, and 11) are negative for cancer. The visceral pleura is invaded by the cancer, but the parietal pleura is not involved; therefore, this is a stage IB lung cancer.

The patient tolerates the procedure well, although intensive postoperative respiratory support is required to assist with the clearing of secretions. The patient recovers uneventfully and is discharged on the sixth postoperative day.

Presentation

A 40-year-old man with no significant past medical history is referred by a primary medical physician for evaluation of an abnormal chest x-ray finding. The patient reports an episode of chest pain accompanied by fever and mild dyspnea 3 years ago. Antibiotics and analgesics were prescribed at that time, which resulted in significant improvement. At this time, the patient experiences wheezing and a dry cough upon lying flat. He was evaluated by a pulmonologist who recommended inhalers. With inhaler therapy, the symptoms did not improve, and the cough became productive of thick white sputum, occasionally blood tinged.

Chest X-rays

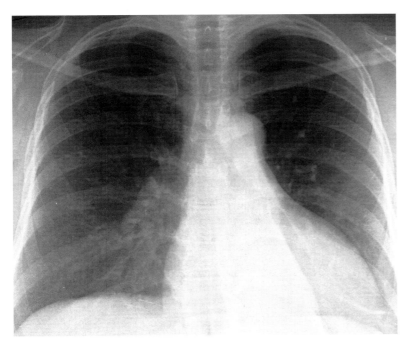

Figure 54-1

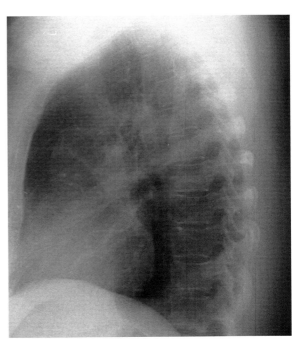

Figure 54-2

Chest X-ray Report

Dense perihilar consolidation is identified in the retrocardiac region, most likely representing left lower lobe atelectasis. Underlying mass cannot be excluded. There are no pleural effusions. The heart is not enlarged. ▨

Recommendation

Computed tomography (CT) scans of the chest.

▨ CT Scans

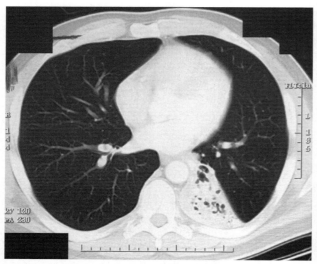

Figure 54-3

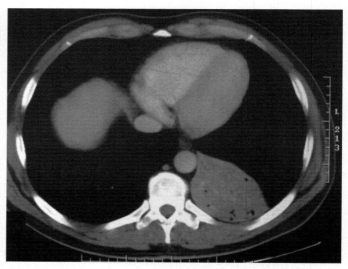

Figure 54-4

CT Scan Report

Left lower lobe consolidation and atelectasis with evidence of bronchiectasis. An atypical pneumonia is suspected, but radiographically, an occult endobronchial lesion cannot be excluded. ▨

Discussion

The differential diagnosis of lobar collapse includes both benign and malignant etiologies. Presenting symptoms can include cough, wheezing, fever, chest pain, and hemoptysis. Often, patients are initially treated with antibiotics and bronchodilators, which fail to provide symptomatic improvement.

Radiographic evidence of lobar collapse includes displacement of the fissures, decreased aeration with opacification of the collapsed lobe, elevation of the ipsilateral hemidiaphragm, displacement of the hilum, and compensatory overinflation of the remaining lung. The trachea and mediastinum may also shift toward the side of the collapsed lobe. Lobar collapse can result from endobronchial tumors and from extrinsic compression of the airway by peribronchial adenopathy or by tumor. Tumors of the airway may be primary or secondary; primary tumors are benign or malignant. Tumors in the tracheobronchial tree, which can present with lobar atelectasis, include squamous papillomas, carcinoid tumors, adenoid cystic carcinomas, mucoepidermoid tumors, and lung cancers. When endobronchial disease is present, bronchoscopy has more than a 90% diagnostic yield.

Recommendation

Flexible bronchoscopy.

Bronchoscopy Findings

At flexible bronchoscopy, the left lower lobe orifice is completely obstructed by a firm, whitish tumor. The tumor extends toward the upper lobe bronchus. There are no other abnormalities of the tracheobronchial tree. The biopsy specimen is interpreted on histologic evaluation as mucoepidermoid carcinoma. ▪

Recommendation

Left thoracotomy and resection.

Discussion

Options for the management of endobronchial disease include dilation with a rigid bronchoscope, pneumatic dilation, or in the case of a foreign body, removal with a snare or forceps. Alternative therapy includes lasers (argon; potassium, titanium, oxide phosphate [KTP]; carbon dioxide; neodymium:yttrium-aluminum-garnet [Nd-YAG]), with or without photodynamic therapy and electrocautery. The treatment of choice for mucoepidermoid tumors located within the tracheobronchial tree without evidence of metastatic disease remains surgical resection. Conservation of lung parenchyma is favored for low-grade mucoepidermoid carcinoma found in the airway. Because of its location within the proximal airway, these tumors are often amenable to a bronchoplastic resection.

Operative Findings

The patient is intubated with a double-lumen tube and placed in a right lateral decubitus position. A muscle-sparing thoracotomy is performed through the fifth interspace. Palpation reveals the lower lobe to be chronically consolidated, with some small abscesses, but the tumor itself is about 2 cm in size and located peribronchially. The pulmonary artery and vein branches are divided in the standard fashion. Because of the extent of tumor in the airway, stapling of the airway is not possible, and the bronchus is opened just distal to the left upper lobe bronchus. Bronchotomy confirms the lesion in the airway, and the remainder of the bronchus is opened circumferentially. The tumor slides out of the proximal airway, and examination reveals that the tumor arises from the distal airway but does not involve the bronchus at this level. Purulent material drains from the distal airway. The left lower lobe is removed, and the frozen section of the bronchial margin is negative for tumor. The bronchus is closed using polyglycolic acid interrupted sutures, and a mediastinal lymph node dissection is performed. Final pathology demonstrates a high-grade mucoepidermoid tumor with no lymph node involvement.

Discussion

Mucoepidermoid tumors are uncommon lesions arising from the excretory ducts of the tracheobronchial tree. These tumors constitute less than 0.2% of all lung neoplasms. Most of these tumors occur distal to the carina but within the mainstem and lobar bronchi. Histologically, the tumors are salivary gland–like tumors and are classified as low or high grade. Low-grade tumors consist of columnar mucus-secreting cells, whereas high-grade tumors consist mostly of squamous cells with only a few mucus-secreting cells. Tobacco use does not increase the risk for mucoepidermoid carcinoma. Radiographically, these tumors present with lobar collapse similar to carcinoid tumors. Diagnosis is most often made by a bronchoscopic biopsy. Treatment of the lesions is surgical resection with clear margins whenever possible. These lesions can be treated with sleeve resections and other bronchoplastic techniques to conserve lung parenchyma. A lymph node dissection should be included in the intraoperative management.

Prognosis is excellent in patients with low-grade tumors, but studies have shown increased mortality for the high-grade tumors. Survival is lower in patients with positive margins of resection. The role of adjuvant therapy is not well defined.

Presentation

A 59-year-old man is referred to your office with right shoulder pain. Past medical history is significant for dyspnea on moderate exertion (two flights of stairs) and pneumonia 5 years previously that required hospitalization. The patient reports no history of trauma but a 40-pack-per-year smoking history. He has worked at a desk job his entire life and has not had any recent travel abroad.

Chest X-rays

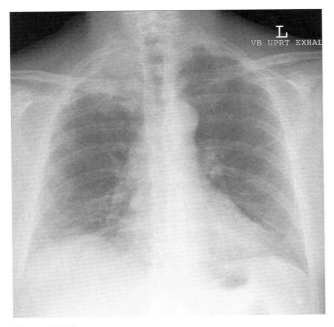

Figure 55-1

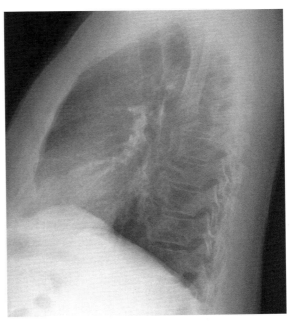

Figure 55-2

Chest X-ray Report

Chest x-rays demonstrate a large lobulated mass involving the right lung apex with apparent destruction of the medial aspect of the third rib on the right side. There is left apical pleural thickening. There are no other parenchymal abnormalities, and the hilum and mediastinum are normal in appearance. This lesion is commonly referred to as Pancoast's tumor. ■

Case Continued

The finding of rib destruction on chest x-ray most often implies a malignant etiology as opposed to an infectious process. History of smoking with an associated lung mass suggests a lung primary as opposed to a primary bone tumor with extension into the lung. Chest computed tomography (CT) scans, which include the liver and the adrenal glands, help to delineate the abnormality in the right lung apex. In addition, CT scans help to assess the right hilum, mediastinum, liver, and adrenals.

CT Scans

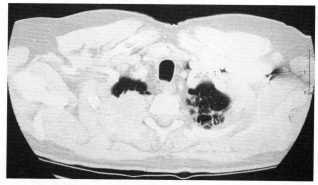

Figure 55-3

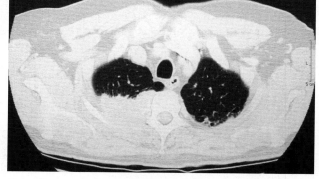

Figure 55-4

CT Scan Report

The CT scans demonstrate a posteriorly based 6-cm × 5-cm mass in the right lung apex associated with destruction of the posterior portion of the right third rib. There is scarring at the left lung apex posteriorly but no other parenchymal abnormalities within either lung. There is no evidence of hilar or mediastinal lymphadenopathy (all lymph nodes smaller than 1 cm in short-axis diameter). The liver and adrenal glands are normal.

Discussion

Tumors of the lung apices can invade the chest wall early in the course of the disease because of the close proximity of the apex of the lung to the chest wall. Patients are symptomatic more often when tumors are located in this area. Invasion of the stellate ganglion is common and results in a Horner's syndrome. Shoulder and arm pain radiating down the C8 to T1 distribution are also common. Pathologic confirmation of the suspected tumor is required because a small number of patients may have small cell carcinoma, which necessitates a different treatment regimen. Bronchoscopy with transbronchial biopsy under fluoroscopic guidance yields a diagnosis in only 10% to 30% of patients. A CT-guided lung biopsy has a high yield in establishing a diagnosis with a low risk for a pneumothorax because the tumor is adherent to the chest wall.

CT-guided Needle Biopsy Report

Malignant cells, poorly differentiated adenocarcinoma with necrosis, rare atypical metaplastic squamous cells, mucinous material, and connective tissue.

Recommendation

Positron-emission tomography (PET) scan and brain magnetic resonance imaging (MRI).

PET Scan Report

A large mass with intense metabolic activity is noted in the apical region of the right lung, SUV of 15. A small focal area of increased metabolic activity is seen in the right paratracheal area with an SUV of 4. No other lesions are seen.

Case Continued

The brain MRI (not shown) does not demonstrate metastatic disease. Although the CT scan of the chest reveals no evidence of mediastinal lymphadenopathy, the PET scan does show uptake (SUV of more than 2.5) in the right lower para- tracheal area (R4) of the mediastinum, which is suggestive of tumor in that region. A mediastinoscopy should be performed to confirm the presence of tumor in this region. If tumor is present in this nodal region, it is classified as stage IIIA (T3 N2 M0), and definitive chemoradiation should be offered to the patient. However, if tumor is not confirmed in this region, the clinical stage is IIA (T3 N0 M0), and the patient should be offered trimodality therapy. This treatment con- sists of induction chemoradiation followed by surgical excision provided that the postinduction restaging reveals either stable or diminished disease.

An outpatient mediastinoscopy shows no evidence of tumor in either the R2 (right upper paratracheal), R4 (right lower paratracheal), station 7 (carinal), or L4 (left lower paratracheal) lymph nodes. The patient is clinically staged as a stage IIA adenocarcinoma of the right lung apex and offered a trimodality therapy. Chemotherapy includes cisplatin and paclitaxel (Taxol) given concurrently with 4,500 cGy of radiation. Surgery is scheduled for 3 to 6 weeks after the completion of induction chemoradiation.

CT Scans after Chemotherapy and Radiation

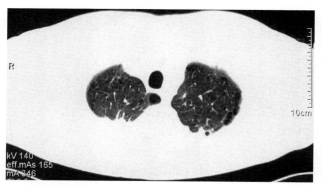

Figure 55-5

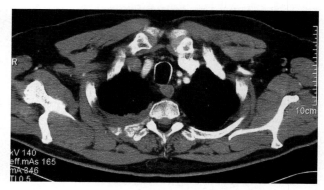

Figure 55-6

CT Scan Report

The CT scans demonstrate an interval decrease in the extent of the right upper lobe mass. There appears to be destructive changes of the posterior right third rib. Centrilobar and paraseptal emphysema are noted. In the left lung, apical thickening is unchanged. There are no new left lung nodules, masses, or consolidations. No interval mediastinal, hilar, internal mammary or axillary lymph node enlargement is present.

Discussion

Pancoast's tumor resection involves removal of the right upper lobe *en bloc* with the involved ribs in addition to one rib above and one rib below the involved rib. A thoracic lymphadenectomy or lymph node sampling is also performed. In cases in which there is pulmonary dysfunction that precludes lobectomy and in cases in which the tumor is more localized, a wedge resection of the upper lobe may also be considered.

Case Continued

A posterolateral thoracotomy is performed. Division of the lower portion of the trapezius and rhomboid major and minor muscles is completed. The chest cavity is entered through the fourth intercostal space to facilitate rib resection. Resectability is determined by inspecting the tumor and the involved ribs as well as lymph node–bearing areas. Suspicious (N2) lymph nodes were removed and sent for frozen section, which did not demonstrate malignant cells. If more than one node is positive for tumor, it is unlikely that the patient will benefit from surgery; however, if only a single N2 station lymph node is positive, the patient may benefit from resection. Assessment of invasion of the subclavian vessels should also be made when tumors are located anteriorly. Care is taken to avoid crossing tumor planes, and every effort is made to resect the ribs at least 2.5 cm away from the area of tumor invasion. The scapula is elevated off the chest wall using a small rib spreader. The involved ribs are then transected anteriorly. Posterior segments of ribs two, three, and four are disarticulated from the vertebral bodies with individual ligation of the neurovascular bundle. The first rib is not involved by the tumor. After the rib resections are completed, the tumor with the attached ribs is retracted into the pleural space, and a standard lobectomy is completed. A thoracic lymphadenectomy is performed as well. The chest wall defect does not require reconstruction because the defect is located beneath the scapula. In the event that more than three ribs are resected, the defect may be patched with prosthetic material. The prosthesis is positioned and sutured with care to avoid injury to the brachial plexus or the subclavian vessels.

Discussion

Adverse prognostic factors of Pancoast's tumor include (a) subclavian vessel involvement, (b) vertebral body destruction by the cancer, (c) positive N1 and N2 lymph nodes, (d) incomplete resection, and (e) wedge resection. However, extended resection techniques, the anterior surgical approach, and neoadjuvant therapy have somewhat modified these factors. The recently described anterior approach for an apical cancer invading the subclavian vessels has been demonstrated to provide satisfactory results. Neoadjuvant therapy consisting of chemotherapy in combination with radiation minimizes a possibility of an incomplete resection and also can sterilize positive N2 lymph nodes. Complete vertebral body resection with prosthetic reconstruction and stabilization has recently been described. Lobectomy is the procedure of choice unless compromised pulmonary functions mandate a lesser resection.

The time-honored standard of therapy of Pancoast's tumor is preoperative radiation followed by resection. Radiation therapy dose is 4,000 to 4,500 cGy, and if distant disease is not present, resection is carried out 4 weeks after completion of radiation. Chemoradiation consists of a similar dose of radiation combined with cisplatin-based chemotherapy. A complete resection is possible in 75% of patients with a projected 5-year survival of 35% to 40%. Recent reports tend to favor preoperative chemoradiation over radiation alone.

Presentation

A 22-year-old woman is admitted through the emergency department with an episode of severe upper gastrointestinal bleeding. The patient has a known history of cavernous transformation of the portal and splenic veins but has been non-compliant with propanolol treatment. The bleeding is controlled with a Minnesota tube and transfusion of 4 units of blood. Endoscopy and sclerotherapy of bleeding varices are performed. The patient is scheduled for a gastric devascularization procedure. The following is the admission chest x-ray.

▨ Chest X-ray

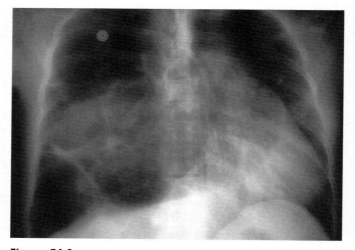

Figure 56-1

Chest X-ray Report

The chest film demonstrates a hyperinflated right lung with mediastinal shift to the left and atelectasis of the left lung. ▨

Case Continued

Upon further questioning, the patient states that the pulmonary abnormality had been recognized 3 years earlier with her first episode of gastrointestinal bleeding. Before that time, she states that she exercised daily. Since then, she complains that she has been having worsening dyspnea on exertion and occasional blood-streaked sputum. Computed tomography (CT) scans of the chest are recommended.

CT Scans

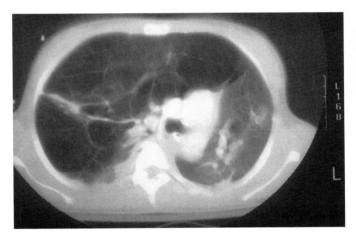

Figure 56-2

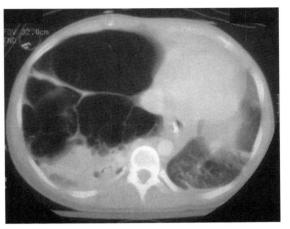

Figure 56-3

CT Scan Report

The CT scans demonstrate diffuse cystic changes throughout the right lung, with some sparing of the apex of the right upper lobe. There is consolidation of the right lower lobe. The mediastinum is shifted to the left with atelectasis of the left lung.

Case Continued

Concerns are raised about the patient's ability to tolerate a gastric devascularization procedure. Pulmonary functions tests are obtained that reveal a forced expiratory volume in 1 second (FEV$_1$) of 1.08 L and a diffusing capacity of lung for carbon monoxide (D$_{LCO}$) 50% of predicted value. A quantitative perfusion scan was obtained.

Quantitative Perfusion Scan

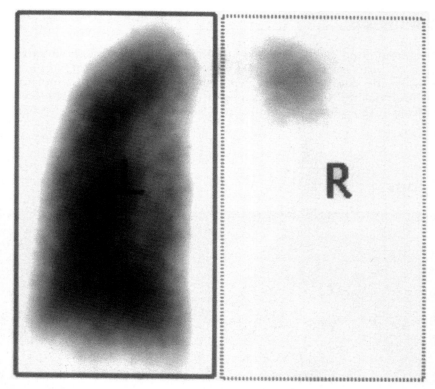

Figure 56-4

Perfusion Scan Report

The scan shows 82% of the pulmonary blood flow going to the left lung and 18% to the right. Based on these findings, the plan is made for a right middle and lower lobectomy, attempting to salvage the right upper lobe, which radiographically appears atelectatic.

Surgical Approach

The patient is approached through a right posterolateral thoracotomy, entering the chest through the fifth intercostal space. The latissimus dorsi is divided but the serratus anterior spared, and the rib is transected posteriorly but not removed. This incision provides better exposure compared with a muscle-sparing incision because the mediastinum is shifted toward the left and, despite the use of a double-lumen endotracheal tube, the lung does not deflate to any considerable extent. Intraoperatively, the entire right lung is determined to be abnormal, with minimal sparing of the parenchyma in the right upper lobe. There are no identifiable fissures present, and there are multiple, clot-filled cysts in the posterior aspect of the lung. The resection is facilitated by the use of positive end-expiratory pressure (PEEP) on the left lung to help shift the mediastinum back toward the right side. A right pneumonectomy is performed.

Right Lung

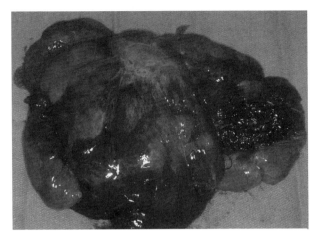

Figure 56-5

Pathologic Findings

The pathologic findings are consistent with congenital cystic adenomatoid malformation involving all three lobes of the right lung. There is evidence of recent hemorrhage within the cysts. ▪

Case Continued

The postoperative chest x-ray shows the left lung to be well expanded and without evidence of cystic disease. After surgery, the patient requires another sclerotherapy procedure and is discharged home on the eleventh postoperative day.

Discussion

Congenital cystic adenomatoid malformation (CCAM) represents a spectrum of cystic and solid abnormalities of the lung. The disease is characterized by the absence of mature alveoli and, in their place, a proliferation of bronchiolar tubular structures. These structures are lined by ciliated columnar epithelium, interspersed with cysts and a disorganized connective tissue stroma. There is an absence of bronchial mucoserous glands and cartilaginous plates.

The symptoms correlate with the pathologic findings. When the lung is mostly solid, the result is a stillborn infant or premature infant born with fetal anasarca, ascites, and maternal polyhydramnios. This has been classified as type III CCAM. Type II contains a mixture of solid and cystic elements, with the near-term infant presenting with respiratory distress.

Patients with mostly cystic lesions (type I) can present as infants, children, or adults, most often with recurring episodes of pneumonia. In most patients, only a single lobe is involved. The differential diagnosis in an infant includes congenital diaphragmatic hernia and congenital lobar emphysema.

In the infant, surgical resection is directed toward relieving the symptoms of respiratory distress caused by compression of the contralateral lung. In the older child or adult, resection is performed as a consequence of recurrent pneumonia. A recommendation has been made to resect all cystic adenomatoid malformations at the time of diagnosis because malignant tumors have been identified in children with this congenital abnormality.

Presentation

A 32-year-old woman is referred to you by her primary care physician with complaints of chest discomfort for the past 2 weeks. She is otherwise a healthy, non-smoking woman with no significant past medical history. Physical examination is unremarkable. The patient presents to your office with the following chest x-rays.

Chest X-rays

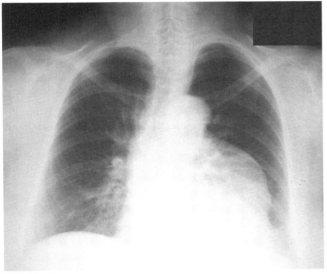

Figure 57-1

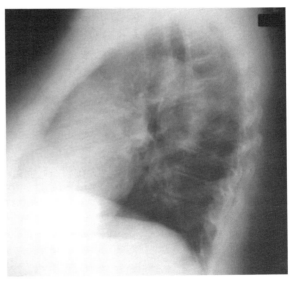

Figure 57-2

Chest X-ray Report

The chest x-rays demonstrate a large mass in the left chest. The left heart border is obscured by the mass. On the lateral x-ray, the mass is anterior to the heart. There are no lesions in the lung fields, and there is no evidence of pleural effusion.

Recommendation

The computed tomography (CT) scan is an accurate and reliable method to evaluate the mediastinum and lungs. A standard protocol for CT scanning of the chest includes contiguous images from the lung apices to the adrenal glands with inclusion of the liver. Intravenous contrast is recommended to define vascular structures in the chest and their relationship to any detected abnormalities.

CT Scan

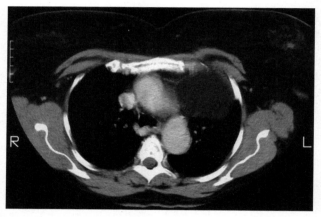

Figure 57-3

CT Scan Report

The CT scan demonstrates a left-sided anterior mediastinal mass in proximity to the arch of the aorta. The mass appears to be well circumscribed with a cystic component. There is no obvious invasion of mediastinal structures or of the adjacent lung parenchyma. The lung fields are free of abnormalities, and there is no pleural effusion. The liver and adrenals are normal. Calcification is noted in the mass.

Recommendation

Magnetic resonance imaging (MRI) can further delineate the relationship of the mass to adjacent vascular structures. MRI of the chest is not particularly beneficial for evaluating the lung parenchyma but does provide excellent soft tissue characterization along with vascular enhancement.

MRIs

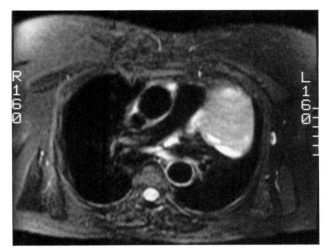

Figure 57-4

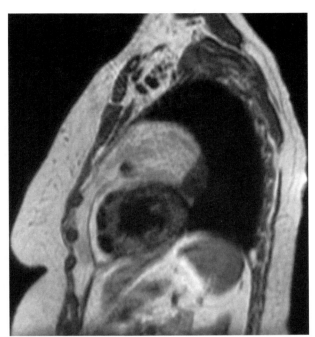

Figure 57-5

MRI Report

The MRIs demonstrate an anterior mediastinal mass not involving the aortic arch or any other vascular structures. ▨

Discussion

The mediastinum is divided into three compartments: the anterior, middle, and posterior. The common lesions in the anterior mediastinum include goiters, thymic cysts and thymomas, lymphomas, and germ cell tumors originating from embryonic cell rests. More rare tumors that can present in the anterior mediastinum include parathyroid adenomas, lipomas, hemangiomas, and metastatic tumors.

Patients presenting with an anterior mediastinal mass may be asymptomatic or have symptoms of chest pain, cough, or dyspnea. The absence of symptoms can suggest that the lesion is a benign neoplasm. A large goiter can cause stridor with associated dyspnea; thymomas are associated with myasthenia gravis and other systemic manifestations; and lymphomas are usually asymptomatic with possible fever, night sweats, weight loss, and rarely, pruritus. Malignant germ cell tumors are rare in women and present with symptoms associated with compression of the airway, esophagus, or great vessels. Benign teratomas are usually asymptomatic but can present with anterior chest pain, cough, and dyspnea.

The CT scan can assist in providing an accurate clinical impression. Lesions that contain fluid in the anterior mediastinum include goiters, thymic cysts, and teratomas. Lesions that contain calcium include goiters, thymomas, and granulomatous inflammatory lesions. The MRI study is only obtained if vascular structures need assessment or sagittal or coronal views would be helpful in planning a surgical procedure. Ultrasonography can define fluid-filled structures and can define an area for specific percutaneous aspiration. Radionuclide studies would include thyroid scanning, which must be done before a CT scan with contrast enhancement. However, the thyroid scan frequently does not show the extent of the mediastinal extension of the goiter and is usually only obtained when the diagnosis is doubtful. The thallium-technetium scan can be of benefit in identifying a mediastinal parathyroid adenoma.

Serum α-fetoprotein (AFP) and human chorionic gonadotropin (hCG) should be obtained to assist in the diagnosis of nonseminomatous germ cell tumors. Biopsy is recommended for large mediastinal masses that invade contiguous structures or appear to be unresectable. Needle aspiration biopsy may provide inadequate material when poorly differentiated malignancies are present, and core needle biopsy is usually recommended to obtain more tissue. Anterior mediastinotomy is an appropriate diagnostic surgical technique to provide adequate tissue for precise histologic verification of the neoplasm. The video-assisted thoracic surgery (VATS) technique can also be used for mediastinal tumor biopsy. If the anterior mediastinal tumor is potentially resectable and serum markers are not elevated, surgical excision is recommended. Mediastinoscopy is only of benefit if a large tumor extends far superiorly in approximation to the sternal notch.

Surgical Approach

Median sternotomy with resection of the anterior mediastinal mass is recommended. The anterior sternal approach provides access to both sides of the mediastinum and adjacent vascular structures. Involved lung tissue can easily be resected if required. This patient could be considered for a left thoracotomy because the tumor does project somewhat into the left chest. However, sternotomy is the recommended approach for most anterior mediastinal tumors. Small anterior mediastinal neoplasms or cystic structures can be considered for resection by the VATS technique. However, this approach is not recommended for larger tumors or suspected benign teratomas, which have associated peritumor fibrosis.

The patient undergoes median sternotomy with excision of the mass. The dissection is made somewhat difficult by rather extensive fibrotic reaction around the tumor, but all major structures are preserved. The final pathologic diagnosis is a benign teratoma.

Discussion

Mature teratomas are the most common type of germ cell tumor in the mediastinum and approximately 50% to 75% of cases. The benign teratoma has an equal incidence in men and women, whereas malignant primary mediastinal germ cell tumors are rare in women. Most germ cell tumors in men present in the testes, and 10% present at extragonadal sites, including the mediastinum, retroperitoneum, and pineal gland. Cells responsible for these tumors arise from germinal cells that migrate into the mediastinum from the urogenital ridge during embryologic life. In young men with a large anterior mediastinal tumor, marked elevation of AFP or hCG (greater than 300 ng/mL) is diagnostic of a nonseminomatous germ cell tumor, and confirmatory biopsy is not required. The pure mediastinal seminoma can become quite large and is a slow-growing neoplasm. About 10% of patients with a pure seminoma have an elevated serum hCG level. The serum AFP should always be normal with a pure mediastinal seminoma. Elevation of AFP indicates the presence of a nonseminomatous component. Malignant nonseminomatous tumors include embryonic carcinoma, endodermal sinus tumor, choriocarcinoma, and the mixed germ cell tumor. Primary mediastinal seminomas have an approximate 90% cure rate, and recommended treatment is chemotherapy. Nonseminomatous germ cell tumors are treated with combination chemotherapy with surgical resection for residual disease if serum markers are decreased.

Teratomas are the most common germ cell tumor of the anterior mediastinum. They are cystic and well circumscribed and can become quite large. They frequently contain cystic areas that can contain mucoid material as well as hair and other tissue, such as skin, bone, gastrointestinal mucosa, and teeth. Calcification may be present in about 30% of benign teratomas. These tumors classically contain ectodermal, endodermal, and mesenchymal tissue. Recurrence does not occur after complete resection, and long-term prognosis is excellent. The surgeon must always be prepared for a difficult dissection because of the often-dense adhesions associated with these lesions.

case 58

Presentation

A 65-year-old woman is referred to you with symptoms of cough and upper chest and shoulder pain. She denies fever, weight loss, and hemoptysis. She reports a 50-pack-per-year smoking history. On physical examination, blood pressure in the right arm is 120/80 mm Hg, there is no supraclavicular adenopathy, and the lung fields are clear to auscultation and percussion. The patient has a full range of motion of the right arm and hand. Blood chemistries are within normal limits.

Recommendation

The differential diagnosis for this includes pulmonary and mediastinal neoplasm. Chest wall abnormalities must also be considered. Inflammatory pulmonary disease should have associated systemic manifestations. A chest x-ray is an appropriate initial study.

Chest X-rays

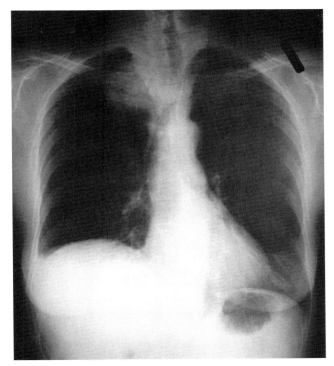

Figure 58-1

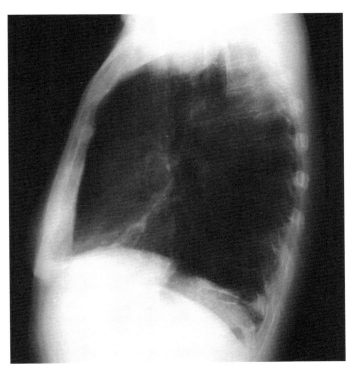

Figure 58-2

Chest X-ray Report

The chest x-rays reveal a mass in the upper right chest with possible compression of the trachea. The lateral chest x-ray shows the mass to be located anteriorly at the level of costosternal junction. Computed tomography (CT) scans are recommended for further anatomic delineation.

CT Scans

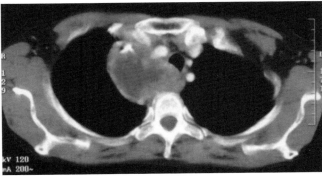

Figure 58-3

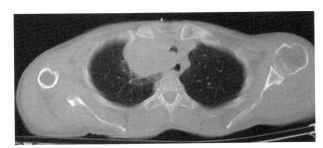

Figure 58-4

CT Scan Report

CT scans of the chest demonstrate a large anterior medial mass with central necrosis, which displaces the trachea to the left side and also is adjacent to the esophagus. Evaluation of all levels of the CT scans demonstrates compression and possible invasion of the subclavian artery and subclavian vein. No obvious enlarged mediastinal lymph nodes are seen.

Discussion

The radiologic appearance of the mass is suspicious for an anterosuperior sulcus lung cancer. Clinical staging is necessary to determine the histology of the mass and to define the extent of the cancer. Bronchoscopy with associated brushings and transbronchial biopsy can frequently fail to reveal a histologic diagnosis of cancer because of the more peripheral location of the lesion. Transthoracic needle aspiration biopsy provides a high incidence of histologic diagnosis. Mediastinoscopy is indicated to rule out metastasis to mediastinal lymph nodes because their positive involvement carries a very poor prognosis. Mediastinoscopy is recommended in all patients with superior sulcus tumors. The CT scans rule out the presence of neoplasm in the liver and adrenal glands. The patient has no central nervous system symptoms, and brain scan is not necessary. Magnetic resonance imaging (MRI) examination can be helpful in evaluating the brachial plexus when associated arm and hand symptoms are present. It can also define vascular involvement.

Recommendation

Transthoracic needle biopsy to establish the diagnosis of cancer with subsequent mediastinoscopy and bronchoscopy.

Results

The transthoracic needle biopsy reveals squamous cell carcinoma. On mediastinoscopy, biopsy of level 4 lymph nodes reveals no evidence of cancer. The bronchoscopic examination demonstrates deviation of the trachea and normal right main-stem and right upper lobe bronchi.

Discussion

Contraindications to surgical resection of a superior sulcus tumor include the presence of distant metastatic cancer, N2 disease, and extensive invasion of the brachial plexus, trachea, esophagus, or vertebral bodies. Involvement of the subclavian vessels is not a contraindication to a surgical approach. There is some controversy about the best therapeutic approach to the superior sulcus tumor. Recommendations vary from the surgical approach alone, surgery followed by radiation, preoperative radiation, or preoperative chemotherapy and radiation. Recent reports indicate that neoadjuvant chemoradiation followed by surgical resection can achieve improved results. The best prognosis is achieved in patients who have a complete resection without evidence of mediastinal lymph node involvement; 5-year survival rates in these patients approach 35%. High-dose radiation therapy has been advocated by some, but local recurrent rates are high, and long-term survival rates are lower than those after surgery.

This patient has no evidence of metastatic disease but has primarily an anterosuperior sulcus tumor with compression of the trachea and esophagus. Neoadjuvant chemoradiation is recommended to provide a better opportunity for a complete resection. Patients who are deemed inoperable should receive high-dose radiation. Preoperative chemotherapy is carboplatin based, and radiation approximates 4,000 to 5,000 cGy. After completion of therapy, extent of disease is reassessed with a CT scan and a positron-emission tomography (PET) scan. Progression of disease can indicate inoperability.

Case Continued

The patient receives neoadjuvant chemotherapy and 4,500 cGy of radiation. After the neoadjuvant treatment, the patient is restaged with a repeat CT scan and PET scan.

◼ Repeat CT Scan and PET Scan

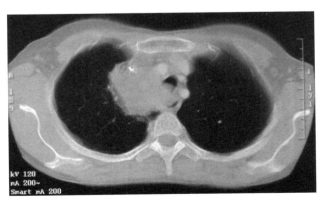

Figure 58-5

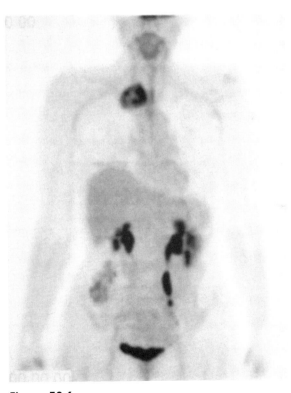

Figure 58-6

CT Scan and PET Scan Report

The tumor demonstrates minimal decrease in size. There is no evidence of distant disease on the PET scan or evidence of new mediastinal lymph node involvement. ▒

Discussion

The CT scan has identified the anterior location of this superior sulcus tumor with possible involvement of the subclavian artery and subclavian vein. The C7 to T1 root of the brachial plexus may also be involved. The surgeon must consider an anterior approach for this neoplasm. Dartavelle has described the transclavicular approach for the anterosuperior sulcus tumor. A cervical incision along the sternocleidomastoid muscle is performed that extends horizontally below the clavicle out to the deltopectoral groove. Appropriate musculature is removed from the clavicle and first rib, and assessment of the neoplasm is carried out. If the lesion is thought to be resectable, the medial half of the clavicle is removed. This exposure permits resection of the subclavian vein if necessary; the subclavian artery can also be resected and reconstituted by appropriate grafting techniques. The pulmonary resection can be accomplished through this anterior approach with some difficulty. If necessary, a posterolateral thoracotomy can subsequently be carried out to complete the pulmonary resection or removal of the tumor from the vertebral body. It is imperative not to injure the long thoracic nerve in order to avoid rotation of the shoulder anteriorly, which will cause significant functional discomfort. A second recommended approach is the hemi-clamshell technique, which is a partial sternotomy with extension into the fourth intercostal space anteriorly. The medial half of the clavicle is removed for enhanced exposure of the subclavian vessels and brachial plexus. Involved ribs can also be removed through this exposure. Other modifications of these incisions have been described. The surgical techniques are difficult, and the surgeon must be familiar with all modifications and aspects of these various incisions. Complications include hemothorax, chylothorax, and muscle paralysis of the forearm and hand, Horner's syndrome, and spinal fluid leakage. Postoperative recovery is long term, and frequent arm and shoulder rehabilitation is necessary.

Case Continued

An anterior surgical approach is taken using the hemi-clamshell technique. The medial half of the clavicle is resected. It is necessary to resect the subclavian vein, but the subclavian artery is preserved. Sharp dissection is necessary to remove the tumor from the lateral wall of the trachea and esophagus. Prevertebral fascia is removed in continuity with the tumor. A deep wedge resection of the upper lobe is accomplished by stapling technique. Postoperative complications include swelling of the right arm and right-sided vocal cord paralysis.

Pathology Report

Resected mediastinal lymph nodes are negative for evidence of cancer, and residual active squamous cancer is present in the specimen. Significant necrosis had occurred from the preoperative chemoradiation. ▒

index of cases

selected readings

Case 1. Nonseminomatous Germ Cell Tumor

Murphy BR, Breeden ES, Donohue JP, et al. Surgical salvage of chemorefractory germ cell tumors. *J Clin Oncol* 1993;11(2):324–329.

Takeda S, Miyoshi S, Ohta M, et al. Primary germ cell tumors in the mediastinum: a 50-year experience at a single Japanese institution. *Cancer* 2003;97 (2):367–376.

Wright CD, Kesler KA. Surgical techniques and outcomes for primary nonseminomatous germ cell tumors. *Chest Surg Clin N Am* 2002;12(4):707–715. Review.

Case 2. Segmentectomy

Jones DR, Stiles BM, Denlinger CE, et al. Pulmonary segmentectomy: results and complications. *Ann Thorac Surg* 2003;76(2):343–348; discussion 348–349.

Martini N, Bains MS, Burt ME, et al. Incidence of local recurrence and second primary tumors in resected stage I lung cancer. *J Thorac Cardiovasc Surg* 1995;109(1):120–129.

Warren WH, Faber LP. Segmentectomy versus lobectomy in patients with stage I pulmonary carcinoma. Five-year survival and patterns of intrathoracic recurrence. *J Thorac Cardiovasc Surg* 1994;107 (4):1087–1093; discussion 1093–1094.

Case 3. Epiphrenic Diverticulum

Allen MS. Treatment of epiphrenic diverticula. *Semin Thorac Cardiovasc Surg* 1999;11(4):358–362. Review.

Benacci JC, Deschamps C, Trastek VF, et al. Epiphrenic diverticulum: results of surgical treatment. *Ann Thorac Surg* 1993;55(5):1109–1113; discussion 1114.

Nehra D, Lord RV, DeMeester TR, et al. Physiologic basis for the treatment of epiphrenic diverticulum. *Ann Surg* 2002;235(3):346–354.

Case 4. Echinococcal Disease

Aggarwal P, Wali JP. Albendazole in the treatment of pulmonary echinococcosis. *Thorax* 1991;46(8): 599–600.

Crausaz PH. Surgical treatment of the hydatid cyst of the lung and hydatid disease of the liver with intrathoracic evolution. *J Thorac Cardiovasc Surg* 1967;53(1):116–129. Review.

Sharma SK, Eggleston FC. Management of hydatid disease. *Arch Surg* 1969;99(1):59–63.

Case 5. Spontaneous Pneumothorax

Baumann MH. Treatment of spontaneous pneumothorax. *Curr Opin Pulm Med* 2000;6(4):275–280. Review.

Baumann MH, Strange C, Heffner JE, et al. AACP Pneumothorax Consensus Group. Management of spontaneous pneumothorax: an American College of Chest Physicians Delphi consensus statement. *Chest* 2001;119(2):590–602. Review.

Ferraro P, Beauchamp G, Lord F, et al. Spontaneous primary and secondary pneumothorax: a 10-year study of management alternatives. *Can J Surg* 1994;37(3):197–202.

Mahfood S, Hix WR, Aaron BL, et al. Reexpansion pulmonary edema. *Ann Thorac Surg* 1988;45(3): 340–345. Review.

Sherman SC. Reexpansion pulmonary edema: a case report and review of the current literature. *J Emerg Med* 2003;24(1):23–27. Review.

Case 6. Atypical Carcinoid

Arrigoni MG, Woolner LB, Bernatz TE. Atypical carcinoid tumors of the lung. *J Thorac Cardiovasc Surg* 1972;64:413.

Filosso PL, Ruffini E, Oliaro A, et al. Long-term survival of atypical bronchial carcinoids with liver metastases, treated with octreotide. *Eur J Cardiothorac Surg* 2002;21(5):913–917.

Hage R, de la Riviere AB, Seldenrijk CA, et al. Update in pulmonary carcinoid tumors: a review article. *Ann Surg Oncol* 2003;10(6):697–704. Review.

Wilkins EW Jr, Grillo HC, Moncure AC, et al. Changing times in surgical management of bronchopulmonary carcinoid tumor. *Ann Thorac Surg* 1984;38(4):339–344.

Case 7. Thyroid Goiter

Ozdemir A, Hasbahceci M, Hamaloglu E, et al. Surgical treatment of substernal goiter. *Int Surg* 2000;85 (3):194–197.

Souza JW, Williams JT, Ayoub MM, et al. Bilateral recurrent nerve paralysis associated with multinodular substernal goiter: a case report. *Am Surg* 1999;65 (5):456–459. Review.

Wright CD, Mathisen DJ. Mediastinal tumors: diagnosis and treatment. *World J Surg* 2001;25(2): 204–209. Review.

Case 8. CT-guided Needle Biopsy

Berquist TH, Bailey PB, Cortese DA, et al. Transthoracic needle biopsy: accuracy and complications in relation to location and type of lesion. *Mayo Clin Proc* 1980;55(8):475–481.

Calhoun P, Feldman PS, Armstrong P, et al. The clinical outcome of needle aspirations of the lung when cancer is not diagnosed. *Ann Thorac Surg* 1986; 41(6):592–596.

Gress FG, Savides TJ, Sandler A, et al. Endoscopic ultrasonography, fine-needle aspiration biopsy guided by endoscopic ultrasonography, and computed tomography in the preoperative staging of non–small-cell lung cancer: a comparison study. *Ann Intern Med* 1997;127(8 Pt 1):604–612.

Case 9. Zenker's Diverticulum and Diverticulopexy

Balaji NS, Peters JH. Minimally invasive surgery for esophageal motility disorders. *Surg Clin North Am* 2002;82(4):763–782. Review.

Gutschow CA, Hamoir M, Rombaux P, et al. Management of pharyngoesophageal (Zenker's) diverticulum: which technique? *Ann Thorac Surg* 2002;74(5): 1677–1682; discussion 1682–1683.

Ibrahim IM. Zenker diverticulum. *Arch Surg* 2003; 138(1):111.

Case 10. Lung Transplant and Tracheal Stent

Cassivi SD, Meyers BF, Battafarano RJ, et al. Thirteen-year experience in lung transplatation for emphysema. *Ann Thorac Surg* 2002;74:1663–1670.

Chhajed PN, Malouf MA, Tamm M, et al. Ultraflex stents for the management of airway complications in lung transplant recipients. *Respirology* 2003;8(1): 59–64.

Lonchyna VA. Single lung transplantation. *Thorac Cardiovasc Surg* 1999;4:142–161.

Lonchyna VA, Arcidi JM Jr, Garrity ER Jr, et al. Refractory post-transplant airway strictures: successful management with wire stents? *Eur J Cardiothorac Surg* 1999;15(6):842–849; discussion 849–850.

Meyers BF, Patterson GA. Chronic obstructive pulmonary disease: bullectomy, lung volume reduction surgery, and transplantation for patients with chronic obstructive pulmonary disease. *Thorax* 2003;58:634–638.

Susanto I, Peters JI, Levine SM, et al. Use of balloon-expandable metallic stents in the management of bronchial stenosis and bronchomalacia after lung transplantation. *Chest* 1998;114(5): 1330–1335.

Case 11. Mesothelioma

Van Ruth S, Baas P, Zoetmulder F. Surgical treatment of malignant pleural mesothelioma. *Chest* 2003;123:551–561.

Waller DA. Role of surgery in the diagnosis and treatment of malignant pleural mesothelioma. *Curr Opin Oncol* 2003;15:39–43.

Zellos L, Sugarbaker DJ. Current surgical management of malignant pleural mesothelioma. *Curr Oncol Rep* 2002;4:354–360.

Case 12. Achalasia and Esophageal Myotomy

Balaji NS, Peters JH. Minimally invasive surgery for esophageal motility disorders. *Surg Clin North Am* 2002;82(4):763–782.

Bloomston M, Fraiji E, Boyce HW Jr, et al. Preoperative intervention does not affect esophageal muscle histology or patient outcomes in patients undergoing laparoscopic Heller myotomy. *J Gastrointest Surg* 2003;7(2):181–188.

Zaninotto G, Costantini M, Portale G, et al. Etiology, diagnosis, and treatment of failures after laparoscopic Heller myotomy for achalasia. *Ann Surg* 2002; 235(2):186–192.

Case 13. Osteosarcoma

Athanassiadi K, Kalavrouziotis G, Rondogianni D, et al. Primary chest wall tumors: early and long-term results of surgical treatment. *Eur J Cardiothorac Surg* 2001;19(5):589–593.

Picciocchi A, Granone P, Cardillo G, et al. Prosthetic reconstruction of the chest wall. *Int Surg* 1993; 78(3):221–224. Review.

Ryan MB, McMurtrey MJ, Roth JA. Current management of chest-wall tumors. *Surg Clin North Am* 1989;69(5):1061–1080. Review.

Case 14. Adenoid Cystic Carcinoma

Gaissert HA. Primary tracheal tumors. *Chest Surg Clin N Am* 2003;13(2):247–256.

Grillo HC. The history of tracheal surgery. *Chest Surg Clin N Am* 2003;13(2):175–189.

Mathisen DJ. Tracheal tumors. *Chest Surg Clin N Am* 1996;6(4):875–898. Review.

Case 15. Broncholithiasis

Arrigoni MG, Bernatz PE, Donoghue FE. Broncholithiasis. *J Thorac Cardiovasc Surg* 1971;62(2): 231–237.

Faber LP, Jensik RJ, Chawla SK, et al. The surgical implication of broncholithiasis. *J Thorac Cardiovasc Surg* 1975;70(5):779–789.

Olson EJ, Utz JP, Prakash UB. Therapeutic bronchoscopy in broncholithiasis. *Am J Respir Crit Care Med* 1999;160(3):766–770.

Trastek VF, Pairolero PC, Ceithaml EL, et al. Surgical management of broncholithiasis. *J Thorac Cardiovasc Surg* 1985;90(6):842–848.

Vix VA. Radiographic manifestations of broncholithiasis. *Radiology* 1978;128(2):295–299.

Case 16. Parathyroid Adenoma

Banzo I, Pena FJ, Allende RH, et al. MIBI SPECT and radioguided surgery in the accurate location of a posterior mediastinal parathyroid adenoma. *Clin Nucl Med* 2003;28(7):584–586.

Kao CL, Chou FF, Chang JP. Minimal invasive surgery for resection of parathyroid tumor in the aortopulmonary window. *J Cardiovasc Surg (Torino)* 2003;44(1):139–140.

O'Herrin JK, Weigel T, Wilson M, et al. Radioguided parathyroidectomy via VATS combined with intraoperative parathyroid hormone testing: the surgical approach of choice for patients with mediastinal parathyroid adenomas? *J Bone Miner Res* 2002;17 (8):1368–1371.

Ott MC, Malthaner RA, Reid R. Intraoperative radioguided thoracoscopic removal of ectopic parathyroid adenoma. *Ann Thorac Surg* 2001;72(5): 1758–1760.

Rubello D, Casara D, Fiore D, et al. An ectopic mediastinal parathyroid adenoma accurately located by a single-day imaging protocol of Tc-99m pertechnetate-MIBI subtraction scintigraphy and MIBI-SPECT-computed tomographic image fusion. *Clin Nucl Med* 2002;27(3):186–190.

Case 17. Video-assisted Thoracic Surgery (VATS) Lobectomy

Gharagozloo F, Tempesta B, Margolis M, et al. Video-assisted thoracic surgery lobectomy for stage I lung cancer. *Ann Thorac Surg* 2003;76(4):1009–1014; discussion 1014–1015.

Koizumi K, Haraguchi S, Hirata T, et al. Lobectomy by video-assisted thoracic surgery for lung cancer patients aged 80 years or more. *Ann Thorac Cardiovasc Surg* 2003;9(1):14–21.

Walker WS, Codispoti M, Soon SY, et al. Long-term outcomes following VATS lobectomy for non–small cell bronchogenic carcinoma. *Eur J Cardiothorac Surg* 2003;23(3):397–402.

Case 18. Barrett's Esophagus

Ferguson MK, Durkin A. Long-term survival after esophagectomy for Barrett's adenocarcinoma in endoscopically surveyed and nonsurveyed patients. *J Gastrointest Surg* 2002;6(1):29–35.

Ferguson MK, Naunheim KS. Resection for Barrett's mucosa with high-grade dysplasia: implications for prophylactic photodynamic therapy. *J Thorac Cardiovasc Surg* 1997;114(5):824–829.

Romagnoli R, Collard JM, Gutschow C, et al. Outcomes of dysplasia arising in Barrett's esophagus: a dynamic view. *J Am Coll Surg* 2003;197(3):365–371.

Case 19. Aspergilloma

Battaglini JW, Murray GF, Keagy BA, et al. Surgical management of symptomatic pulmonary aspergilloma. *Ann Thorac Surg* 1985;39:512.

Robinson LA, Reed EC, Galbraith TA, et al. Pulmonary resection for invasive aspergillus infections in immunocompromised patients. *J Thorac Cardiovasc Surg* 1995;109:1182.

Varkey B, Rose HD. Pulmonary aspergilloma: a rational approach to treatment. *Am J Med* 1976;61: 626.

Case 20. Malignant Pleural Effusion

Antunes G, Neville E, Duffy J, Ali N. BTS guidelines for the management of malignant pleural effusions. Pleural Diseases Group, Standards of Care Committee, British Thoracic Society. *Thorax* 2003;58 Suppl 2:ii29–38.

Henry M, Arnold T, Harvey J. BTS guidelines for the management of spontaneous pneumothorax. Pleural Diseases Group, Standards of Care Committee, British Thoracic Society. *Thorax* 2003;58 Suppl 2:ii39–52.

Ohm C, Park D, Vogen M, et al. Use of an indwelling pleural catheter compared with thorascopic talc pleurodesis in the management of malignant pleural effusions. *Am Surg* 2003;69(3):198–202.

Porcel JM, Vives M. Etiology and pleural fluid characteristics of large and massive effusions. *Chest* 2003;124(3):978–983.

Spiegler PA, Hurewitz AN, Groth ML. Rapid pleurodesis for malignant pleural effusions. *Chest* 2003; 123(6):1895–1898.

Case 21. Leiomyoma

Choong CK, Meyers BF. Benign esophageal tumors: introduction, incidence, classification, and clinical features. *Semin Thorac Cardiovasc Surg* 2003; 15(1):3–8. Review.

Samphire J, Nafteux P, Luketich J. Minimally invasive techniques for resection of benign esophageal tumors. *Semin Thorac Cardiovasc Surg* 2003;15(1): 35–43. Review.

Taniguchi E, Kamiike W, Iwase K, et al. Thoracoscopic enucleation of a large leiomyoma located on the left side of the esophageal wall. *Surg Endosc* 1997; 11(3):280–282.

Case 22. Bronchogenic Cyst

Coselli MP, de Ipolyi P, Bloss RS, et al. Bronchogenic cysts above and below the diaphragm: report of eight cases. *Ann Thorac Surg* 1987;44(5):491–494.

Martinod E, Pons F, Azorin J, et al. Thoracoscopic excision of mediastinal bronchogenic cysts: results in 20 cases. *Ann Thorac Surg* 2000;69(5):1525–1528.

McAdams HP, Kirejczyk WM, Rosado-de-Christenson ML, et al. Bronchogenic cyst: imaging features with clinical and histopathologic correlation. *Radiology* 2000;217(2):441–446.

Case 23. Congenital Lobar Emphysema

Olutoye OO, Coleman BG, Hubbard AM, et al. Prenatal diagnosis and management of congenital lobar emphysema. *J Pediatr Surg* 2000;35(5):792–795.

Ozcelik U, Gocmen A, Kiper N, et al. Congenital lobar emphysema: evaluation and long-term follow-up of thirty cases at a single center. *Pediatr Pulmonol* 2003;35(5):384–391.

Tander B, Yalcin M, Yilmaz B, et al. Congenital lobar emphysema: a clinicopathologic evaluation of 14 cases. *Eur J Pediatr Surg* 2003;13(2):108–111.

Case 24. Non–Small Cell Lung Cancer

Cerfolio RJ, Ojha B, Bryant AS. The role of FDG-PET scan in staging patients with nonsmall cell carcinoma. *Ann Thorac Surg* 2003;76:861–866.

Myrdal G, Lambe M, Gustafsson G. Survival in primary lung cancer potentially cured by operation: influence of tumor stage and clinical characteristics. *Ann Thorac Surg* 2003; 75:356–363.

Warren WH, Faber LP. Segmentectomy versus lobectomy in patients with stage I pulmonary carcinoma. *J Thorac Cardiovasc Surg* 1994;107:1087.

Case 25. Esophageal Perforation

Ferguson MK, Reeder LB, Olak J. Outcome after failed initial therapy for rupture of the esophagus or intrathoracic stomach. *J Gastrointest Surg* 1997;1(1): 34–39.

Muir AD, White J, McGuigan JA, et al. Treatment and outcomes of esophageal perforation in a tertiary referral centre. *Eur J Cardiothorac Surg* 2003;23(5): 799–804.

Reeder LB, DeFilippi VJ, Ferguson MK. Current results of therapy for esophageal perforation. *Am J Surg* 1995;169(6):615–617.

Case 26. Blastomycosis

Chapman SW, Bradsher RW Jr, Campbell GD Jr, et al. Practice guidelines for the management of patients with blastomycosis. Infectious Diseases Society of America. *Clin Infect Dis* 2000;30(4): 679–683.

Goldman M, Johnson PC, Sarosi GA. Fungal pneumonias. The endemic mycoses. *Clin Chest Med* 1999;20(3):507–519. Review.

Martynowicz MA, Prakash UB. Pulmonary blastomycosis: an appraisal of diagnostic techniques. *Chest* 2002;121(3):768–773.

Wheat LJ, Goldman M, Sarosi G. State-of-the-art review of pulmonary fungal infections. *Semin Respir Infect* 2002;17(2):158–181. Review.

Case 27. Lymphoma

Cohen AJ, Thompson L, Edwards FH, et al. Primary cysts and tumors of the mediastinum. *Ann Thorac Surg* 1991;51:378.

Coleman CN, Picozzi VJ Jr, Cox RS, et al. Treatment of lymphoblastic lymphoma in adults. *J Clini Oncol* 1986;4:1628.

Rendina EA, Venuta F, De Giacomo T, et al. Comparative merits of thoracoscopy, mediastinoscopy, and mediastinotomy for mediastinal biopsy. *Ann Thorac Surg* 1994;57(4):992–995.

Case 28. Pulmonary Artery Sarcoma

Bacha EA, Wright CD, Grillo HC, et al. Surgical treatment of primary pulmonary sarcomas. *Eur J Cardiothorac Surg* 1999;15(4):456–460.

Galea J, Manche A. Pulmonary artery sarcoma. *J Thorac Cardiovasc Surg* 2002;123(3):581.

Genoni M, Biraima AM, Bode B, et al. Combined resection and adjuvant therapy improves prognosis of sarcomas of the pulmonary trunk. *J Cardiovasc Surg (Torino)* 2001;42(6):829–833.

Kim JH, Gutierrez FR, Lee EY, et al. Primary leiomyosarcoma of the pulmonary artery: a diagnostic dilemma. *Clin Imaging* 2003;27(3):206–211.

Mayer E, Kriegsmann J, Gaumann A, et al. Surgical treatment of pulmonary artery sarcoma. *J Thorac Cardiovasc Surg* 2001;121(1):77–82.

Case 29. Esophageal Adenocarcinoma and Ivor Lewis Esophagectomy

Bartels HE, Stein HJ, Siewert JR. Respiratory management and outcome of non-malignant tracheobronchial fistula following esophagectomy. *Dis Esophagus* 1998;11(2):125–129.

Hulscher JB, van Sandick JW, de Boer AG, et al. Extended transthoracic resection compared with limited transhiatal resection for adenocarcinoma of the esophagus. *N Engl J Med* 2002;347(21):1662–1669.

Iannettoni MD, Whyte RI, Orringer MB. Catastrophic complications of the cervical esophagogastric anastomosis. *J Thorac Cardiovasc Surg* 1995;110 (5):1493–1500.

Case 30. Empyema

Anstadt MP, Guill CK, Ferguson ER, et al. Surgical versus nonsurgical treatment of empyema thoracis: an outcomes analysis. *Am J Med Sci* 2003;326(1): 9–14.

Roberts JR. Minimally invasive surgery in the treatment of empyema: intraoperative decision making. *Ann Thorac Surg* 2003;76(1):225–230; discussion 229–230.

Thourani VH, Lancaster RT, Mansour KA, et al. Twenty-six years of experience with the modified eloesser flap. *Ann Thorac Surg* 2003;76(2):401–405; discussion 405–406.

Case 31. Typical Carcinoid

Mezzetti M, Raveglia F, Panigalli T, et al. Assessment of outcomes in typical and atypical carcinoids according to latest WHO classification. *Ann Thorac Surg* 2003;76(6):1838–1842.

Okike N, Bernatz P, Woolner LB. Carcinoid tumours of the lung. *Ann Thorac Surg* 1976;50:52.

Schreurs AJ, Westermann CJ, van den Bosch JM, et al. A twenty-five-year follow-up of ninety-three resected typical carcinoid tumors of the lung. *J Thorac Cardiovasc Surg* 1992;104(5):1470–1475.

Case 32. Neurofibroma

Bousamra M, Haasler GB, Patterson G, et al. A comparative study of thoracoscopic versus open removal of benign neurogenic mediastinal tumors. *Chest* 1996;109:1461–1465.

Cirino LMI, de Campos JRM, Fernandez PP, et al. Diagnosis and treatment of mediastinal tumors by thoracoscopy. *Chest* 2000;117:1787–1792.

Fahimi H, Casselman FP, Mariani MA, et al. Current management of postoperative chylothorax. *Ann Thorac Surg* 2001;71:448–450.

Han PP, Dickman CA. Thoracoscopic resection of thoracic neurogenic tumors. *J Neurosurg* 2002;96(3 Suppl):304–308.

Reeder LB. Neurogenic tumors of the mediastinum. *Semin Thorac Cardiovasc Surg* 2000;12(4): 261–267. Review.

Ricci C, Rendina EA, Venuta F, et al. Diagnostic imaging and surgical treatment of dumbbell tumors of the mediastinum. *Ann Thorac Surg* 1990;50(4): 586–589.

Shadmehr MB, Gaissert HA, Wain JC, et al. The surgical approach to "dumbbell tumors" of the mediastinum. *Ann Thorac Surg* 2003;76:1650–1654.

Case 33. Pneumonectomy

al-Kattan K, Cattalani L, Goldstraw P. Bronchopleural fistula after pneumonectomy with a hand suture technique. *Ann Thorac Surg* 1994;58(5): 1433–1436.

Ferguson MK, Karrison T. Does pneumonectomy for lung cancer adversely influence long-term survival? *J Thorac Cardiovasc Surg* 2000;119(3): 440–448.

Koong HN, Pastorino U, Ginsberg RJ. Is there a role for pneumonectomy in pulmonary metastases? International Registry of Lung Metastases. *Ann Thorac Surg* 1999;68(6):2039–2043.

Case 34. Esophageal Adenocarcinoma and Transhiatal Esophagectomy

Donington JS, Miller DL, Allen MS, et al. Tumor response to induction chemoradiation: influence on survival after esophagectomy. *Eur J Cardiothorac Surg* 2003;24(4):631–637; discussion 636–637.

Goldberg M, Farma J, Lampert C, et al. Survival following intensive preoperative combined modality therapy with paclitaxel, cisplatin, 5-fluorouracil, and radiation in resectable esophageal carcinoma: a phase I report. *J Thorac Cardiovasc Surg* 2003;126(4): 1168–1173.

Makary MA, Kiernan PD, Sheridan MJ, et al. Multimodality treatment for esophageal cancer: the role of surgery and neoadjuvant therapy. *Am Surg* 2003;69(8): 693–700; discussion 700–702.

Mariette C, Finzi L, Fabre S, et al. Factors predictive of complete resection of operable esophageal cancer: a prospective study. *Ann Thorac Surg* 2003;75(6):1720–1726.

Spector SA, Livingstone AS, Franceschi D, et al. Neoadjuvant and adjuvant chemotherapy without radiation for esophageal cancer. *J Surg Res* 2003;114(2): 277.

Case 35. Palliative Laser Stent Treatment

Morris CD, Budde JM, Godette KD, et al. Palliative management of malignant airway obstruction. *Ann Thorac Surg* 2002;74(6):1928–1932; discussion 1932–1933.

Mountain CF. Revision in the international system for staging lung cancer. *Chest* 1997;111: 1710–1717.

Mountain CF, Dresler CM. Regional lymph node classification for lung cancer. *Chest* 1997;111: 1718–1723.

Myrdal G, Gustafsson G, Lambe M, et al. Outcome after lung cancer surgery. Factors predicting early mortality and major morbidity. *Eur J Cardiothorac Surg* 2001;20:694–699.

Nesbitt JC, Putnam JB, Walsh GL, et al. Survival in early-stage non–small cell lung cancer. *Ann Thorac Surg* 1995;60:466–472.

Petrou M, Goldstraw P. The management of tracheobronchial obstruction: a review of endoscopic techniques. *Eur J Cardiothorac Surg* 1994;8(8): 436–441.

Ploeg AJ, Kappetein AP, van Tongeren RB, et al. Factors associated with perioperative complications and long-term results after pulmonary resection for primary carcinoma of the lung. *Eur J Cardiothorac Surg* 2003;23:26–29.

Stephens KE Jr, Wood DE. Bronchoscopic management of central airway obstruction. *J Thorac Cardiovasc Surg* 2000;119(2):289–296.

Venuta F, Rendina EA, De Giacomo T, et al. Nd:YAG laser resection of lung cancer invading the airway as a bridge to surgery and palliative treatment. *Ann Thorac Surg* 2002;74(4):995–998.

Wood DE. Management of malignant tracheobronchial obstruction. *Surg Clin North Am* 2002;82 (3):621–642.

Wood DE, Lin YH, Vallieres E, et al. Airway stenting for malignant and benign tracheobronchial stenosis. *Ann Thorac Surg* 2003;76(1):167–172; discussion 173–174.

Case 36. Foramen of Morgagni Hernia

Al-Salem AH, Nawaz A, Matta H, Jacobsz A. Herniation through the foramen of Morgagni: early diagnosis and treatment. *Pediatr Surg Int* 2002;18(2–3): 93–97.

Angrisani L, Lorenzo M, Santoro T, et al. Hernia of foramen of Morgagni in adult: case report of laparoscopic repair. *JSLS* 2000;4(2):177–181. Review.

Hinshaw LJ, Collins J. Foramen of Morgagni hernia. *Semin Roentgenol* 2002;37:3–4.

Thomas GG, Clitherow NR. Herniation through the foramen of Morgagni in children. *Br J Surg* 1977; 64(3):215–217.

Case 37. Radiation Pneumonitis

Deasy JO, Bradley J, El Naqa I, et al. Risk of radiation pneumonitis classified via dosimetric parameters. *Int J Radiat Oncol Biol Phys* 2003;57(2 Suppl): S412.

Magana E, Crowell RE. Radiation pneumonitis successfully treated with inhaled corticosteroids. *South Med J* 2003;96(5):521–524.

Wang JY, Chen KY, Wang JT, et al. Outcome and prognostic factors for patients with non–small cell lung cancer and severe radiation pneumonitis. *Int J Radiat Oncol Biol Phys* 2002;54(3):735–741.

Case 38. Thymic Carcinoma

Chahinian AP. Chemotherapy of thymomas and thymic carcinomas. *Chest Surg Clin N Am* 2001;11 (2):447–456. Review.

Chung DA. Thymic carcinoma—analysis of nineteen clinicopathological studies. *Thorac Cardiovasc Surg* 2000;48(2):114–119. Review.

Goh MH, Liu XY, Goh YS. Anterior mediastinal masses: an anaesthetic challenge. *Anaesthesia* 1999; 54(7):670–674. Review.

Loehrer PJ Sr, Wick MR. Thymic malignancies. *Cancer Treat Res* 2001;105:277–302. Review.

Narang S, Harte BH, Body SC. Anesthesia for patients with a mediastinal mass. *Anesthesiol Clin North America* 2001;19(3):559–579. Review.

Case 39. Squamous Cell Carcinoma of the Esophagus

Beitler AL, Urschel JD. Comparison of stapled and hand-sewn esophagogastric anastomoses. *Am J Surg* 1998;175(4):337–340.

Lam TC, Fok M, Cheng SW, et al. Anastomotic complications after esophagectomy for cancer. A comparison of neck and chest anastomoses. *J Thorac Cardiovasc Surg* 1992;104(2):395–400.

Orringer MB, Marshall B, Iannettoni MD. Eliminating the cervical esophagogastric anastomotic leak with a side-to-side stapled anastomosis. *J Thorac Cardiovasc Surg* 2000;119(2):277–288.

Case 40. Intralobar Sequestration

Collin PP, Desjardins JG, Khan AH. Pulmonary sequestration. *J Pediatr Surg* 1987;22(8):750–753.

Halkic N, Cuenoud PF, Corthesy ME, et al. Pulmonary sequestration: a review of 26 cases. *Eur J Cardiothorac Surg* 1998;14(2):127–133.

Kravits RM. Congenital malformations of the lung. *Pediatr Clin North Am* 1994;41(3):453–472. Review.

Case 41. Bullous Disease

Divisi D, Battaglia C, Di Francescantonio W, et al. Giant bullous emphysema resection by VATS. Analysis of laser and stapler techniques. *Eur J Cardiothorac Surg* 2002;22(6):990–994.

Fabian T, Federico JA, Ponn RB. Fibrin glue in pulmonary resection: a prospective, randomized, blinded study. *Ann Thorac Surg* 2003;75(5):1587–1592.

Jackson MR. Fibrin sealants in surgical practice: an overview. *Am J Surg* 2001;182(2 Suppl):1S–7S. Review.

Meyers BF, Patterson GA. Chronic obstructive pulmonary disease. 10: Bullectomy, lung volume reduction surgery, and transplantation for patients with chronic obstructive pulmonary disease. *Thorax* 2003;58(7):634–638. Review.

Case 42. Histoplasmosis

Camacho MT, Edelman M, Rozenblit A, et al. Mediastinal histoplasmosis causing massive hematemesis. *J Thorac Cardiovasc Surg* 1996;111(6): 1283–1286.

Kauffman CA. Pulmonary histoplasmosis. *Curr Infect Dis Rep* 2001;3(3):279–285.

Prager RL, Burney DP, Waterhouse G, et al. Pulmonary, mediastinal, and cardiac presentations of histoplasmosis. *Ann Thorac Surg* 1980;30(4):385–390.

Case 43. Synchronous Lung Nodules

Billing PS, Miller DL, Allen MS, et al. Surgical treatment of primary lung cancer with synchronous brain metastases. *J Thorac Cardiovasc Surg* 2001;122 (3):548–553.

Hollaus PH, Wurnig PN, Pridun NS. The natural history of recurrence after bronchoplastic procedures for non–small cell lung cancer. *Ann Thorac Surg* 2003;76(2):363–369.

Rea F, Zuin A, Callegaro D, et al. Surgical results for multiple primary lung cancers. *Eur J Cardiothorac Surg* 2001;20(3):489–495.

Vansteenkiste JF, De Belie B, Deneffe GJ, et al. Leuven Lung Cancer Group. Practical approach to patients presenting with multiple synchronous suspect lung lesions: a reflection on the current TNM classification based on 54 cases with complete follow-up. *Lung Cancer* 2001;34(2):169–175.

Case 44. Achalasia and Esophagectomy

Banbury MK, Rice TW, Goldblum JR, et al. Esophagectomy with gastric reconstruction for achalasia. *J Thorac Cardiovasc Surg* 1999;117(6):1077–1084.

Bruley des Varannes S, Scarpignato C. Current trends in the management of achalasia. *Dig Liver Dis* 2001;33(3):266–277.

Goldblum JR, Whyte RI, Orringer MB, Appelman HD. Achalasia. A morphologic study of 42 resected specimens. *Am J Surg Pathol* 1994;18(4):327–337.

Orringer MB, Stirling MC. Esophageal resection for achalasia: indications and results. *Ann Thorac Surg* 1989;47(3):340–345.

Waters PF, Pearson FG, Todd TR, et al. Esophagectomy for complex benign esophageal disease. *J Thorac Cardiovasc Surg* 1988;95(3):378–381.

Case 45. Hamartoma

Cardillo G, Regal M, Sera F, et al. Videothoracoscopic management of the solitary pulmonary nodule: a single-institution study on 429 cases. *Ann Thorac Surg* 2003;75(5):1607–1611; discussion 1611–1612.

Decamp MM Jr. The solitary pulmonary nodule: aggressive excisional strategy. *Semin Thorac Cardiovasc Surg* 2002;14(3):292–296.

Fletcher JW. PET scanning and the solitary pulmonary nodule. *Semin Thorac Cardiovasc Surg* 2002; 14(3):268–274.

Ost D, Fein AM, Feinsilver SH. Clinical practice. The solitary pulmonary nodule. *N Engl J Med* 2003; 348(25):2535–2542.

Tan BB, Flaherty KR, Kazerooni EA, Iannettoni MD; American College of Chest Physicians. The solitary pulmonary nodule. *Chest* 2003;123(1 Suppl):895–965.

Case 46. Tuberculosis

Mault JR, Pomerantz M. Mycobacterium tuberculosis and other mycobacteria. *Chest Surg Clin N Am* 1999;9(1):227–238, x. Review.

Pomerantz BJ, Cleveland JC Jr, Olson HK, et al. Pulmonary resection for multi-drug resistant tuberculosis. *J Thorac Cardiovasc Surg* 2001;121(3):448–453.

Sung SW, Kang CH, Kim YT, et al. Surgery increased the chance of cure in multi-drug resistant pulmonary tuberculosis. *Eur J Cardiothorac Surg* 1999;16(2):187–193.

Case 47. Pleural Fibroma

Cardillo G, Facciolo F, Cavazzana AO, et al. Localized (solitary) fibrous tumors of the pleura: an analysis of 55 patients. *Ann Thorac Surg* 2000;70(6): 1808–1812.

Chamberlain MH, Taggart DP. Solitary fibrous tumor associated with hypoglycemia: an example of the Doege-Potter syndrome. *J Thorac Cardiovasc Surg* 2000;119(1):185–187.

Magdeleinat P, Alifano M, Petino A, et al. Solitary fibrous tumors of the pleura: clinical characteristics, surgical treatment and outcome. *Eur J Cardiothorac Surg* 2002;21(6):1087–1093.

Nonaka M, Kadokura M, Takaba T. Benign solitary fibrous tumor of the parietal pleura which invaded the intercostal muscle. *Lung Cancer* 2001;31(2–3): 325–329.

Case 48. Zenker's Diverticulum with Previous Left Carotid Endarterectomy

Gutschow CA, Hamoir M, Rombaux P, et al. Management of pharyngoesophageal (Zenker's) diverticulum: which technique? *Ann Thorac Surg* 2002;74(5): 1677–1682.

Mirza S, Dutt SN, Irving RM. Iatrogenic perforation in endoscopic stapling diverticulotomy for pharyngeal pouches. *J Laryngol Otol* 2003;117(2):93–98.

Sideris L, Chen LQ, Ferraro P, et al. The treatment of Zenker's diverticula: a review. *Semin Thorac Cardiovasc Surg* 1999;11(4):337–351.

Case 49. Pneumatocele

Hall RA, Salhany KE, Lebel E, et al. Fungal pulmonary abscess in an adult secondary to hyperimmunoglobulin E (Job's) syndrome. *Ann Thorac Surg* 1995;59(3):759–761.

Lui RC, Inculet RI. Job's syndrome: a rare cause of recurrent lung abscess in childhood. *Ann Thorac Surg* 1990;50(6):992–994.

Shamberger RC, Wohl ME, Perez-Atayde A, et al. Pneumatocele complicating hyperimmunoglobulin E syndrome (Job's Syndrome). *Ann Thorac Surg* 1992; 54(6):1206–1208. Review.

Case 50. Thymoma

Baraka A. Anesthesia and critical care of thymectomy for myasthenia gravis. *Chest Surg Clin N Am* 2001;11(2):337–361. Review.

Lopez-Cano M, Ponseti-Bosch JM, Espin-Basany E, et al. Clinical and pathologic predictors of outcome in Thymoma-associated myasthenia gravis. *Ann Thorac Surg* 2003;76(5):1643–1649.

Singhal S, Shrager JB, Rosenthal DI, et al. Comparison of stages I–II thymoma treated by complete resection with or without adjuvant radiation. *Ann Thorac Surg* 2003;76(5):1635–1642.

Case 51. Ewing's Sarcoma

Cotterill SJ, Ahrens S, Paulussen M, et al. Prognostic factors in Ewing's tumor of bone: analysis of 975 patients from the European Intergroup Cooperative Ewing's Sarcoma Study Group. *J Clin Oncol* 2000; 18(17):3108–3114.

de Alava E, Pardo J. Ewing tumor: tumor biology and clinical applications. *Int J Surg Pathol* 2001;9(1): 7–17.

Paulussen M, Ahrens S, Dunst J, et al. Localized Ewing tumor of bone: final results of the cooperative Ewing's Sarcoma Study CESS 86. *J Clin Oncol* 2001;19 (6):1818–1829.

Paulussen M, Frohlich B, Jurgens H. Ewing tumour: incidence, prognosis and treatment options. *Paediatr Drugs* 2001;3(12):899–913.

Sailer SL. The role of radiation therapy in localized Ewing's Sarcoma. *Semin Radiat Oncol* 1997;7(3): 225–235.

Case 52. Pericardial Cyst

Cangemi V, Volpino P, Gualdi G, et al. Pericardial cysts of the mediastinum. *J Cardiovasc Surg (Torino)* 1999;40(6):909–913.

Kutlay H, Yavuzer I, Han S, et al. Atypically located pericardial cysts. *Ann Thorac Surg* 2001;72(6): 2137–2139.

Takeda S, Miyoshi S, Minami M, et al. Clinical spectrum of mediastinal cysts. *Chest* 2003;124(1): 125–132.

Case 53. Pulmonary Function Test

Ferguson MK, Reeder LB, Mick R. Optimizing selection of patients for major lung resection. *J Thorac Cardiovasc Surg* 1995;109(2):275–281; discussion 281–283.

Ohno Y, Hatabu H, Takenaka D, et al. CT-guided transthoracic needle aspiration biopsy of small (< or = 20 mm) solitary pulmonary nodules. *AJR Am J Roentgenol* 2003;180(6):1665–1669.

Sekine Y, Iwata T, Chiyo M, et al. Minimal alteration of pulmonary function after lobectomy in lung cancer patients with chronic obstructive pulmonary disease. *Ann Thorac Surg* 2003;76(2): 356–361; discussion 362.

Case 54. Mucoepidermoid Carcinoma

Breyer RH, Dainauskas JR, Jensik RJ, et al. Mucoepidermoid carcinoma of the trachea and bronchus: the case for conservative resection. *Ann Thorac Surg* 1980;29(3):197–204.

Heitmiller RF, Mathisen DJ, Ferry JA, et al. Mucoepidermoid lung tumors. *Ann Thorac Surg* 1989;47(3):394–399.

Watterson KG, Wisheart JD. Tracheobronchial mucoepidermoid carcinoma in childhood with a ten-year follow-up. *Eur J Cardiothorac Surg* 1990;4(2): 112–113.

Case 55. Pancoast's Tumor

Arcasoy SM, Jett JR. Superior pulmonary sulcus tumors and Pancoast's syndrome. *N Engl J Med* 1997;337(19):1370–1376. Review.

Detterbeck FC. Changes in the treatment of Pancoast tumors. *Ann Thorac Surg* 2003;75(6):1990–1997. Review.

Urschel HC Jr. Superior pulmonary sulcus carcinoma. *Surg Clin North Am* 1988;68(3):497–509.

Case 56. Congenital Cystic Adenomatoid Malformation

Browdie D, Todd D, Agnew R, et al. The use of "nonanatomic" pulmonary resection in infants with extensive congenital adenomatoid malformation of the lung. *J Thorac Cardiovasc Surg* 1993;105(4): 732–736.

Sugiyama M, Honna T, Kamii Y, et al. Management of prenatally diagnosed congenital cystic adenomatoid malformation of the lung. *Eur J Pediatr Surg* 1999;9(1):53–57.

Waszak P, Claris O, Lapillonne A, et al. Cystic adenomatoid malformation of the lung: neonatal management of 21 cases. *Pediatr Surg Int* 1999;15(5–6): 326–331.

Case 57. Teratoma

Adkins RB Jr, Maples MD, Hainsworth JD. Primary malignant mediastinal tumors. *Ann Thorac Surg* 1984;38(6):648–659.

Knapp RH, Hurt RD, Payne WS, et al. Malignant germ cell tumors of the mediastinum. *J Thorac Cardiovasc Surg* 1985;89(1):82–89.

Moran CA, Suster S. Primary germ cell tumors of the mediastinum: I. Analysis of 322 cases with special emphasis on teratomatous lesions and a proposal for histopathologic classification and clinical staging. *Cancer* 1997;80(4):681–690.

Case 58. Superior Sulcus Tumor

Alifano M, D'Aiuto M, Magdeleinat P, et al. Surgical treatment of superior sulcus tumors: results and prognostic factors. *Chest* 2003;124(3):996–1003.

Suntharalingam M, Sonett JR, Haas ML, et al. The use of concurrent chemotherapy with high-dose radiation before surgical resection in patients presenting with apical sulcus tumors. *Cancer J* 2000;6(6):365–371.

subject index

Note: Page numbers followed by *f* indicate figures; those followed by *t* indicate tables.